Back to Basics

FOUNDATIONS

OF HEALTHCARE

MANAGEMENT

Back to Basics

Basics

FOUNDATIONS

OF HEALTHCARE

MANAGEMENT

Health Administration Press, Chicago, Illinois

05 04 03 02 01   5 4 3 2 1

Library of Congress Cataloging-in-Publication Data

Back to basics : foundations of healthcare management.
        p.   cm.
    Includes bibliograhical references.
    ISBN 1-56793-140-5 (alk. paper)
        1. Health services administration.   2. Hospitals—Administration.
        3. Leadership.   I. Health Administration Press.
    RA971 .B136 2000
    362.1'068—dc21

                                                    00-059692
                                                    CIP

The paper used in this publication meets the minimum requirements of American National Standard for Information Sciences—Permanence of Paper for Printed Library Materials, ANSI Z39.48-1984.™

Health Administration Press
A division of the Foundation of the American College of Healthcare Executives
1 North Franklin Street, Suite 1700
Chicago, IL 60606-3491
(312) 424-2800

Contents

Fundamentals of
Healthcare Management

Healthcare executives today face challenges as varied as meeting complex regulatory requirements, determining how to structure services in a competitive environment, and communicating with a diverse workforce about organizational change. Meeting these challenges requires a heady mix of technical knowledge, strategic foresight, and interpersonal skills.

In an era so crowded with disparate challenges, executives need to rely on a solid foundation of excellence in the basics of healthcare management. Drawing largely from material published by Health Administration Press, this book brings together the best introductions to these management basics.

PLANNING

The importance of planning cannot be overestimated in a rapidly changing and highly competitive environment. In the chapter "Strategic Planning for Healthcare Organizations," Alan M. Zuckerman, FACHE, explains the importance of planning today and lays out a four-phase process for effective planning. F. Douglas Scutchfield, M.D.; Joel M. Lee, Dr.P.H.; and Steven T. Fleming, Ph.D., show how planning must involve a clear understanding of the population served to ensure that the organization meets the needs of that population. "Epidemiology and the Planning Function" thoroughly reviews different kinds of healthcare planning, including strategic planning, marketing planning, and community health planning, and applies the tools of epidemiology to that planning.

WORKING WITH PHYSICIANS

Hospitals and health systems must have a strong relationship with physicians to succeed, yet that relationship has been a challenge for economic, cultural, and other reasons. The development of integrated delivery systems, with primary care physicians as entry points, has created new dimensions—not always positive ones—to the relationship. In "The Challenges of Physician–Health System Partnerships," Craig E. Holm, CHE, clarifies the essential nature of this relationship in the context of the current demands of the healthcare system.

PERFORMANCE MANAGEMENT AND IMPROVEMENT

The movement toward continuous quality improvement, outcomes measurement, and public accountability has placed measuring and improving performance center stage in healthcare management. John R. Griffith, FACHE, explains the basic tools and processes necessary to continuously improve care and services in his chapter, "Measuring Performance."

FINANCIAL MANAGEMENT

Sister Irene Krause's famous quote, "No margin, no mission," succinctly captures the importance of effective financial management in healthcare. Facing constricting payment rates, complex financial arrangements with payers and others, the need to generate capital for strategic initiatives, and harsh penalties for mismanagement, executives need to develop and execute effective financial plans or face organizational detriment. "Planning and Budgeting," by Louis C. Gapenski, Ph.D., addresses perhaps the most important of all healthcare finance activities. This chapter explains the central concepts and explains how planning and budgeting can be used to help control operations.

INFORMATION MANAGEMENT

Managing operational, clinical, and financial information is essential to ensuring high-quality care and service. Additionally, the very high cost of information systems and the high risk associated with inadequate systems make a basic knowledge of information management all the more necessary for executives, as does the influx of new technology and applications such as computer-based patient records and e-commerce. In "Information Technology Today," Charles J. Austin, Ph.D., and Stuart B. Boxerman, D.Sc., offer a succinct overview of how information technology and the changing healthcare environment interact.

EVALUATION AND DECISION MAKING

More than ever, healthcare managers must make decisions based on fact. That fact must not only establish a cause for action, but must predict its effect on a variety of stakeholders. In addition, the results of decisions must be measured and evaluated to determine level of success. This process occurs within a complex environment in which an organization's political situation may have as much influence over decisions as does systematic evaluation. In "Evaluation and the Decision-Making Process," James E. Veney, Ph.D., and Arnold D. Kaluzny, Ph.D., present a framework for incorporating evaluation into decision making, including needs assessment, program implementation, and outcomes assessment.

LEGAL AND ETHICAL DECISION MAKING

Increasing government scrutiny of the business practices of healthcare organizations is perhaps the most tangible aspect of law in healthcare management today; but it is only one of many legal challenges healthcare executives face. Credentialing, antitrust, malpractice, access to care, termination of care, and a host of other legal issues touch a healthcare organization's activities on a daily basis. Rather than present a too-brief overview of all these issues, this book will address just one salient issue in the chapter "Healthcare Fraud and Abuse," by J. Stuart Showalter, J.D.

HEALTH POLICY ANALYSIS

Healthcare executives' efforts to provide the best possible care to their communities are strongly influenced by government policy; fallout from the Balanced Budget Act and the flurry of activity to meet the Health Insurance Portability and Accountability Act are only the most recent examples. Recognizing this reality, healthcare executives are well advised to understand not only the policymaking process, but also how they can influence that process and use their knowledge of health policy in organizational planning. These are subjects of the chapter "Influencing Public Policy Environments," by Beaufort B. Longest, Jr., Ph.D, FACHE.

GOVERNANCE

A healthcare organization's governing body can help ensure an effective strategic direction or can expend effort with disappointing results both to the board members and the staff who work with that board. The crucial strategic decisions the healthcare organizations must make today require that boards function at the peak of their ability. The chapter "Universal Truths About

Governance," by J. Larry Tyler, FACHE, and Errol Biggs, Ph.D., FACHE succinctly identifies the key qualities of effective healthcare governance and the CEO's role in helping to ensure that a board embodies those qualities.

MARKETING

Marketing has become increasingly important in healthcare as organizations have needed to find ways to structure, price, and promote services to enhance competitive position. The chapter "The Meaning of Marketing," by Eric N. Berkowitz, Ph.D., discusses the components of healthcare marketing and how they can be implemented within an organization and within the healthcare system.

MANAGING ALLIANCES

Healthcare management today is not a strictly intraorganizational activity. In recent years, organizations increasingly have formed strategic alliances that may even find former competitors collaborating. Identifying appropriate partners, structuring the alliance, and managing the alliance are complex tasks, requiring the ability to understand and respond to needs of the community, the market, and the alliance partners. In the chapter "Strategic Alliances," Howard S. Zuckerman, Ph.D.; Arnold D. Kaluzny, Ph.D.; and Thomas C. Ricketts III, Ph.D., explain the basics of how alliances are formed to meet their varied objectives.

HUMAN RESOURCES MANAGEMENT

Typically among the largest employer in a community, a healthcare organization thrives or fails according to its ability to plan for, hire, train, compensate, and motivate its workforce. In his chapter "Human Resources System," John R. Griffith, FACHE, explains the purpose and functions of a human resources system, along with such issues as the makeup of a human resources department and its information needs.

MANAGING CHANGE

If words were brickbats, the one that has hit healthcare executives the hardest and the most often is "change." To a large extent, an executive's success today can be measured by how well he or she manages change, both personally and as an organization leader. In his article "Managing Change," Thomas A. Atchison, Ed.D., does not just exhort change; he explains how to measure and manage the intangibles, such as culture and morale, on which successful change rests.

TEAM MANAGEMENT

Inextricably linked to managing change and arguably the single most important skill of a leader is the ability to draw people together and motivate them to reach a common goal. In his chapter "Working Together," Carson F. Dye, FACHE, defines two key elements of managing a team: cohesiveness and conflict. The chapter defines these elements of team interaction—including the benefits and drawbacks of each—and presents suggestions on how a healthcare leader can engender collaboration while managing conflict.

CAREER MANAGEMENT

Healthcare executives would do a disservice to themselves, their organizations, and their fields if all their attention were turned outward. Successful executives must not only manage organizations; they must manage their own careers. In "Managing Your Career in the Era of Uncertainty," J. Larry Tyler, FACHE, offers tips on the career paths available in the various settings and amid the various changes in healthcare delivery.

No single book can do justice to the intricacies of all these fundamental healthcare management topics. However, the editors hope this collection will raise awareness among executives about these fundamentals, generate new ideas for management and leadership, and draw readers to further examination of the specific skill or subject most pressing for their efforts to improve the health of society.

Strategic Planning for Healthcare Organizations: Planning Amid Turmoil

Alan M. Zuckerman, FACHE

No industry in the 1990s experienced such phenomenal growth and environmental turbulence as the U.S. healthcare delivery system. Since 1980, healthcare expenditures have quadrupled and now represent about 14 percent of the gross domestic product.[1] Factor in the reversal of economic incentives, a technological revolution, regulatory changes, eroding public trust, and government-led reform initiatives with healthcare's exponential growth, and turmoil is the term that best describes what today's healthcare providers are facing.

With the amount and pace of change showing no signs of abating, the greatest challenge facing healthcare managers today is to plan amid the chaos. Pummeled by pressures to reduce costs, improve quality, assume economic risk, and broker affiliations, providers can easily lose sight of strategies needed to position organizations for long-term success, particularly when healthcare has become one of the most complex and dynamic industries in the country. The large number of healthcare organizations that are failing, and the flurry of mergers, acquisitions, and alliances, are indicators of the massive restructuring that is occurring.

Strategic planning is a well-tested approach that is experiencing a resurgence among organizations that must develop forward-looking, feasible

Editor's Note: This chapter is from Chapter 1 of *Healthcare Strategic Planning* by Alan M. Zuckerman, 1998, HAP strategies, or face potential demise. Healthcare providers have typically been slow to use modern management techniques, such as strategic planning, in favor of maintaining the status quo and weathering environmental changes.[2] But a heightened sense of urgency is emerging for providers who realize they can and must manage their services more efficiently and effectively. The public perception that mismanagement of resources by healthcare organizations has contributed, at least in part, to skyrocketing costs will not be swayed by soft-sell marketing campaigns. And employers, insurance companies, and government agencies are not likely to ease up on their demands for more input into how, where, and by whom healthcare services are provided.

This chapter will define what healthcare strategic planning is, present an overview of the planning process and environment, and discuss why strategic planning is critical to the success of all providers in the twenty-first century.

STRATEGIC PLANNING IS . . .

The concept of strategy has roots in both political and military history, from Sun Tzu to Euripides.[3] The Greek verb *stratego* means "to plan the destruction of one's enemies."[4] Many terms associated with strategic planning, such as objective, mission, strength, and weakness, were developed by or used in the military.[5]

A number of definitions have evolved to pinpoint the essence of strategic planning. According to Duncan, Ginter, and Swayne (1995), "strategic planning is the set of processes used in an organization to understand the situation and develop decision-making guidelines (the strategy) for the organization."[6] Campbell (1993) adds the concept of measurement to his definition: "Strategic planning refers to a process for defining organizational objectives, implementing strategies to achieve those objectives, and measuring the effectiveness of those strategies."[7] Evashwick and Evashwick (1988), including the concepts of vision and mission in their definition, define strategic planning as "the process for assessing a changing environment to create a vision of the future, determining how the organization fits into the anticipated environment based on its institutional mission, strengths, and weaknesses; and then setting in motion a plan of action to position the organization accordingly."[8]

Strategic planning has been used in the business sector for the past 50 years. The concept of planning, programming, and budgeting systems was introduced in the late 1940s and early 1950s and used only sparingly by business and government.[9] In the 1960s and 1970s, leading firms, such as General Electric, practiced strategic planning, promoting the merits of providing a framework beyond the 12-month cycle and a systematic approach to managing business units.[10] Strategic planning in the 1980s and 1990s has been based on corporate market planning, which emphasizes maximizing profits through identification of a market segment and development of strategies to control that segment.[11] Today more than 97 percent of the top 100 industrial companies in the United States report using strategic planning activities.[12]

Strategic planning has been used by healthcare organizations somewhat sporadically since the 1970s, and it has been oriented toward providing services and meeting the needs of the population. Prior to the 1970s, hospitals were predominately independent and not-for-profit, and healthcare planning was usually conducted on a local or regional basis by state, county, or municipal governments. Other elements of the healthcare system were nearly universally far smaller and less organizationally complex than hospitals and, until recently, evidenced little need or desire for formal strategic planning.

The use of strategic planning has waned during recent years with reengineering and total quality management (TQM) rising in popularity as quick fixes for lagging financial performance. While reengineering and TQM are powerful tools for reshaping individual processes, these efforts often overlook how to manage the processes once they have been improved and fail to focus on strategic issues, such as the organization's position in the market. TQM and reengineering also often fail to consider environmental issues, improving a process to compete in an environment that no longer exists.[13]

Cost consciousness takes precedence today. The external and competitive forces that prompted businesses to adopt strategic planning are now being felt full-force by the healthcare industry. Strategic planning must now focus on determining if there is consumer demand for specific services and assessing whether the organization has the resources to provide these services. This broader planning focus, in which market and service information is integrated with financial analyses, must include an openness to buying or brokering products and services, rather than relying on internal development.[14] According to Spiegel and Hyman (1991), "in essence health care providers move from a service-based orientation to a profit-motivated one, from serving a general public regardless of internal needs and profits to a selective population that will guarantee organizational survival through generating profits."[15] Planners must also determine how to work with other providers to survive financially and fulfill the organization's mission.

THE STRATEGIC PLANNING PROCESS

Many variations of a strategic planning model have emerged in both the business and healthcare sectors, but the basic model has remained relatively unchanged since its inception. Two similar versions of strategic planning emerged in the 1980s. Sorkin, Ferris, and Hudak (1984) presented their basic steps of strategic planning:

- scan the environment;
- select key issues;
- set mission statements and broad goals;
- undertake external and internal analyses;
- develop goals, objectives, and strategies for each issue;
- develop an implementation plan to carry out strategic actions; and
- monitor, update, and scan.[16]

Simyar, Lloyd-Jones, and Caro (1988) tailored the process to healthcare strategic planning:

- identify the organization's current position, including present mission, long-term objectives, strategies, and policies;
- analyze the environment;
- conduct an organizational audit;
- identify the various alternative strategies based on relevant data;
- select the best alternative;
- gain acceptance;
- prepare long-range and short-range plans to support and carry out the strategy; and
- implement the plan and conduct an ongoing evaluation.[17]

For the purposes of this book, these various steps of strategic planning have been synthesized into the four stages illustrated in Figure 2.1. The first stage is the situation analysis that focuses on the question of where are we now, and includes four activities:

1. organizational review, including mission, philosophy, and culture;
2. external assessment of the market structure and dynamics;
3. internal assessment of distinctive characteristics; and
4. evaluation of competitive position, including advantages and disadvantages.

The goal of situation analysis is to determine which factors are subject to the organization's control, and how the organization will be affected by external forces.

The second stage of the planning process is strategic direction, followed by the third stage of strategy formulation. Stages two and three address the question, Where should we be going? The main activity of the strategic direction stage is to develop a future strategic profile of the organization by examining alternative futures, mission, vision, and key strategies. Strategy formulation, stage three, establishes goals and objectives for the organization.

Figure 2.1 Strategic Planning Approach

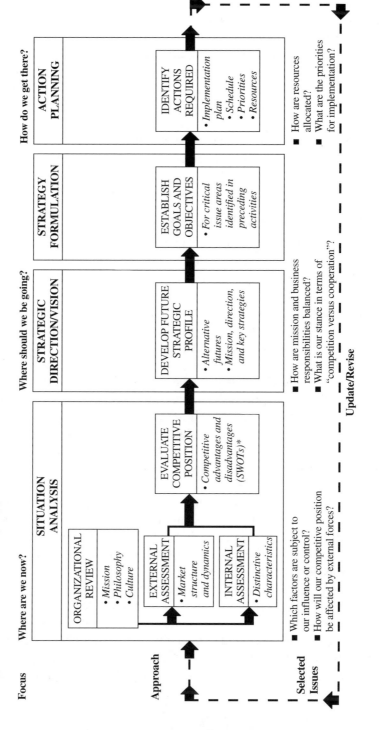

*SWOTs = strengths, weaknesses, opportunities, threats.

The purpose of these stages of the planning process is to determine what broad, future direction is possible and desirable, and what, generally, the organization is going to target as its future scope of services and position.

The fourth and final stage is action planning, determining how we get there. This stage involves identifying the actions needed to implement the plan. Key activities include setting a schedule, determining priorities, and allocating resources to ensure implementation. While implementation needs to occur as soon as possible after completion of the plan, if not actually during this final stage, a return to the initial stages and updating of the plan, at least in part, ensures that strategic planning becomes an ongoing activity of the organization. Each of these stages will be discussed in detail in the following chapters.

THE STRATEGIC PLANNING ENVIRONMENT

While the definitions of strategic planning may seem relatively basic and straightforward and the process a clear-cut sequence of activities, effective strategic planning is an intricate process of self-examination, forecasting the future, fleshing out problems and determining solutions, choosing a course of action into potentially unknown territory, and then bringing the plan to life. The process becomes even more daunting considering the past influences that have shaped healthcare organizations and the pressures that lie ahead.

Other than technological advances, the most sweeping changes affecting healthcare organizations have been in the payment environment. Since 1966, four phases of the payment environment have emerged.[18] The end of the 1960s was a calm, prosperous environment for healthcare organizations with an abundant fee-for-service and cost-plus-reimbursement system. During this "entitlement" phase, as implementation of Medicare and Medicaid generated surging demand, healthcare organizations had little need for strategic planning.

From 1972 to 1982, the payment system was relatively stable, but some strategy was needed to maximize reimbursement and create cost reports that justified expenses to payors. This "growth without limit" phase found providers playing catch up as the increasing demand exceeded the supply. The result was rampaging inflation.

By the mid-1980s, the federal government's 20-year involvement in healthcare planning was rescinded. President Ronald Reagan, the American Hospital Association, the American Medical Association, and others claimed that stimulating competition, rather than relying on federal regulation, would more effectively contain medical costs. A prospective payment system using diagnosis-related groups (DRGs) for reimbursement, the proliferation of managed care, and the shift of much inpatient care to the ambulatory setting were viewed as more promising alternatives for holding down costs than reliance on certificate-of-need and rate regulation.[19] During this period, proprietary providers emerged as a significant influence in healthcare delivery, taking advantage of unrestrained growth in demand and considerable potential for profitability brought on by DRGs and scale economy opportunities.

The past ten years have undoubtedly been the most turbulent for the healthcare industry. The prospective payment system has shifted providers' mindsets from quality healthcare at any cost to cost containment. The proliferation of managed care systems such as preferred provider organizations (PPOs) and health maintenance organizations (HMOs) has spurred growth of integrated healthcare delivery. These developments, along with peer review organizations that serve as quality and utilization watchdogs, have fueled a competitive environment in which many healthcare organizations find themselves in a tailspin.

Regulation, competition, and the consolidated purchasing power of public and private payors have resulted in what many people are labeling "bare bones" reimbursement. Healthcare organization incomes have been dropping due to lower reimbursement, decreasing demand in some sectors, and high fixed costs. As healthcare organizations lose patient volume, the losses come directly off the bottom line because costs do not drop in proportion to lower admissions. A 1993 survey by the Healthcare Financial Management Association attests to the pressures facing hospital executives. According to 32 percent of survey respondents, declining margins is the most significant challenge facing chief executive officers (CEOs) of hospitals.[20]

Trends for the Future

The future healthcare environment shows no signs of being "kinder and gentler" to providers. A number of trends on the horizon will affect providers and their decisions about the future.

Providers will assume increasing risk for underutilization and overutilization of services.

Economic risk is shifting from insurance companies and employers to providers. Comprehensive systems will assume risk for a defined population group, and will be paid a fixed fee per covered life. By keeping the group of covered lives healthy, and providing and controlling a full continuum of services for their patients, providers will reduce utilization and, ultimately, costs. The philosophical shift from building volume by increasing admissions, tests, and procedures, to keeping a population healthy and reducing utilization will not come easily.

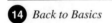

Only unique or geographically isolated providers will remain independent.
Providers in the healthcare system of the future will be closely aligned. Partnerships, alliances, mergers, and consolidations are the watchwords for healthcare providers of the future. Adversarial relationships will lead to failure.

Healthcare reform is occurring parallel to, and in spite of, state and federal healthcare reform initiatives.
Universal insurance coverage, healthcare purchasing groups, and other reform measures may eventually develop. In the meantime, many providers are reforming themselves. Legislation may simply formalize changes already occurring.

Technological advances will enhance and challenge healthcare delivery.
Existing and developing technology has enormous potential to improve efficiency and productivity, but often at a high price. Use of technology may increase operational costs and drain resources if the value of the technology is not proven to reduce staffing or resource utilization.

Providers must manage excess capacity.
As inpatient and specialist utilization continues to drop and many services move beyond the traditional institutional setting, providers must cope with the burden of excess capacity. Consolidating or closing down services and reallocating resources to provide services that maintain or improve economic viability are imperatives facing providers.

Limitations on reimbursement for high-cost services will stimulate continued growth of ambulatory care services and increase demand for post-acute options.
With continued emphasis on cost containment, providing services on an outpatient basis will be a viable, cost-saving option for providers. Home healthcare, skilled nursing centers, and rehabilitation facilities will help healthcare organizations downstage patients out of costly acute care settings. Primary care, including dramatically increased use of physician extenders, will continue as a substitute for specialty medical services.

As healthcare moves toward an all managed care system, the number of physicians needed will drop dramatically, which will result in an oversupply of physicians, particularly specialists.
The oversupply of physicians may have lasting effects on the quality, availability, and costs of healthcare. Options for physicians include planning early

retirement, practicing in underserved communities, and seeking retraining as primary care physicians.

WHY STRATEGIC PLANNING?

With the chaos pervading the healthcare field, many executives and not-for-profit boards may wonder if it is possible to plan effectively or plan at all given the uncertainty ahead. Indeed, many providers are *not* conducting comprehensive strategic planning. Research shows that many providers fail to evaluate the environment in which they operate. A study by Zallocco and Joseph (1991) evaluated 13 activities considered to be a part of strategic market planning.[21] The three activities categorized as environmental analysis (market analysis, competitive analysis, and general consumer surveys) were performed by less than half of the hospitals surveyed.

Many healthcare organizations that have undertaken strategic planning experienced problems that jaded their leaders to the value of planning. Several problems are typically encountered during the strategic planning process.

Failing to involve the appropriate people in the process

The CEO typically serves as the strategic leader while development and selection of the strategy is the role of line managers who must bring the plan to life. Involvement of physician and community leaders is also essential to ensure widespread support for the plan.

Conducting strategic planning independently of financial planning

If financial considerations are excluded from the strategic plan, strategies may never become a reality. Sound strategic planning will include financial screening of strategic options.

Failing to develop consensus on the organization's internal and external environment

Planning participants will become polarized if agreement is not reached on the current position of the organization and the existing and future operating environment.

Falling prey to paralysis of analysis

The fast-paced healthcare market demands that providers respond to opportunities and threats without extensive delays. Many providers are lulled into a sense of security when they are planning and squander time over endless fine-tuning and revisions. When exhaustive planning takes over, very little change or progress occurs.

Not addressing the critical issues

The most pressing issues may not be addressed because the board and other planning participants assume the organization's leaders are handling these problems. If no one is prepared to initiate discussions of key issues, strategic plans focus on minor topics and ignore the most critical and threatening ones.

Assuming that once objectives are established they will take care of themselves

Failure to implement a strategic plan is one of the most common flaws of the planning process. Staff may be overwhelmed with managing day-to-day crises, leaving little time to implement strategic objectives. The objectives may also lack precision, so that ensuing activities lack direction.

So why should providers conduct comprehensive strategic planning? Why not rely on ad hoc planning based on educated guesses and intuition? Healthcare organizations may have historically survived using less formalized approaches to make policy decisions, but today's providers must be more precise in their choices. Mistakes will not only result in lost revenue, but closure.

There are many tangible benefits of strategic planning that continue long after the plan is completed. Duncan, Ginter and Swayne (1995) identified the following benefits of strategic planning[22]; it:

- may improve financial performance;
- provides the organization with self-concept, specific goals, guidance, and consistency of decision making;
- encourages managers to understand the present, plan for the future, and understand when change is vital;
- requires managers to communicate vertically and horizontally;
- improves overall coordination within the organization; and
- encourages innovation and change to meet the challenges of a complex and evolving environment.

According to Nadler (1994), for many organizations the true value lies in the planning process, not the plan. "Most plans have a tremendously fast rate of depreciation. By the time they're printed and bound they've become obsolete. The value of planning is largely in the shared learning, the shared frame of reference, the shared context for those small decisions that get made over time."[23] Indeed changes may occur daily that influence a strategic plan, and new ideas may surface once the plan is complete. A successful strategic plan enables providers to establish a consistent, articulated direction for the future. But it is also a living document that must be monitored and revised to meet both anticipated and unanticipated needs of the organization and the market, whether these changes are related to managed care, integrated delivery, healthcare reform, systems development, technological advances, or other challenges on the horizon.

NOTES

1. Bureau of the Census. 1995. *Statistical Abstract of the United States*. Washington, D.C.
2. Duncan, W. J., P. M. Ginter, and L. E. Swayne. 1995. *Strategic Management of Health Care Organizations*. Boston: PWS-Kent Publishing Company, p. 17.
3. Ibid.
4. Bracker, J. 1980. "The Historical Development of the Strategic Management Concept." *Academy of Management Review* 5 (2): 219–24.
5. Duncan, Ginter, and Swayne.
6. Ibid.
7. Campbell, A. B. 1993. "Strategic Planning in Health Care: Methods and Applications." *Quality Management in Health Care* 1 (4): 13.
8. Evashwick, C. J., and W. T. Evashwick. 1988. "The Fine Art of Strategic Planning." *Provider* 14 (4): 4–6.
9. Webster, J. L., W. R. Reif, and J. S. Bracker. 1989. "The Manager's Guide to Strategic Planning Tools and Techniques." *Planning Review* 17 (6): 5.
10. Ibid.
11. Spiegel, A. D., and H. H. Hyman. 1991. *Strategic Health Planning: Methods and Techniques Applied to Marketing and Management*. Norwood, NJ: Ablex Publishing Corporation.
12. Klein, H. E., and R. E. Linneman. 1984. "Environmental Assessment: An International Study of Corporate Practice." *The Journal of Business Strategy* 5, 66–75.
13. Garvin, D. A. 1995. "Leveraging Processes for Strategic Advantage." *Harvard Business Review* 73 (5): 80.
14. Goldman, E. F., and K. C. Nolan. 1994. *Strategic Planning in Health Care: A Guide for Board Members*. Chicago: American Hospital Publishing, Inc.
15. Spiegel and Hyman, p. 8.
16. Sorkin, D. L., N. B. Ferris, and J. Hudak. 1984. "Strategies for Cities and Counties." In *A Strategic Planning Guide*. Washington, D.C.: Public Technology, Inc.
17. Simyar, F., J. Lloyd-Jones, and J. Caro. 1988. "Strategic Management: A Proposed Framework for the Health Care Industry." In *Strategic Management in the Health Care Sector: Toward the Year 2000*, edited by F. Simyar and J. Lloyd-Jones, 6–17. Englewood Cliffs, NJ: Prentice Hall.
18. Eastaugh, S. R. 1992. "Hospital Strategy and Financial Performance." *Health Care Management Review* 17 (3): 20.
19. Spiegel and Hyman.
20. Cerne, F. 1993. "Strategic Shakeup." *Hospitals* 67 (7): 28.
21. Zallocco, R. L., and W. B. Joseph. 1991. "Strategic Market Planning in Hospitals: Is It Done? Does It Work?" *Journal of Health Care Marketing* 11 (1): 5–11.
22. Duncan, Ginter, and Swayne, p. 9.
23. Nadler, D. A. 1994. "Collaborative Strategic Thinking." *Planning Review* 22 (5): 30.

Epidemiology and the Planning Function

F. Douglas Scutchfield, M.D.; Joel M. Lee, Dr.P.H.; and Steven T. Fleming, Ph.D.

Ms. Findcare, the head of social services, sends a memo to Mr. Jones in which she reports a number of complaints regarding the coordination of care for the elderly population, particularly those with Alzheimer's disease. She questions whether the ongoing strategic plan is addressing the current or future needs of Medicare enrollees. What kinds of epidemiologic data need to be collected to assess the needs and services required by both current and potential elderly enrollees?

Although most individuals have personal plans, and most organizations have formal planning documents, the commonplace use of the term "planning" focuses on an informal concept. A variety of explanations exist for the professional construct of planning, which is described as:

- making current decisions in light of their future effects;
- a means to assess the future and make provision for it;
- making current choices to influence the future;
- guidance of change;
- deciding in advance what to do, how to do it, when to do it, and who is to do it;

Editor's Note: This chapter is from Chapter 7 of *Managerial Epidemiology* by Steven T. Fleming, F. Douglas Scutchfield, and Thomas C. Tucker, 2000, HAP

- the design of a desired future and of effective ways of bringing it about;
- the ability to control the future consequences of present actions; and
- a process that involves making and evaluating each of a set of interrelated decisions before action is required.

The healthcare organization should include epidemiologic measurement in the planning process, regardless of which of these descriptions is embraced. Decisions about where the organization is going, how to guide the organization through change, and the design of a desired future, must include an assessment of healthcare markets, specifically in terms of the kinds of morbidity that customers have in the present or will have in the future. The purpose of this chapter is to describe ways to incorporate epidemiologic concepts and measurement into the process of community and institutional planning. We discuss the history of health planning in section one, distinguish among various types of health planning in section two, and consider community health planning in the third section, with a particular focus on the tools and benchmarks of planning, such as *Healthy People 2000*. Section four deals with institutional planning, and a strategic planning model is elaborated in section five. In the final section of this chapter we describe healthcare marketing, relate the marketing and planning processes, and discuss the prominent role that epidemiology should play in both processes.

HISTORY OF HEALTH PLANNING

Planning in healthcare has a reasonably long history. Early planning efforts focused on hospital bed need with various models, dating back to the 1920s, based on beds per 1,000 population in a service area. The evolution of hospital bed planning is useful as an example of the increased sensitivity of the resource planning method over time. In 1921, Hoge (1958) developed a model for bed ratio per 25 percent of estimated prevalence of illness. However, he did not address hospital occupancy rate or geographic location. By the late 1920s, additional models were developed to address differences in hospital service areas, including variation in urban/rural populations, contagious disease, pediatrics, maternity, chronic illness, and convalescent care. In 1933, the Committee on the Cost of Medical Care and Lee and Jones (1933) reported estimated illness incidence and prevalence figures by medical diagnostic category, using U.S. Public Health Service and industrial data. Expert physician judgment was used to estimate resource requirements based on past experience, not on future demand. The subsequent evolution of bed planning included the designation of service centers or "areas of study" hospitals and the use of population death ratios as measures of bed need.

When the Second World War ended, the inadequacy of total hospital beds in the United Sates became a pressing concern. In light of this, the Hill-Burton Hospital Survey and Construction Act of 1946 was enacted into federal law to inventory bed supply requirements and to promote hospital construction. The legislation was designed to (1) address the need for additional rural hospital beds, (2) coordinate public and private health services, (3) increase efficiency of the system through the control of new equipment and facilities where use would be insufficient, and (4) establish regionalized service areas. The Hill-Burton Act provided funding for construction costs for short-term general hospital beds, with service area population density and current bed occupancy as criteria for project funding. Hill-Burton also included policies to address the setting of priorities by states, prohibition of discrimination in facility access and use, and the provision of services at no cost to indigent patients. As a part of that legislation, states were required to develop a hospital plan that delineated how and where hospitals were to be constructed. At that time, total estimates indicated a need for 165,000 additional hospital beds in the United States. In 1964, amendments to the Hill-Burton act dropped uniform beds-per-1,000 population rates and directed states to address community context in setting priorities for funding. Under Hill-Burton, the connection between epidemiologic measures and resource use was done at the macro level with population density as the measure of need, rather than morbidity profiles, as was the case in the earlier Lee and Jones (1933) report.

Federally mandated health services planning continued in the establishment of the Regional Medical Program in 1966 to address cancer, heart disease, and stroke through the establishment of regionalized programs covering the entire United States. The Partnership for Health Act of 1967 (Comprehensive Health Planning) established regional health plans and reviewed funded projects for appropriateness. The Social Security Amendments of 1972, section 1122, provided state agency review of proposals to use federal funds for projects with a cost greater than $100,000. The National Health Planning and Resources Development Act of 1974 consolidated the Hill-Burton, Regional Medical Program, Comprehensive Health Planning, and Section 1122 legislation and authorized a $1 billion, three-year program for health planning and resource development. This legislation was very ambitious: it created an administrative and voluntary board that represented consumers, health providers, and payers at the state level and in health service areas across the United States. In exchange for federal financial support, states were required to establish state health planning laws, including certificate-of-need laws. The regional Health Systems Agencies (HSAs) were responsible for the development of a long-range health plan for their area, the health system plan (HSP), and annual plans to implement the HSP called the annual implementation plan (AIP). They were also responsible for initial certificate-of-need review for the states and for the approval of local federal grants designed to improve or change the healthcare system. Funding for the federal legislation was phased out in the early 1980s, although some HSAs continued to operate for a period of time as local support and private contributions for their operation attempted to replace the federal funding. Certificate-of-need legislation has also been revised or repealed in many states. The proximate causes of the demise of this most ambitious law was underfunding of specific aspects of the law, questions about efficacy, and—most significantly—the notion that the healthcare system should be deregulated to respond to market forces.

The idea of health planning, however, did not entirely disappear with the departure of the National Health Planning and Resource Development Act. During this period of transition, many healthcare organizations, in an effort to comply with legislative mandates, created positions for planners. The need for organizations to plan still existed. Not even the collapse of certificate-of-need legislation, for example, could affect the needs of hospitals to respond to consumer demand for new services. Many hospitals recognized the usefulness of planning and retained their planners after the federal and state mandates ended. It appears that hospitals found value in planning activities and redefined the responsibilities of staff to include the functions of planning and marketing in a competitive environment. Interest in planning has also been promoted by the recent focus by managers on total or continuous quality improvement, as evidenced by the recent establishment of Baldrige National Quality Awards in Health Care and the Ernest D. Codman Quality Award of the Joint Commission on Accreditation of Health Care Organizations. Nevertheless, the planning function in health organizations retains many of the health planning methods and functions that were used by Health Systems Agencies and other legislatively mandated public planning organizations. In fact, most large American hospitals will have some administrator with the notion of planning in his or her title, such as vice president for development and planning.

It should be clear that, to some degree, each of these planning programs embraced epidemiologic concepts and measurement. Even the early Hoge model (1958) was based on an estimate of the prevalence of disease, as was the Lee-Jones report (1933). The Regional Medical Program focused specifically on the top three causes of mortality: heart disease, cancer, and stroke. The health services agencies funded by the National Health Planning and Resources Development Act were steeped in epidemiologic data as they developed the long-range health plans for their local areas.

In assessing the efficacy of these formalized planning efforts, we need to address a variety of questions. Was the construction or purchase of unneeded services prevented? Do healthcare organizations currently make decisions in accordance with plans? Is the public better served by the healthcare system? Has money been saved? It is difficult to evaluate these questions because we have no way of measuring the number of projects that were considered and then dropped after conscientious internal review. Other public programs with active planning components have included examination of the Graduate National Medical Advisory Commission and the *Healthy People* series.

PLANNING: DEFINITIONS AND DISTINCTIONS

Peddecord (1998) has defined planning as "a future-oriented systematic process of determining a direction, setting a goal and taking actions to achieve that goal." Planning is essential to all managerial functions, and perhaps it is one of the most important activities in which those who are responsible for a healthcare program or activity engage. A plan sets a course of action. It describes the direction that an organization is pursuing and the ways in which it will go about the process of achieving positive outcomes. Without a plan the manager will not know what to do in pursuit of an objective, how to accomplish results along the way, and when the final objective has been achieved.

Most planning proceeds from the model of planning, implementation, and evaluation, and leads to further planning. Planning involves not only the technical aspects that form the major focus of this chapter, but also the social processes that drive it forward. Planning is rarely done by an individual; it most often is done in organizations or communities of individuals and organizations with an interest—as stakeholders—in the work and in the results of that organization.

Typically a plan consist of five components, although the order may vary:

1. *Ends:* specification of outcomes in goals and objectives;
2. *Means:* selection of policies, programs, procedures, and practices by which objectives and goals are to be pursued;
3. *Resources:* determination of the types and amounts of resources required, the ways in which they will be generated or acquired, and their allocation to activities;
4. *Implementation:* design and organization of decision-making procedures so that the plan can be carried out; and
5. *Control:* design of a procedure for anticipating or detecting errors in the plan, or plan failures, and for preventing or correcting problems on a continuing basis.

A major distinction in planning is whether the planning is being carried out at the institutional level or the community level. **Institutional planning** is in some ways easier given the institution's hierarchical structure. And, theoretically, all are looking out for the institution's best interest. On the other hand, **community health planning** involves many institutions and organizations, each with its own vested interest and agenda. The major effort in community health planning is to recognize that each organization has its own agenda. The challenge is to harmonize plans so that all are accommodated to one final outcome. Table 3.1 illustrates the major distinctions between community and institutional planning.

Whether health planning is community or institution based, five significant categories or levels of planning exist. Strategic, operational, and tactical planning all focus on the organization as it defines its future direction and implementation. The first and most general of these three categories is **strategic planning**, which has a comprehensive scope and a long-range time line; it is the most relevant for application, as in defining the future structure of the organization. Strategic planning is usually done at the upper levels of the organization's governing body and senior staff, and frequently has a three- to five-year time line. A strategic plan normally will include four components that prescribe all aspects of planning:

Vision: clear identification of the most successful view of the organization in the very long run;

Mission: encapsulated purpose of the organization and its reasons for existing;

Goals: broad statements of the achievements required for fulfillment of the organzation's mission; and

Objectives: specific measurable outcomes linked to the goal statements.

Clearly, an organization should incorporate epidemiologic concepts and measurement into the strategic planning process. Suppose the vision of a healthcare organization is to be recognized for excellence in patient care, education, and research. "Excellence" in patient care is an undefined benchmark for which there are some epidemiologic measures, such as case-fatality rates or risk-adjusted mortality measures. Alternatively, the vision statement may envision assisting "people in taking responsibility for their own health by actively promoting wellness and facilitating healing" (Duncan, Ginter, and Swayne 1995). The foundation here for wellness, obviously, is the vast body of epidemiologic literature that identifies risk factors such as diet, smoking, and other wellness-enhancing or disease-promoting behaviors. Suppose the mission statement claims an interest in health status improvement for people in a defined geographic area. The mission statement presumes that one can measure health status improvement in a geographic region through epidemiologic measures such as mortality and morbidity rates. Goals and objectives can be defined specifically in epidemiologic terms such as reducing neonatal mortality, the rates of nosocomial infection, risk-adjusted surgical mortality rates for cardiovascular disease, early- versus late-stage diagnosis of cancer, and so on.

A second level of planning is **operational planning**, which has a functional scope. Although its time range is shorter and more functional, operational planning continues to address the organization's broadest levels of operation, such as financial planning. Other levels of planning are more functional. Tactical or operational planning is normally conducted at the unit level and has a much shorter time range. Its application focuses on the more routine activities of a department, such as the scheduling of staff to accommodate seasonal variations in demand. **Tactical planning** is generally carried out throughout the organization and concerns itself with the achievement of mission, vision, goals, and objectives on a day-to-day basis. It usually has a much shorter time horizon than strategic plans and is concerned with the nuts and bolts of running an organization.

Two additional levels of planning—project/program planning and contingency planning—address more specific aspects of organizational operation. **Project** or **program planning** addresses very specific activities of the organization. Its application is the design and management of a specific activity of the organization, such as construction of a new facility or service. The scope and time frame for this type of planning varies with the activity and is sometimes managed by an external construction company. A final category of planning is **contingency planning**. A contingency plan addresses the possible but not certain occurrence of a specific future event such as a disaster, unplanned weather, a union strike, or an epidemic. Scope varies, and the time line of the event is normally short, but decisions must be made immediately if the event occurs. As a result, contingency plans are developed in advance to ensure preparedness for these events. A recent problem with healthcare planning has been that of a turbulent and uncertain environment, which has made it difficult to plan a number of years into the future while, at the same time, many operational tasks require a great deal of time to complete. Rapid environmental change makes it difficult to plan for the evolution of managed care. An example would be limiting a strategic plan time horizon to a few years while implementation of an operational plan, such as a marketing strategy, may require just as many years to achieve the enrollment critical to self-sufficiency. Despite these limitations, planning remains essential, and

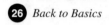

Table 3.1 Institutional Versus Community Planning

Selected Characteristics, Attributes, or Steps in a Planning Process	*Institutional*	*Community-Based*
Main focus or reason for planning	Furthering that organization's goals: profit, survival, improving services to the market that is served	Concerned with the health and welfare of an entire defined population (e.g., cross-institutional planning, safety net planning)
Who does planning? Which organizations or groups?	All organizations, both public and private, must plan for institutional success or survival	Health and public welfare agencies, public school districts, community- based organizations with broad mandates
Are strategic issues (issues that relate to the core concerns or values of the business or community) addressed?	Yes, but only within the context of the organization's goals	Yes, but terms such as *community* or *health system* may be used
Short time frame (months)	Yes	Community planning may need to be rapid; some planning goes on for years
Long time frame (years)	Yes	Yes
Need for political savvy	Essential in large organizations—many factions must be reconciled	Essential—many groups must be satisfied or dealt with; self interest of groups may make consensus difficult or impossible
Information needs and use	Information from inside and outside the organization is needed	Information may be complex and from many sources—difficult to find information for some concerns
Examples of management science or planning techniques used	Budgets, operations research, cost analysis, models, statistical process control may be useful for program or operational plans	Group management techniques and nominal group process may be useful

continued

Table 3.1   *Continued*

Selected Characteristics, Attributes, or Steps in a Planning Process	Institutional	Community-Based
Assessment of needs	Usually termed "marketing" or "market research" in an institution situation	Often done in a community context: which services are needed and by whom, and so forth
Implementation: operational planning and program planning	Most planning done at this level by supervisors, workers	Not an emphasis— institutions that have resources usually do implementation
Results or outputs of the planning process	Organizations develop action plans, business plans, or program plans to implement programs, finance operations, raise money	Community-based planning groups may not have an organizational base or resources but may provide recommendations to policymakers and organizations that provide services
Emphasis on written documents	May be little emphasis on the written plan per se—more emphasis on policies, procedures, action plans, budgets, or business plans that implement the agreed-upon strategy	Well-detailed plans may be needed to communicate to those who can influence public policy or implement action

Source: Peddecord, K. M. 1998. "Public Health Management Tools Planning." In *Maxcy-Rosenau-Last: Public Health and Preventive Medicine, 14th ed.*, edited by R. B. Wallace and B. N. Doebbeling. Stamford, CT: Appleton & Lang.

each level of planning has an individual and specific function in healthcare. These functions are complementary: the performance of each planning function is required to maximize organizational performance.

Regardless of whether planning is done on the community or institutional level, and regardless of the level of planning that involves the professionals, the first step in developing an effective plan is to collect and analyze data regarding the present situation and the future. These data can be quantitative or qualitative, or both. For example, in addressing tuberculosis, quantitative data for planning might include the number of patients in the community who have active tuberculosis or the population at risk. These data are usually statistical in nature and can be manipulated through use of the epidemiological and biostatistical tools at the planner's disposal to address trends or conduct comparisons to other areas. Qualitative data, on the other hand, is not necessarily statistical. For example, the results of a focus group that has considered a question cannot be statistically manipulated. These results, however, are very useful data with an important role in planning; they can provide important insights to the planning process. Another type of qualitative data is key informant surveys, which are generally open-end discussions with major community leaders or stakeholders. Again, key informants are not a "random sample," and this type of survey does not lend itself to the usual epidemiological and statistical techniques available to the health planner. Again, this does not diminish the value of the data, it just limits their manipulation.

COMMUNITY HEALTH PLANNING TOOLS AND BENCHMARKS

It is important in any planning process to have benchmarks. One of the most frequently used tools in community health planning is the Healthy People series. In 1979, *Healthy People*, the surgeon general's report on health promotion and disease prevention, was released. This monograph did several things: first, it established a series of goals that we, as a nation, should achieve in the year 1990. These goals were related to decreased mortality, by age group, for those up to 65 years of age, and they related to morbidity for those over 65:

Life Stage	1990 Target
Infants	35% lower death rate/9 deaths per 1,000 live births
Children	20% lower death rate/34 per 100,000
Adolescents/Young Adults	20% lower death rate/93 per 100,000
Adults	25% lower death rate/400 per 100,000
Older Adults	20% fewer days of restricted activity

The monograph also identified 15 priority programs, under the rubrics of health promotion, preventive services, and health protection.

Immediately following the release of this report, the Centers for Disease Control and Prevention, along with the federal Office of Disease Prevention and Health Promotion, convened a series of working groups. These groups had the charge to create specific objectives tied to the 15 priority areas that would help track our ability to achieve the life stage goals. Their report, published in 1980, was titled *Promoting Health/Preventing Disease*;

Objectives for the Nation and presents materials in the following standard format:

- Nature and extent of the problem
- Prevention and promotion measures
- Specific national objectives for
  - Improved health status
  - Reduced risk factors
  - Improved public/professional awareness
  - Improved services/protection
  - Improved surveillance
- Principal assumptions underlying the objective
- Data necessary for tracking the objective

The process worked well, and as 1990 approached, the U.S. Department of Health and Human Services created a working group to establish objectives for the year 2000. In 1990, the next in the series of prevention benchmarks was published, *Healthy People 2000*, which had three major goals:

- Increase the span of healthy life for all Americans
- Reduce health disparities among Americans
- Achieve access to preventive services for all Americans

As with the 1990 objectives, the priority areas were grouped into a series of three principal areas (health promotion, health protection, and preventive services), each with health status objectives, risk reduction objectives and service/protection objectives. To illustrate, here are examples from one priority area, tobacco.

Health status objective:	Reduce coronary heart disease deaths to no more than 100 per 100,000 people.
Risk reduction objective:	Reduce cigarette smoking to a prevalence of no more than 15 percent among those aged 20 and older.
Service and protection objectives:	Increase to at least 75 percent the proportion of worksites with a formal smoking policy that prohibits or severely restricts smoking in the workplace.

A logical question is, How well are we doing with these measures? Table 3.2 shows the 1977 baseline level on life stage objectives, the 1980 targets, where we finally ended up in 1990, the 1987 baseline, 2000 targets, and the status in a midcourse review done in 1992. Apparently, we were successful in exceeding the target in children, and we met the target in infants and adults; we were unsuccessful, however, in meeting the target for young people. We appeared to be doing very well with children again in this last decade as we nearly met the target for this age group only two years into the 1990s. Table 3.2 also shows how we were doing, in the midcourse 1995 review, in meeting the objectives target and the targets for minority populations.

The objectives for the year 2010 were released in January 2000. They are available on the web at http://web.health.gov/healthypeople. Table 3.3 compares priority areas for each of the three *Healthy People* series. Although new areas of interest are included in the more recent series (e.g., HIV disease), many of the priority areas remain the same: tobacco use, sexually transmitted diseases, nutrition, and so on.

It is obvious with this discussion that data systems must be designed and developed to track the objectives in the various reports. Such systems usually include vital statistics tracking systems. They may include special studies, such as the Behavioral Risk Factor Survey (BRFS) surveillance system that the CDC and the states use to track the various risk factors for disease. With all of its data sources, the major way that data are presented and reported has to do with both incidence and prevalence. In addition, traditional descriptive epidemiology is used to define the time, place, and person variables associated with the various objectives.

Several planning tools have been developed for use in community health planning activities. One of the most used tools—the one most linked to *Healthy People 2000*—is *Healthy Communities 2000: Model Standards*. This tool has been developed by the American Public Health Association (APHA) in conjunction with the CDC and several national public health organizations (1991). Table 3.4 shows how *Healthy Communities* can be used to tie local benchmarks to the national benchmarks contained in *Healthy People 2000* for

Table 3.2 Progress on Life-Stage Objectives, 1995

	*Year 1990 Targets**			*Year 2000 Targets**		
Age Group	*1977 Baseline*	*1990 Target*	*1990 Final*	*1987 Baseline*	*2000 Target*	*1992 Status*
Infants (age < 1)	1,412	900	908	1,008	700	852
Children (age 1–14)	42.3	34	30.1	33.7	28	28.8
Young people (age 15–24)	114.8	93	104.1	97.8	85	95.6
Adults (age 25–64)	532.9	400	400.4	426.9	340	394.7

*Deaths per 100,000 population

Source: Adapted from U.S. Department of Health and Human Services, Public Health Service. 1996. *Healthy People 2000: Midcourse Review and 1995 Revisions.* Washington DC: Government Printing Office.

tobacco use. The elimination of tobacco is one of eight model standard goals under health promotion. This goal can be accomplished by health status, risk reduction, and services/protection objectives that allow local communities to target dates for completion of each objective, and by indicators to measure success. According to Table 3.4, each community specifies a time (with year 2000 as the target) when tobacco-related mortality and morbidity, CHD, lung cancer, and COPD mortality rates will meet *Healthy People 2000* objectives. Moreover, a number of risk reduction objectives can be targeted, such as the prevalence rates of smoking and smoking cessation, as indicated in the table. *Healthy Communities 2000: Model Standards* encourages a consensus process to involve community leaders in the development of local goals, outcome and process objectives, and implementation plans to achieve the agreed-on objectives.

Another more recent tool, the *Healthy People 2010 Toolkit*, has been developed by the Public Health Foundation. Like *Healthy People 2010*, the tool kit is available on the World Wide Web at http://www.health.gov/healthypeople/state/toolkit. It identifies seven action areas:

- Building the foundation: leadership and structure
- Identifying and securing resources
- Identifying and engaging community partners
- Setting health priorities and establishing objectives
- Obtaining baseline measures, setting targets, and measuring progress
- Managing and sustaining the process
- Communicating health goals and objectives

Each of these seven areas includes

- a brief explanation and rationale;
- a checklist of major activities;
- tips for success;
- national and state examples to illustrate *Healthy People* processes in action;
- recommended "Hot Picks" of resources for more information; and
- planning tools easily adapted to state or local needs.

Obviously, epidemiology becomes important in the areas related to setting priorities and objectives and in obtaining baseline data and tracking progress. Again, it is traditional descriptive epidemiology and the concepts of disease prevalence and incidence that form the base of this community health planning process.

Table 3.3 Priority Areas for *Healthy People*

Category	1990	2000	2010
Health Promotion (1990; 2000) Promote Healthy Behaviors (2010)	Smoking cessation Misuse of alcohol/drugs Improved nutrition Exercise and fitness Stress control	Tobacco Alcohol and other drugs Nutrition Physical activity/Fitness Family planning Mental health/Disorders Violent/Abusive behavior Education/Community programs	Tobacco use Nutrition and overweight Physical activity/Fitness
Health Protection (1990; 2000) Promote Health and Safe Communities (2010)	Toxic agent control Occupational safety/Health Accidental injury control Infectious agent control	Food and drug safety Occupational safety/Health Unintentional injuries Environmental health Oral health	Education and Community-based programs Food safety Occupational safety and Health Injury/Violence protection Environmental health Oral health
Preventive Services (1990; 2000) Prevent and Reduce Diseases/Disorders (2010)	Immunizations Family planning Pregnancy and infant care Sexually transmitted diseases High blood pressure control	Immunization and Infectious diseases Maternal and infant health Sexually transmitted diseases HIV infection Heart disease and stroke Cancer Diabetes and chronic disabling conditions	Immunization and Infectious diseases Sexually transmitted diseases HIV Heart disease and stroke Cancer Diabetes

continued

Table 3.3 *Continued*

Category	1990	2000	2010
			Chronic kidney disease
			Disability and secondary conditions
			Mental health and mental disorders
			Respiratory diseases
			Substance abuse
			Arthritis, osteoporosis, and chronic back conditions
Improved Systems for Personal and Public Health (2010)			Medical product safety
			Family planning
			Public health infrastructure
			Maternal/Infant/Child health
			Access to quality health services
			Health communication
			Vision and hearing

Source: U.S. Department of Health and Human Services. 1991. *Healthy People 2000: National Health Promotion and Disease Prevention Objectives*. Pub. No. (PHS) 91–50212. Washington, DC: Government Printing Office.; *Healthy People*. 1979. Pub. No. (PHS) 79-55071. Washington, DC: Government Printing Office; http://web.health.gov/healthypeople/prevagenda/focus.htm.

Table 3.4 Model Standards Objectives and Indicators for Some
Tobacco-Related Health Status and Risk-Reduction Objectives

Category	Objectives	Indicator
Tobacco-Related Mortality	By ———reduce deaths due to tobacco-related diseases to no more than ———per 100,000 people *Model standards note*: Tobacco-related deaths include 20 diseases based on the Surgeon General's Report	Tobacco-related diseases death rate
Tobacco-Related Morbidity	By ———reduce morbidity due to tobacco-related diseases to no more than ———per 100,000 people *Model standards note*: Tobacco-related deaths include 20 diseases based on the surgeon general's report	a. Hospital days b. Disability days c. Costs
Deaths from Coronary Heart Disease	By ———(2000) reduce coronary heart disease deaths to no more than ———(100) per 100,000 people. (Age-adjusted baseline: 135 per 100,000 in 1987)	CHD death rate
Deaths from Lung Cancer	By ———(2000) slow the rise in lung cancer deaths to achieve a rate of no more than ———(42) per 100,000 people. (Age-adjusted baseline: 37.9 per 100,000 in 1987) *Model standards note*: Because this objective as stated is to slow the rise in deaths, the target rate is higher than the baseline rate.	Lung cancer death rate
Deaths from Chronic Obstructive Pulmonary Disease	By ———(2000) slow the rise in deaths from chronic obstructive pulmonary disease to achieve a rate of no more than ———(25) per 100,000 people. (Age-adjusted baseline: 18.7 per 100,000 in 1987)	COPD death rate
Prevalence of Cigarette Smoking	By ———(2000) reduce cigarette smoking to a prevalence of no more than ———(15) percent among people age 20 and older. (Baseline: 29 percent in 1987, 32 percent for men and 27 percent for women)	Percent smoking cigarettes

continued

Table 3.4 *Continued*

Category	Objectives	Indicator
Smoking Cessation During Pregnancy	By ——(2000) increase smoking cessation during pregnancy so that at least ——(60) percent of women who are cigarette smokers at the time they became pregnant quit smoking early in pregnancy and maintain abstinence for the remainder of their pregnancy. (Baseline: 39 percent of white women ages 20–44 quit at any time during pregnancy in 1985)	Percent who quit smoking during pregnancy

Source: Adapted from American Public Health Association. 1991. *Healthy Communities 2000 Model Standards: Guidelines for Community Attainment of the Year 2000 National Health Objectives.* Washington, DC: American Public Health Association.

Another useful health planning tool is the Planned Approach to Community Health (PATCH). Developed by the CDC to focus on issues of chronic disease prevention, this model proceeds through a series of phases as well:

- Community mobilization
- Data collection and organization
- Health priorities selection
- Interventions
- Evaluation

An important point regarding PATCH is its explicit inclusion of evaluation in its methodology. As was pointed out at the beginning of this chapter, planning is part of a circular process that includes planning, implementation, and evaluation, and the sum of the process, in turn, leads to further planning.

The final model for discussion here is the Assessment Protocol for Excellence in Public Health (APEX/PH). This model was developed by the National Association for City and County Health Officers to assist local health departments in effectively planning, implementing, and evaluating programs designed to improve the health status of their communities. Health departments, however, are not the only settings in which the model has been used. APEX consists of three components:

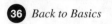

- Organization capacity assessment
- Community process
- Completing the cycle

The organizational capacity assessment is designed to identify strengths and weaknesses in the health department's capacity to carry out the programs that will be identified by the community to improve health status. The health department director and senior staff carry out the assessment. This first APEX component looks at issues such as a program's authority to operate and manage major administrative areas such as finance and human resources.

The second component involves the creation of a community group to identify health problems, set priorities, and establish the health status objectives they wish to achieve. Generally the local group's objectives can follow the national objectives set out in *Healthy People 2000*, or the group can use *Healthy Communities 2000* to develop objectives. The major output of this process is the creation of a community health plan that is data driven and that represents the concerns of the community.

Finally, completing the cycle describes the implementation of that community health plan. This involves putting the results of the organizational assessment and the community health plan together and implementing the program. It allows the health department to better manage itself as the department contributes to the improvement of the community's health status. The steps in APEX/PH are outlined in Figure 3.1.

Effective planning is essential to organizational success. It is imperative to give clear direction about where the organization or community is headed.

Figure 3.1 Assessment Protocol for Excellence in Public Health (APEX/PH) Steps

- Prepare for organizational capacity assessment
- Score indicators for importance and current status
- Identify strengths and weaknesses
- Analyze and report strengths
- Analyze weaknesses
- Rank problems in order of priority
- Develop and implement action plans
- Institutionalize the assessment process

Source: Centers for Disease Control and Prevention (CDC). 1991. *APEX(PH) Assessment Protocol for Excellence in Public Health*. Bethesda, MD: CDC.

The goals and objectives must be clear and, in the case of health programs, accurate knowledge must be present to identify and describe the major community health problems that need to be addressed. This is true whether you are discussing health planning for the community or your institution's health planning. It is imperative that the tools of descriptive epidemiology play a part in identifying major health problems, and the use of time, place, and person descriptors of these health problems allows for the most effective planning. The ability to set priorities is influenced substantially by the burden of disease and its impact on the community: again, questions for epidemiology. Finally, it is important to remember that planning is part of the plan-implement-evaluate cycle: epidemiology is useful in the evaluation effort, as well.

A number of health planning tools exist that can assist managers in the planning effort. These tools are well proven and many are experienced in their use. The successful planner will be familiar with them and their use in a variety of settings.

INSTITUTIONAL PLANNING

In healthcare organizations, planning tends to be done the way it has always been done. This is a consequence of several factors: staff do what they know and what they have experience doing, and they do what they are told to do, frequently by people who have similar previous work experiences. As a result, planning is frequently limited. In ways similar to theories of management, many proponents have advocated "one best way to plan," rather than recognizing that planning is situational. Issues of planning can be addressed on a positive or a normative basis. **Positive theory**, descriptive about what currently exists, makes predictions based on precedent, whereas **normative theory** addresses values and questions of future possibilities. There are four basic models of planning theory: rational/comprehensive, mixed scanning, incremental, and radical planning (Berry 1974).

Rational/Comprehensive planning seeks to consider the broadest view of the environment and its complexity. Basically the method identifies all opportunities for possible action by decision makers, identifies each consequence of each possible action, and selects the action that should result in the preferred set of consequences. The method seeks to consider data concerning all resources for technical decisions, and it works well if the future is stable, clear trends exist, values are implicit, and efficiency is the highest goal. Rational/Comprehensive planning is relevant to issues such as the development of a long-range master plan or the definition of specific health services in a particular community.

Incremental planning, a second method, involves conducting successive comparisons of options where the means to achieve outcomes are not considered. Incremental planning is most appropriate in addressing applied problems such as scarce resources, where there is an emphasis on workability and agreement on policy, and where conflicting values exist or compromise is important. Incremental planning is relevant to issues such as long-term situations where change is gradual, such as budget. A third method is **mixed scanning**, which creates a situational blend of the first two strategies using incremental decisions that lead to a fundamental issue. Mixed scanning permits a detailed examination of some aspects of a plan, along with limited detail in other areas; it is particularly applicable in a rapidly changing environment, where decision making requires flexibility. Mixed scanning is appropriate for issues such as the operation of a complex medical center. The fourth planning strategy, **radical planning**, emphasizes innovation and spontaneity and considers experimentation as a component of the learning process to achieve innovation. Radical planning may be most applicable to the resolution of an issue such as establishment of a new type of health program.

A STRATEGIC PLANNING MODEL

A strategic plan is a useful and necessary tool in corporate strategy development—but it is not (nor should it be) the end objective. Strategic planning seeks to define the organization and its future with an emphasis on designing and bringing about a desired future rather than designing and implementing programs to achieve specific objectives.

Although a variety of approaches to strategic planning exist, they are all based on a generalized concept. This can be illustrated by Figure 3.2, from the accounting firm of Coopers & Lybrand. This model seeks to divide the strategic planning process into four sets of activities that answer four specific questions:

- Where are we now?
- Where should we be going?
- How should we get there?
- Are we getting there?

These questions focus on the activities of planning. For example, to answer the question "Where are we now?" a situational analysis is required where participants must collect and assemble data that address the organization's environment and operations. This leads to an assessment, such as a strengths/weaknesses/opportunities/threats (SWOT) analysis, and concludes with the establishment of a set of issues and challenges for the organization.

Figure 3.2 Strategic Planning Model

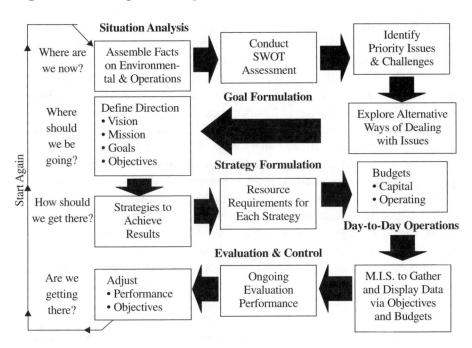

Source: Adapted from Keck, R. K., Jr. 1986. "Strategic Planning in the Health Care Industry: Concentrate on the Basics." *Health Care Issues* (September), reprinted in *Handbook of Business Strategy 1985/1986 Yearbook*, Coopers & Lybrand.

The question "Where should we be going?" can be answered with goal formulation, including an exploration of alternative strategies, and the development of organizational direction in the form of statements of vision, mission, goals, and objectives. Strategy formulation answers the question "How should we get there?" The exercise includes development of strategies or actions to achieve goals and an assessment of the resources needed to achieve each strategy goal (including budgets). Following the strategic implementation of operations, planners address evaluation and control through the final question, "Are we getting there?" The monitoring that this entails requires the collection and analysis of data, followed by the use of this performance feedback to adjust the organization's goals—and the management of operations to achieve these outcomes. This continuous process then is repeated from the beginning, using evaluation data as input for the next situational analysis and further refinement of the strategic planning process. This model breaks down a complex process of decision making into workable segments, but it requires a great deal of time and effort nevertheless. One must bear in mind, throughout the process, that in developing such a plan, the objective is not to write a plan, but to get something accomplished—to take action now regarding the future direction and profitability of the organization

All of these activities are informed by the collection of epidemiologic data. Morbidity profiles, for instance, describe the "Where are we now?" question. For a hospital, this might include case-mix measures or a breakdown of patients by DRGs. Physician practices could characterize patient mix by Current Procedure Terminology (CPT) code or the Resource-Based Relative Value Scale (RBRVS), in the case of Medicare Patients. The "Where should we be?" question requires the organization to describe the service population (both current and potential) in terms of need. Descriptors of need would include both current morbidity burden (measured by the incidence and prevalence of disease) and future morbidity burden. Future need can be estimated based on demographics, as well as the burden of risk factors that can lead to disease, such as the prevalence of smoking, obesity, high blood pressure, and so on. The "How should we get there?" question may also require epidemiologic input, to the extent that alternative patient care or treatment strategies exist, or that "best care" strategies, practice guidelines, or critical pathways need to be collected and implemented. Obviously, the "Are we getting there?" question requires epidemiologic input. It is particularly important in the healthcare sector that performance be measured in terms of patient care as well as financial outcomes.

Suppose, for example, a managed care organization is engaged in the strategic planning process. The organization has described "where they are" in terms of DRG and CPT profiles and notices a relatively high proportion of cardiovascular disease among the enrolled population. Epidemiologic data are collected on service area, in general, which confirms a high prevalence of cardiovascular disease, as well as cardiovascular risk factors such as smoking and obesity. The organization decides to address the "Where should we be?" question by focusing specifically on cardiovascular disease, among other things. The question of how to get there is somewhat more complex; it involves many decisions, such as whether or not to promote prevention through smoking cessation and weight reduction programs. Epidemiologic studies may provide useful insight into this decision-making process.

MARKETING

An organization's most precious asset is its relationship with customers as defined in terms of quality, service, and price. Although many view marketing as advertising, it is a far more complex set of activities. At the most basic level, marketing can be defined as an exchange between two parties to satisfy the needs of both: in the case of healthcare, an exchange of health services for appropriate compensation. Traditional marketing can be described by the **four Ps** of marketing: product, place, price, and promotion. **Product** or service defines the activity of the organization and can be described, for healthcare, as the set of activities focused on particular diagnoses, such as acute myocardial infarction. Alternatively, product/service can be described as the benefits the service provides to the patient, such as relief from pain or anxiety or help in achieving a longer life.

Place or location refers to how the product or service will be delivered to the patient. This marketing concept refers not simply to location, but to other factors such as operating hours, referral mechanisms, and enablers and barriers to access based on both external market segmentation and internal operational factors. The third measure, **price** or fees, addresses not only the charge for the service (which usually is not paid by the patient), but everything that the organization requires the patient to go through to use the service. Price links revenue and consumer satisfaction, as it controls a potential conflict of interest between providing the highest-quality prod-uct and increasing revenue. **Promotion** includes activities to acquaint the prospective patient with the organization and the services it offers. Promotion is a matter of communicating information between an organization and a market; it describes the means by which the patient becomes aware of the services offered and develops an interest in using one or more of the services. Strategic concepts in marketing include product differentiation, price competition, market segmentation by socioeconomic variables, product segmentation for different populations, and mass marketing/advertising. A subcategory of marketing, with a direct relationship to healthcare, is known as social marketing, which focuses on behavior (e.g., on changing health behaviors such as smoking or diet).

Although planning and marketing are closely related both conceptually and operationally (MacStravic 1977), it is the former that has received more considerable attention in terms of governmental policy: note the litany of health planning legislation reviewed earlier in the chapter (Lee 1989). "Planning presents a method for design and management of change, while marketing offers design and management of exchange relations with impor-tant publics" (Lee 1989). Clearly, both planning and marketing are informed by epidemiologic measures. A critical stage of planning is environmental assessment (or needs assessment), in which the organization or agency attempts to characterize the needs of the population served. In the case of healthcare, this must involve morbidity profiles, described specifically in terms of the incidence and prevalence rates of acute and chronic disease. Marketing strategies should also incorporate epidemiologic measures. Product definition, for instance, depends to some degree on descriptions of need. The development of a women's health "product" should be defined on the basis of dimensions of need in this area, much of which is epidemiologically derived—the prevalence of breast and ovarian cancer, for instance. Strategies with regard to place include an assessment of barriers to access. These barriers may be recognized, to some degree, on the basis of epidemiologic measures, the high incidence of cervical cancer among women in eastern Kentucky, for example. Promotional activities may include motivational messages, based in part on epidemiologic studies. Primary prevention, such as cancer screening, can be promoted by encouraging clients to consider the advantages of early- versus late-stage diagnosis in terms of survival studies. Social marketing has clear epidemiologic roots to the extent that behaviors, such as smoking, diet, and sexual behaviors, have been epidemiologically linked to morbidity.

CONCLUSION

Earlier we described planning as making assessments and provision for the future, or as making current choices to influence the future, which may involve guiding the process of change. We have demonstrated the need and the means by which both community and institutional planning should be intimately acquainted with epidemiologic measures. *Healthy People 2000* for example, groups objectives in terms of health status objectives (measured in terms of disease-specific mortality rates, for instance) and risk reduction objectives (measured in terms of reducing the prevalence of a risk factor among the population). With institutional planning, questions regarding the current and future position or role within a health service market require both internal and external assessment processes that thrive on valid epidemiologic measures. Finally, to the extent that planning and marketing are flip-sides of the same coin, organizations would benefit by using epidemiology to describe the morbidity and risk factor burden of current and potential markets, and by using epidemiologic studies to facilitate the promotion of healthcare products to the consumer.

Case Study 3.1: Eastern Kentucky Health

Eastern Kentucky Health (EKH) is a fictitious IPA model health maintenance organization that serves patients in a number of counties in southeastern Kentucky. EKH has entered into partnership with several local communities to meet *Healthy People 2000* objectives, but it is struggling with a number of priority areas dealing with tobacco use, obesity, hypertension, and related mortality (refer to Table 3.5):

1. What are the kinds and sources of data that need to be collected to make rational planning decisions?
2. What kinds of interventions should EKH consider to address the key priority areas?
3. How might EKH market these programs to the enrolled population?

Case Study 3.2: Poudre Valley

Poudre Valley is a profitable hospital in Fort Collins, Colorado with a 90 percent market share and a 7 percent operating margin, according to a report by Fitch IBCA, a New York-based credit rating agency. Lower Medicare reimbursement under the balanced budget act is likely to continue to eat away at those earnings, according to Fitch. But Stacey, Poudre Valley Health System CEO, says planning for the new campus began three years ago, and that the lower reimbursement isn't a reason to back out of the plan. "We've known for some time that rates are going down. It's important for us to be as diversified as possible and have opportunities in outpatient medicine," he says.

Construction on the building is already under way. The facility will include a catheter lab, an ambulatory surgery center, a radiology diagnostic center, and an oncology diagnostic center. Total costs will run to $55 million, Stacey says.

The physicians are equity partners in each of these joint ventures and will pay between one-third and half the cost of the new project. That lessens the capital strain on the hospital, but also cuts into its profits, which are divided according to ownership, but Stacey says the tradeoff is well worth it.

"It really ties (the doctors) into cost containment," he says. (*Preemptive strike*: Part of what drove the deals, according to Stacey, was the knowledge that if the hospital didn't partner with the doctors and help build them new facilities, the doctors could build competing facilities.) Stacey adds, "We think this strategy allows us to maintain access to revenue streams that we otherwise might have lost." (Saphir 1999).

1. Describe the kinds of planning activity that preceded the decision to invest $55 million in the new facilities.
2. What kinds of epidemiologic data should have been collected to inform this decision-making process?
3. What are the advantages and disadvantages of having physicians as equity partners?
4. To what extent should physicians be a source of epidemiologic data?
5. What other sources of epidemiologic data could be collected?

Table 3.5 Mortality Rates, Smoking, and Obesity

Category	Baseline (1987)	Kentucky (1998)**	United States (1998)**	2000 Goal
Cigarette Smoking				
High school education, adults	34%	36%	23%	20%
Blue collar workers, adults	36%	40%	29%	20%
White, adults		31%	23%	
Blacks, adults	34%	26%	23%	18%
Women of reproductive age*	29%	28% (women)	21% (women)	12%
Pregnant women‡	25%	28% (women)	21% (women)	10%
Obesity				
Adolescents	15%†	36%	32%	15%
Adults	26%†			20%
Low-income women	37%†			25%
Black women	44%†			30%
Reduce coronary heart disease mortality (per 100,000)	135			100
Slow the rise in lung cancer mortality (per 100,000)§	47.9			53
Slow the rise in COPD mortality (per 100,000)§	18.7			25

*Baseline for women 18–44; †Baseline is 1976–1980; ‡1985 baseline.

§ The objective is to slow the rise; the rate in 2000 is projected to be higher than the goal.

**Source:* Behavioral Risk Factor Surveillance System.

***United States National

Source: American Public Health Association. 1991. *Healthy Communities 2000 Model Standards: Guidelines for Community Attainment for the Year 2000 National Health Objectives.* Washington, DC: APHA.

REFERENCES

American Public Health Association (APHA). 1991. *Healthy Communities 2000 Model Standards: Guidelines for Community Attainment of the Year 2000 National Health Objectives*. Washington, DC: APHA.

Berry, D. E. 1974. "The Transfer of Planning Theories to Health Planning Practice." *Policy Sciences* 5: 343–61.

Centers for Disease Control and Prevention (CDC). 1991. *APEX(PH) Assessment Protocol for Excellence in Public Health*. Bethesda, MD: CDC.

Duncan, W. J., P. M. Ginter, and L. E. Swayne. 1995. *Strategic Management of Health Care Organizations*. Malden, MA: Blackwell Publishers.

Hoge, V. M. 1958. "Hospital Bed Needs: A Review of Developments in the United States." *Canadian Journal of Public Health* 49 (1): 1–8.

Keck, R. K., Jr. 1986. "Strategic Planning in the Health Care Industry: Concentrate on the Basics." *Health Care Issues* (September), reprinted in *Handbook of Business Strategy 1985/1986 Yearbook*, Coopers & Lybrand.

Lee, J. M. 1989. "Marketing in Health Services Administration." In *Handbook of Human Services Administration*, edited by J. Rabin and M. Steinhauser. New York: Marcel Decker.

Lee, R. I., and L. W. Jones. 1933. *The Fundamentals of Good Medical Care*. Publication of the Committee on the Costs of Medical Care, No. 22. Chicago: University of Chicago Press.

MacStravic, R. E. 1977. *Marketing Health Care*. Germantown, MD: Aspen Systems.

Peddecord, K. M. 1998. "Public Health Management Tools Planning." In *Maxcy-Rosenau-Last: Public Health and Preventive Medicine, 14th ed.*, edited by R. B. Wallace and B. N. Doebbeling, Stamford, CT: Appleton & Lang.

Saphir, A. 1999. "Erector Set." *Modern Healthcare* 29 (49): 50.

U.S. Department of Health and Human Services, Public Health Service. 1996. *Healthy People 2000: Midcourse Review and 1995 Revisions*. Washington, DC: Government Printing Office.

U.S. Department of Health and Human Services. 1991. *Healthy People 2000: National Health Promotion and Disease Prevention Objectives*. Pub. No. (PHS) 91–50212. Washington, DC: Government Printing Office.

———. 1980. *Promoting Health/Preventing Disease: Objectives for the Nation*. Washington, DC: Government Printing Office.

———. 1979. *Healthy People*. Pub. No. (PHS) 79-55071. Washington, DC: Government Printing Office.

The Challenges of Physician–Health System Partnerships

Craig E. Holm, CHE

Physicians and hospitals have long coexisted as the key players in the healthcare delivery system. Relationships between them have been characterized by bonds of codependency, ranging from fierce independence to loose collaborations to complete hospital acquisition of physician practices. Each side has struggled with the harsh reality that neither can thrive without the existence and support of the other.

Physician-hospital affiliations have experienced variable success through the years as the effectiveness of a wide spectrum of models has been tested, largely driven by the potential for securing financial viability. In many cases, hospitals and health systems have pursued affiliations with physicians with the goal of maintaining their existing infrastructure and retaining or increasing referrals. These initiatives have had the appearance of trying to shelter physicians from the maelstrom of upheaval in the industry but have often proved to be control mechanisms that reflect little foresight and understanding of what physicians want and need or of the long-term effects of the affiliation for both parties.

Physicians' avid interest in maintaining autonomy over clinical decisions while securing their financial futures is nurtured by the value of their decisions to patients' well-being and the many years of training their profession demands. Clinical autonomy and income disputes have challenged many physician-hospital partnerships—partnerships that must be grounded by the

Editor's Note: This chapter is from Chapter 1 of *Next-Generation Physician–Health System Partnerships* by Craig E. Holm, 2000, HAP inevitability that the days of lucrative reimbursement and control of the reimbursement process are long gone. Physicians' entrepreneurial nature and their interests in more and better technology and equipment, ample time off, and convenient, accessible facilities have also been factors in the ongoing search for effective physician–health system partnerships.

As conflicts have intensified, a divisive wedge has been driven between physicians and hospitals. But a new urgency is now evident as competition among providers, battles with managed care companies, struggles for market share, tensions between primary care physicians and specialists, and threats from Wall Street—funded, for-profit management corporations have led to all-out warfare to see who will control or be on the receiving end of shrinking provider payments.

Hospitals will not be successful without solid, economically beneficial partnerships with physicians, because physicians control 75 percent of all medical costs within hospitals (Rutledge 1996). The physicians' pivotal position necessitates that physicians take a leading role in balancing the issues of cost, quality, and access in the realigning healthcare system.

As hospitals and physicians strive to provide quality care, the advantages afforded by affiliation and, ultimately, integration, can no longer be ignored. According to the Center for Research in Ambulatory Healthcare Administration (Managed Care Information Center 1998), by 2000, most hospitals and medical groups will have ventured into integrated delivery systems or networks. The study predicts that the number of medical groups that are freestanding will drop from 87 percent in 1994 to 3 percent in 1999. The number of freestanding hospitals is predicted to drop from 78 percent to 5 percent in the same period (Managed Care Information Center 1998).

To make the most of shrinking reimbursement and valuable community resources and to survive the future of healthcare, physicians and hospitals must resolve conflicts and maximize areas of confluence and commonality by collaborating to integrate healthcare services and economic interests. Demands for cost efficiency and measurable outcomes will force hospitals and physicians to overcome their long histories of independence and, at times, dissension and find common ground that will enable them to align into mutually beneficial partnerships and integrated, financially successful systems and networks.

HISTORICAL PERSPECTIVE: HOW DID WE GET HERE?

Relationships between physicians and hospitals have historically been based upon the fundamental premises of independence and separatism. Medical practices were viewed as small, cottage industries and hospitals as large, community-based industries.

During the last 30 years of the twentieth century and particularly during the final decade, physician-hospital relationships nationwide evolved into a curious mix of marginally successful and financially disastrous partnerships.

Hospitals and physicians in the 1970s could be characterized as coexistent and independent—faculty practice plans and hospital-based physicians (e.g., pathologists, radiologists, emergency medicine physicians) were the only common examples of physicians who had been integrated into a system. By the late 1970s, however, early signs of competition emerged as warnings were heeded that the long-standing fee-for-service and cost-plus-reimbursement system might be challenged and that competition for healthcare dollars would increase.

During the 1980s, the notion that physicians and hospitals should consider more formal linkages spurred early integration efforts as competition among providers to align with physician practices intensified. The "alphabet soup" mix of physician-hospital alliances emerged as hospital-linked IPAs (independent practice associations), PHOs (physician-hospital organizations), MSOs (management service organizations), and hospital-affiliated GPWWs (group practices without walls) made their way into healthcare slang.

Intense competition for decreasing reimbursement kept healthcare lawyers, accountants, and consultants busy in the 1990s. The organization of megagroups of physicians, formation of large integrated delivery systems, practice acquisition by health systems, the emergence of closer relationships between physicians and physician practice management and pharmaceutical firms, closure of some hospital medical staffs, and the influence of managed care companies have essentially left physicians with two choices: full integration with a hospital or health system (e.g., practice acquisition and exclusive contracting) or independence. The few options available in between full integration and independence, such as PHOs, have failed to fulfill their promises of providing added value to physicians. Instead, such options often nearly irretrievably damage relationships between physicians and hospitals and leave a legacy of mistrust and jockeying and posturing for control.

The late 1990s witnessed the extent to which physicians have felt frustrated and angered by integrated delivery system and managed care dominance. In June 1999, the American Medical Association (AMA) voted to approve a national union for employed physicians (Reuters Health 1999). The plan authorizes the AMA to establish local negotiating units for physicians in training and hospital medical staff physicians and will affect about 100,000 employed physicians. Private practice physicians are currently not permitted to join unions or to have unions negotiate for them, but the AMA is backing federal and local legislation to remove this restriction and allow the AMA union to offer its services to self-employed physicians (Reuters Health 1999). State and regional organization efforts are currently underway.

CULTURE CLASH

While environmental forces have driven and molded many physician-hospital alliances and affected their degree of success, the vastly divergent cultural backgrounds that physicians and healthcare executives have brought to the bargaining table have also profoundly influenced the structure of the partnerships and their potential for success.

Physicians are highly autonomous and individualistic. Even in group practices they regard themselves as individuals tied together by centralized clinical and management systems (Barnett 1998). Physicians tend to exhibit healthy skepticism and be critical of themselves and others, and their loyalty typically lies with their patients and physician colleagues with whom they have worked for years. In contrast, physicians' relationships with hospital leaders are far more tenuous—a result, in part, of the shorter tenure of hospital administrative staff. Mistrust and concern over control often characterize physician views of hospital and healthcare system leaders, because the skills that have allowed a hospital to run profitably and effectively have not always been successful in meeting the needs and managing the operations of physician partnerships.

Further evidence of this "culture clash" is found in the training backgrounds of those ultimately responsible for physician practices (i.e., physicians) and those primarily responsible for hospital systems (i.e., hospital administrators). Physicians are trained in clinical practice, which demands decision making and management skills that are quite different from those of their hospital administrator colleagues. Understanding these differences helps provide insight into the challenges of developing meaningful and lasting partnerships.

Characteristics of Self-Employed Physicians

According to data from the AMA Socioeconomic Monitoring System (AMA 1998), the number of patient care physicians who are employees has risen fairly rapidly, increasing from 29 percent to 54 percent between 1983 and 1997. Despite this increase, many physicians remain self-employed (i.e., in private practice) and often exhibit many of the characteristics presented below.

- Physicians work independently. Until recently most physicians were leaders of one-physician practices and had a total of two to five employees. Interaction with hospitals was periodic and sporadic, and included such activities as continuing education and other professional relationships, some of which were required for staff privileges and clinical referral relationships. Academic medical center faculty and hospital-based physicians (e.g., anesthesiologists, pathologists, radiologists, and emergency department physicians) are common exceptions that are discussed later in this chapter.

- Physicians make clinical decisions affecting individual patients and business decisions involving only three to six people. The vast majority of decisions made by physicians are clinical and involve individuals and specific disease conditions. Business decisions in physician practices usually lack great complexity when compared to those made in the hospital environment, and affect only a few staff members.

- Physicians make decisions quickly based on the information available. Clinical decisions are made fairly rapidly to accelerate the healing or preventive health process. Although diagnostic tests aid in decision making, a clinical judgement or diagnosis sometimes must be based on less than complete information to expedite decision making about the appropriate treatment plan. It is often appropriate to render a diagnosis quickly based on the availability of the vast majority of the information than to delay a treatment plan until all of the desired information is available. The available timeframe for decision making may be quite short.

- Physicians lack business or management training. Medical school training focuses on the scientific origin of disease and clinical diagnosis and treatment. Training in business and practice development is virtually nonexistent, and is usually gained through "on-the-job" experiences.

- Physicians work in an entrepreneurial, small business environment. Physicians in private practice have the ultimate motivation: to make their practice succeed to protect their personal livelihood, reputation, and status. However, the complexity and magnitude of the variables influencing a successful practice are few in comparison to those that lead to the success or failure of a hospital system. Solo practices usually generate between $200,000 and $750,000 in revenue annually, compared to a hospital system often with annual revenue of several hundred million dollars.

- Physicians often lack consensus-building skills. Because of the small size of many physician practices and the nature of solo leadership, physicians rarely have a chance to develop or test consensus-building skills. Most clinical decisions are made quickly with limited information. In contrast, developing consensus is time-consuming and usually requires thorough investigation of all components of the situation and the underlying rationale is explored from every imaginable perspective to satisfy as many of the affected constituents as possible.

Characteristics of Hospital Administrators

In contrast, hospital administrators are often responsible for one component or for all of a multimillion-dollar business enterprise. Their training, professional behavior, and work environment are usually a striking contrast to that of the typical physician in private practice.

- Hospital administrators facilitate consensus decision making. Most hospital systems are made up of 30 to 40 individual departments, many of which have oversight by a professional manager and a clinical (often a physician) leader. For most major hospital system decisions (e.g., whether to merge or affiliate, development of new programs, development of an annual capital budget), multiple departments are affected and vast resources and professional talent are usually available. In general, to successfully manage a complex enterprise, such as a hospital, administrators must obtain as much input as possible to facilitate consensus decision making.

- Administrators require a comprehensive analysis of the rationale, implications, and process for an issue or problem before making a decision. The reason behind this behavior is linked to the preceding point. Such an approach enables the hospital administrator to make progress in gaining consensus regarding a particular issue, but it also renders the process slow and laborious as every new angle is explored and every approach to an issue is examined. As a result, hospital administrators have a reputation for making decisions slowly and exhibiting bureaucratic behavior. Physicians view this behavior as administrators being unable to make decisions on their own. In reality administrators usually attempt to wait to build consensus and analyze the situation in a comprehensive manner before coming to a conclusion and making a recommendation. However, the healthcare market now requires more expeditious decision making. Complete consensus building has become a luxury. Increasingly, decisions are financially driven rather than based predominantly on consensus.

- Administrators work in teams and primarily in meetings. Patients arrive at a physician's office, are examined by a physician, and depart with a diagnosis and treatment plan. In contrast, hospital administrators conduct most of their business day in a group setting and rely on the power of persuasion, thorough analyses, and convincing arguments to sway others toward a specific course of action. Usually, very little progress toward furthering the course of action occurs in between each meeting.

- Administrators gain extensive business and management training through graduate-level education and hospital management continuing education. The typical training of a hospital administrator is a liberal arts or business undergraduate degree followed by several years of experience and then a two-year graduate program focusing on business or healthcare administration. The hospital administrator then participates in ongoing training in the business approach to healthcare at continuing education seminars. In addition, the administrator often has a supervisor who prepares a professional development plan, including participation in targeted continuing education programs.

- Administrators make business decisions that involve many. The administrator, after a comprehensive evaluation of the issues involved, will eventually make or facilitate a decision. Part of the rationale for involving so many people in the input stages of processing an issue is to ensure that constituencies affected will not be surprised and that they will support the implementation process. Although superiors overturn some decisions by hospital administrators, this rarely happens in the physician practice environment where the physician is the "captain of the ship."

Clearly, the operating environments and cultures of the two groups differ greatly in style, have led to miscommunication and a lack of trust between physicians and hospitals, and have engendered separatism rather than partnerships. However, exceptions to the rule of absolute independence of physicians and hospital systems have occurred, mostly prior to 1990, and varying levels of integration have been achieved. Three of these exceptions are outlined below.

1. Faculty–academic medical center relationship. In this relationship, physicians are employed, usually through a faculty practice plan, to practice within the confines of the organization's academic mission, including education, research, and clinical responsibilities. Often these employed faculty physicians earn tenured, professional status similar to other university faculty. However, these relationships are limited to a relatively small subset of physicians, usually subspecialty physicians whose focus is predominantly teaching or research instead of clinical practice. This exception is generally successful because of the confluence of objectives, notably the shared pursuit by all parties of the academic mission: research, teaching, and clinical care.

2. Physician relations programs. These programs, which exhibit some level of affiliation and collaboration but not necessarily a partnership, continue to be fairly common in the industry. The concept is for personal visitation to physician practices by a hospital management representative (often called a "physician sales representative"). The formal agenda for the visit was historically, "How can ABC Hospital support your practice?" The hidden agenda for these visits was "How can ABC Hospital garner some, all, or more of your inpatient and ancillary referral volumes?" These programs have been prevalent as

vehicles for addressing a major source of conflict between health systems and physician practices—unresolved or unattended hospital operations inefficiencies.

3. Employment or practice acquisition by a hospital system. Before the flurry of primary care physician employment in the 1990s, employment of physicians was mostly limited to hospital-based specialists (e.g., anesthesiologists, radiologists, emergency medicine physicians, intensivists, and pathologists). Often a limited number of other specialists whose practices included a substantial portion of hospital-linked care also had some sort of contractual relationship with a hospital system. Examples of these contractual relationships include medical directorship of medicine or surgery; the intensive care unit; the pathology, emergency medicine, or radiology departments; the vascular laboratory; and the hospital-based gastrointestinal laboratory. The logic for developing these contractual relationships has been to secure and stabilize coverage in those specialties that support all other specialties practicing at the hospital and to pay a stipend in some cases to offset losses in clinical practice revenue resulting from administrative responsibilities. This approach has been used extensively by hospitals because it provides a major area of confluence: hospitals' desire for coverage and physicians' desire for secure, contractual relationships.

These and many other strategies (e.g., MSOs, joint contracting, joint ventures) have been employed to integrate physicians; however, independence has historically been the most common state for physician practices. Hospitals have relied on the attraction of technology and equipment and the loyalty of physicians to focus their practice at a particular hospital. In such a relationship, physicians work in a hospital, refer to a hospital's programs and services, refer to specialists who are affiliated with the hospital, and satisfy the medical staff membership requirements of hospital committee and meeting attendance.

Without formal ties, physicians can easily shift loyalties and practices from one hospital system to another. In Philadelphia, "the three Bs," three well-known orthopedists, Arthur Bartolozzi, Robert Booth, and Richard Balderston, left the Rothman Institute at Pennsylvania Hospital in July 1997 to join Allegheny Health System (Cohen 1999). The corporation owned by the three orthopedists was guaranteed $3.9 million a year in salary plus incentives. Allegheny also agreed to pay for all building upgrades, billing and support staff, and valet parking for patients (Stark 1998). One year later Allegheny filed for bankruptcy and the group took their 4,000 procedures per year back to Pennsylvania Hospital (Business News in Brief 1998).

To combat the potential loss of physicians, hospitals have employed various strategies in an attempt to "bind" physicians. Examples from the late 1980s and early 1990s include:

- Recruitment assistance. This service has typically included the payment (when legally warranted) of recruitment fees, reimbursement for moving expenses for new recruits, and loans for practice start-up expenses. Federal regulators (e.g., the Internal Revenue Service) seem to afford more latitude (so that hospitals do not jeopardize their tax-exempt status) if consideration of these payments is preceded by an evaluation of community need for physicians. The evaluation should objectively demonstrate that the hospital system is supporting, either in the present or projected for the future, the provision of incremental physician supply to an area of demonstrated community need.

- Designation of medical director positions. Sometimes a stipend is provided to a physician who is designated as medical director for a service. Examples include a quality assurance or utilization review medical director and medical director of a clinical program (e.g., cardiology, oncology, home care). The medical director stipend should be a legitimate fair market payment for work required. Such work includes committee meeting attendance, quality review of a program, and other responsibilities. These attempts have generally failed to secure the loyalty of physicians, as demonstrated by the high turnover rate of medical directors and the fact that the linkage is focused on a narrow topic rather than broad based.

PHYSICIAN–HEALTH SYSTEM PARTNERSHIPS IN A COMPETITIVE, MANAGED CARE ENVIRONMENT

The realities of the reimbursement environment have been felt full force by hospitals and health systems in the past five to seven years as physicians and hospitals are attempting to deal with the "common enemy"—managed care payors and their influences. A number of integration strategies, such as MSOs, PHOs, joint ventures, and IPAs, have been attempted to improve practice and health system visibility and have dramatically changed the relationships between hospital systems and physicians. These strategies have experienced some marginal success but in most cases—such as practice acquisition and employment—have led to disastrous financial performance and strained relationships. The growing pains experienced by these physician-hospital relationships include governance and control battles, mistrust about the intentions of each party, huge operating losses, declines in physician productivity and morale, bloated cost structures, and, generally, failed promises.

Despite these failures, a number of compelling rationales remain for continuing to explore and create more effective physician-hospital partnerships:

- Hospitals and physicians are in the same business of healthcare, serving the same customers, in the same communities. Ideally, hospitals and physicians should share responsibility and accountability for the health status of communities they serve. Many potential physician partners represent entities from outside a community whose interests are profit motivated rather than community oriented.

- Hospitals' and physicians' strategic advantages are different but complementary—hospitals can certainly learn about entrepreneurship from physicians and physicians can benefit from hospitals' resources and clout.

- Competition between hospitals and physicians can be a deleterious use of valuable and often shrinking community resources. A common example is the proliferation of independent physician-owned ambulatory surgery centers that have duplicated resources available at hospital operating rooms.

- Physician-hospital partnerships have the potential to generate financial benefits for both parties, including improved market position from the more extensive development of programs and services, the ability to secure managed care contracts, and joint venture opportunities that can increase physician practice incomes while sustaining or maintaining hospital system revenue.

- Hospitals are motivated to create sustainable partnerships with physicians. Hospitals face threats from other hospitals, physician practice management firms, and payors who may attempt to partner with physicians and force hospitals into the role of a vendor or commodity rather than that of a vital component or driver of healthcare delivery in a community. Hospitals also fear that their "loyal" physicians will partner with "nonloyal" physicians.

Recently, more creative and meaningful relationships between systems and physicians have been emerging, and employment is not the only example of a fully integrated relationship. Relationships between physicians and hospital systems are evolving. The limited number of options thought to exist for hospitals and physicians has been expanded to include a variety of relationships that establish sustainable partnerships, provide value to both physicians and hospitals, and reduce conflict.

These evolving relationships and how they affect both physicians and hospitals must be examined. How can hospitals and health systems avoid steep financial losses from physician affiliations? How can physicians benefit from partnerships with hospitals? How can partnerships be structured to enhance the clinical autonomy of physicians and stave off reductions in physician income? How can partnerships create value for the hospital, physicians, patients, and payors?

With increasingly compelling evidence that their futures are inextricably intertwined, hospitals and physicians must aggressively seek new and more creative models for working together—models that are grounded in trust and shared governance and are committed to managing care to enhance quality and control costs, rather than control referrals. In this volatile and unstable period in the healthcare industry, the risks of maintaining the status quo or letting past failures prevent future collaborations are high. Hospitals and physicians with a willingness to break new ground and create more effective alliances will set the standard for physician-hospital partnerships in the next century of healthcare and will become strong competitors in their markets.

REFERENCES

American Medical Association and the Center for Health Policy Research. 1998. *Socioeconomic Characteristics of Medical Practice* 1997/98, 18. Chicago: American Medical Association.

Barnett, A. E. 1998. "Public Physician Practice Management Companies." *Medical Group Management Journal* (May/June): 51.

Business News in Brief. 1998. *Philadelphia Inquirer* September 16: C3

Cohen, M. 1999. "Waiting for Bartolozzi." *Philadelphia Magazine* [Online article. Retrieval 5/14/99]. www.phillymag.com

Managed Care Information Center. 1998. *Top Trends in Physicians' Roles in an Integrated Healthcare Environment*, 2. Pamphlet. Manasquan, NJ: The Managed Care Information Center.

Reuters Health. 1999. "AMA OK's Union for Docs." [Online article. Retrieval 6/99]. www.news.excite.com.

Rutledge, V. R. 1996. "Hospital/Physician Alignment: A Model for Success." *Oncology Issues* 11 (6): 18–20.

Stark, K. 1998. "Allegheny Culture: Privileges and Perks Bankruptcy Neared, But Salaries Soothed." *Philadelphia Inquirer* December 27: A01.

Measuring Performance

John R. Griffith, FACHE

Well-managed healthcare organizations study their open systems environment, develop community-oriented strategies in response, and continuously improve their operating processes. They have a strong customer focus, an emphasis on mission and vision, and a commitment to empowering their operating core. This philosophy leads them to a strategically focused governing board, a service-oriented executive group, and a flexible, decentralized organization.

Continuous improvement requires realistic and convincing analysis of opportunities. To meet these criteria, the decision processes of well-managed healthcare organizations rely heavily on the use of quantitative data covering multiple dimensions of activities.[1] Quantitative information begins as simple counts and measures recorded in the course of events. Rarely will these suffice. Definitions and collection routines are required to ensure accuracy. The original measures are useful only in context of other events, requiring adjustments that must be carefully specified and uniformly administered. And random variation clouds analysis; comparison must acknowledge the limits of accuracy on each measure. The ability to define, acquire, store, retrieve, and analyze these data, to maintain a "source of truth" about the various elements of the organization and its environment, becomes a critical resource. Mastery of performance measurement allows the well-managed healthcare organization to gain a competitive advantage.

Simply put, vast databases, analytic skills, and reporting mechanisms are as important as the physical and human resources for an organization's

Editor's Note: This chapter is from Chapter 6 of The *Well-Managed Healthcare Organization, Fourth Edition,* by John R. Griffith, 1999, HAP

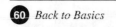

success. This chapter explores the use of numbers in healthcare management. It discusses what they are, where they come from, and how they are analyzed.

PURPOSE OF QUANTITATIVE INFORMATION

The purpose of quantitative information in organizations is to improve the quality of exchanges between the organization and its partners and constituents. Quantitative information allows communication about expectations and performance to be:

- *Explicit.* "High blood pressure" is ambiguous. "Diastolic pressure of 100 mm of mercury" is unambiguous. "High health insurance cost" is ambiguous. "One hundred forty dollars per member per month" is explicit. Removing ambiguity clarifies communication and speeds conclusion of negotiation.
- *Precise.* "Diastolic pressure of 100 +/– 5 mm mercury" and "one hundred forty dollars per member per month guaranteed" are statements of precision. Precision is only possible with quantitative information. The notions of expectations and improvement depend on precision; they are unworkable without it.
- *Efficient.* The concept of blood pressure measurement offers a new order of medical control. The graph in Figure 5.1A conveys quantitative information that actually defines the disease of hypertension. A full explanation of Figure 5.1A would be quite lengthy, but any literate person can see the message—"This patient's blood pressure is trending upwards and is already in the dangerous range." Figure 5.1B shows the same graph, but with different dimensions. Its message is "The cost of our services is trending upward and has already exceeded the amount our customer agreed to pay."
- *Timely.* Information that is explicit, precise, and efficient can be conveyed quickly. The message reaches the person or group that can do something about it in time for them to act.

Rapid learning, quick response, and close tolerances demand numbers because words alone are too ambiguous, too inefficient, and too slow.

KINDS OF QUANTITATIVE INFORMATION

The only disadvantage to the use of quantitative information is the cost of collecting the supporting data. Much of this cost is hidden from the accounting system, but it is real. The solution is to make the data collection as efficient as possible, and the keys to efficient data collection are an understanding of

Figure 5.1   Efficiency Possible with Quantitative Information

A. Patient's Diastolic Blood Pressure

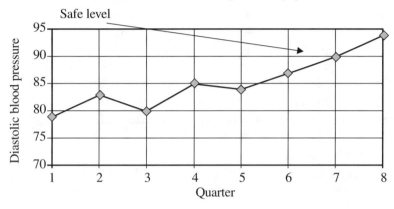

B. Cost of Care per Member per Month

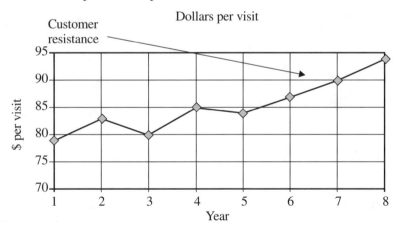

data needs, a systematic scheme for collecting data as a routine part of care activities themselves, and an understanding of the levels of precision required.

Dimensions for Quantitative Performance in Organizations

Figure 5.2 shows the dimensions of information required to measure performance of healthcare activities. They provide a comprehensive description of performance for a function or a final product. They apply to any level of organization, from the work group to an integrated system. Three of these dimensions, demand, cost, and output/productivity, are familiar from the conventional accounting system. They are expanded from the traditional accounting view to reflect all of the areas where expectations can be established. The other three, human resources, quality, and customer satisfaction, are more recent additions, reflecting increased market concerns and improved measurement technology. Conceptually at least, the six dimensions apply to any product or service. A manufacturer or a hairdresser would want to know demand, cost, workers available, sales, quality, customer satisfaction, and profit, but as the detail develops, the measures become unique to healthcare. The six are clearly interrelated, often in precise mathematical terms. If all six are managed, the business is likely to succeed; if even one is overlooked, it is likely to fail.

Input-related measures

Three measurement dimensions relate to the starting points of the exchange. There must always be a demand for service, raw materials, and people to perform the work. Several kinds of measures are needed for each dimension, to support the various kinds of decisions that must be made.

Demand

Measures of demand include requests for service, market share, appropriateness of service, and logistics of service.

Figure 5.2 Dimensions of Healthcare Performance

Input-Oriented	*Output-Oriented*
Demand	Output/Productivity
Requests for service	Treatments or discreet
Market share	Services rendered
Appropriateness of service	Productivity
Logistics of service	(Resources/treatment or service)
Cost/Resources	Quality
Physical counts	Clinical outcomes
Costs	Procedural quality
Resource condition	Structural quality
Human Resources	Customer Satisfaction
Supply	Patient satisfaction
Satisfaction	Referring physician satisfaction
Training	Other customer satisfaction
	Access

- *Requests for service.* The simplest level of demand is the number of patients requesting service. Requests are normally counted on a specific time basis and often segregated by patient characteristic as well as the service itself. Demand can be aggregated by function (**intermediate products**) or episodes of care for individual patients (**final products**). For example, demand for imaging service would be counted by type of examination, patient demographics, diagnosis, referring physician, insurance carrier, and time of request and time filled. Final product demand aggregates where imaging is important include trauma, pneumonia, chronic lung disease, and breast cancer. The parameters recorded are necessary for some part of the service, but they also provide a database for analysis of demand processes.

- *Market share.* The percentage of total demand in a market served by the organization is an important indicator of success. Most organizations strive for increasing **market share**. The measurement of market share requires an estimate of the demand going to other suppliers, a number usually purchased or acquired from an independent source. The imaging department would want to know its market share by insurance carrier, referring physician, and kind of examination to develop a strategy protecting and expanding share.

- *Appropriateness of service.* The goal of healthcare is to provide all appropriate service, but only appropriate service. Counting appropriate demand always requires judgment, either in establishing rules applicable to all cases, or in conducting individual review of specific cases. Various promotional, educational, and management activities are undertaken to minimize inappropriate requests and maximize appropriate ones. Requests received can be counted as appropriate or inappropriate, and strategies devised to discourage inappropriate ones.

  Counting requests that were not received but should have been is more complicated. It involves identifying a population at risk and subtracting the number who requested service. The provider organization must undertake special studies to obtain data on the population at risk. For example, breast cancer screening guidelines were established in 1997 after extensive national debate.[2] Mammography in women under 40 is inappropriate; and mammography in women over 50 is appropriate. (Women 40 to 50 have an option.) Counting women over 50 who did not request a mammography requires identifying and measuring a population at risk, probably using some form of census or household survey, rather than the population seeking services, which would serve for a market share estimate.

- *Logistics of service.* Scheduling systems manage both the demand itself and the resources available to meet it. They make a fundamental contribution to productivity. Few healthcare activities are controlled by the caregiver; most depend on demand. For example, an imaging department would schedule patients to minimize waiting in the facility for service. It might use a sophisticated scheduling system to ensure that emergency patients receive priority, non-emergency patients are treated with minimum delay, and staffing levels are balanced to expected demand. Measures of scheduling would include the delay for patients seeking mammography, by women with an identified lump and women seeking routine examinations; delay for reporting back to referring physician; and measures of the productivity of the staff (examinations per person-hour) and the facility (examinations per machine-hour).

Costs and resources

Resources are counted by physical units, costs, and various measures of condition.

- *Physical units* are units of resource such as worker hours, specific supplies, and items of equipment. They are normally organized by type, labor, supplies, equipment, and other. Physical quantities are important in managing production processes; staffing decisions and care decisions are made about physical resources, not dollar amounts. Most counts of physical units are obtained in the accounting process. Examples are "radiologic technician hours worked," "number of films used," "inventory of film available" and "hours of imaging machine operation."
- *Costs* are economic measures of resources. Physical units are multiplied by a market or transfer price to obtain costs. Costs are recorded in the accounting process at the level of individual purchases. They are routinely aggregated by type and also by characteristic, as variable, semivariable, and fixed, as well as direct and indirect. Costs are recorded and summarized by functional work group and are highly accurate at that level. In the imaging unit, film would be a variable cost, labor a semivariable or fixed one, the equipment fixed. All of these are direct. Resources such as malpractice insurance and support from the executive office are indirect.

  Costs for the component intermediate products, for example, chest films, uterine ultrasounds, skull magnetic resonance examinations, can be identified by special study or by establishing the activity as a responsibility center. Because most clinical work groups do a wide range of activities, unit costs of individual services include a number of estimates that reduce the accuracy of unit costs. Costs for final products and service lines are established by reaggregating unit costs, a process called **activity-based costing**.[3] Well-designed accounting systems now produce activity-based costs that are generally reliable, but caution is necessary for highly sensitive analysis.[4] Breast screening patients would be one final product group; breast cancer patients another.

- *Resource condition measures* are important in some processes. "Fluoroscopy machines more than five years old," "percentage of inventory items out of stock," and "percentage of soft tissue dyes out of date" are examples.

Human resources

Supply measures of human resources count numbers of workers available, by skill level or job classification. As healthcare facilities cross-train personnel, counts of workers with specific training within a skill level become important. The supply measure is not identical to the cost measure because pay will be based on actual work as opposed to availability. Examples would be the number of imaging technicians employed, and the number trained to operate ultrasound machines. These counts would be different from the number working on a given day, or paid for a given day.

Satisfaction measures assess worker and physician satisfaction with all aspects of working conditions. It is important to differentiate among various classes of workers because they have different responses and different supply markets. Physicians may or may not be employees, but they cannot be omitted. Satisfaction affects both retention of current workers and recruitment of future ones.

Output-related measures

Three dimensions of output measures are now in common use. They include counts of activity, productivity measures constructed from output counts and resources, quality-of-care measures, and customer satisfaction measures.

Outputs

- *Treatments or services rendered.* Outputs are units of demand filled, as opposed to requested. The same parameters are useful. Outputs must be counted for all but the most trivial services and are usually captured in a patient invoice prepared by the accounting department. Separate counts of requests and output permit rapid identification of unfilled requests and provide data to ensure that the number remains very small. Once captured, output counts can be aggregated by intermediate products (function) or final products (episodes of care). Accurate identification and counts of output are essential to many quality measures. Studies to improve processes often begin with a comparison of outputs to demand at very specific levels. Imaging might analyze data on women scheduled for breast exams who did not arrive; repeat exams, incidences where the original film was flawed and had to be retaken; and cases of women diagnosed as negative who developed breast lumps shortly after examination.

- *Productivity.* **Productivity** is the ratio of inputs (resources) to outputs, or vice versa. Convenience and tradition cause some ratios to be inverted. It does not matter because:

  inputs/outputs = 1/(outputs/inputs)

  The term "efficiency" is almost synonymous with productivity, but this text will avoid it when specific measures are referenced. Like resources, productivity is measured in both physical and dollar units. Lab tests/hour worked and lab cost/test are productivity measures. So are length of stay (days of care consumed/patient treated) and cost/case (cost of care/patients treated).

  Productivity measures can be calculated for all components of cost (variable, fixed, direct, indirect). Imaging productivity measures include film cost/examination and direct labor cost/examination, facilities cost/exam and indirect cost/exam. Unit costs can also be calculated for marginal costs—the cost that would be incurred if output increased or saved if output declined. Because fixed costs would not change, the marginal cost would be less than the total, or long-run average cost.

  Load and occupancy ratios are productivity measures for fixed resources; they compare the resource used (an output) to the resource available (an input). Bed occupancy (number of patient days of care rendered/number of bed days available) is an example.

  Productivity measures are essential for strategic management because they can be compared to history, competition, and benchmarks. The actual productivity of imaging, cost/examination or personnel hours/examination, can be compared to price, price or cost information from competitors, and the distribution of similar costs in other, non-competing institutions. The actual productivity measures are routinely compared to constraints.

Quality

Quality measures include clinical outcomes measures, procedural quality measures, and structural quality measures, each of which has its own advantages and disadvantages.

- *Clinical outcomes measures.* **Outcomes measures** of the quality of the final product assess aspects of the patient's condition on discharge or conclusion of an episode of illness or care, whether the patient lived or died, got better or not, or achieved a specific recovery. Most are in the form of counts or rates (counts divided by the total population at risk) and are treated as attributes measures. "Perinatal mortality," "heart attack survival," and "hip surgery patients walking after six weeks" are examples. There are four approaches to developing measures:
  1. *Negative results or departures from established expectations*, for example, deaths, hospital-acquired infections, complications, and

adverse effects. The events can be counted individually or aggregated into a general measure.[5] Unexpected laboratory findings on confirmatory studies such as surgical tissue reports and autopsies also fit this group. It is always possible to state these measures in positive terms (i.e., the number or rate achieving the desired goal). A positive statement is preferable except where the failure rate is very low.

2. *Placement at termination of care*, whether home, ambulatory care, home care, other hospital, nursing home, or other. The measure is only appropriate when there is a defined end point to the episode of care, such as discharge from the hospital, transfer back to primary care physician, or simply an anniversary in a chronic disease.

3. *Subjective assessment of condition*, for example, the caregiver's opinion of whether the patient is cured, improved, stable with reduced function, or unstable and deteriorating.

4. *Objective assessment of condition* using various scales of physiological function, such as scales of laboratory values or scales of ability to perform functions of daily living, and any departure from planned course such as readmission, complication, or deterioration.

Data often come from medical records, but special surveys are sometimes necessary. Once outcomes measures are generated, they are available at any level of aggregation, from the individual patient to the entire patient population of the hospital. They can be aggregated only by patient or disease groups; there is no such thing as a clinical outcome from functional services. (The outcome must be related to the entire episode of care; it cannot be attributed to any particular component.) Outcomes measures often require collection of data from beyond the episode of care itself. Special surveys are sometimes required to collect the data. For example, cancer survival is usually assessed five years after treatment.

Using measures of clinical outcomes presents a number of serious problems. Outcomes are difficult to define in some situations, such as terminal care. The measures may not be sensitive, because only very small percentages of patients fail. It is difficult to aggregate diverse measures such as perinatal mortality, orthopedic patients experiencing full recovery, and postoperative infections, into a single index or indicator for an institution. Outcomes depend on many factors, some of which may be beyond the control of the healthcare organization.[6] Perinatal mortality, for example, depends on the health of the mother before and throughout the pregnancy. The number of hip surgery patients walking in six weeks depends on their condition when they requested surgery. Finally, outcomes measures are difficult to relate to potential corrections. For example, if 20 percent of patients fail to walk six weeks after hip surgery, why did they fail? Was it poor surgical technique, poor postoperative care, or factors outside the normal care system, such as inadequate housing or lack of motivation on the patient's part?

Despite their limitations, buyer pressure is strong to use all reasonable outcomes measures in assessing performance.[7,8,9] Some outcomes measures are already required by accreditation agencies, and the number will certainly grow.

- *Procedural quality measures.* These are counts of compliance to accepted clinical practice. "Patients with care plans" and "patients asked to file advance directives" are examples. All functional areas have generally accepted practices and most have established mechanisms to count procedural quality. The measures are often useful in establishing cause of outcomes problems or opportunities for improvement. Statistical analysis can show the relationship between specific process measures and outcomes, identifying the critical elements of a process or function.

- *Structural quality measures.* These are measures of resources present that can be used to infer quality or the lack of it. Many are simple yes/no tallies covering safety equipment, sanitation procedures, and the like. "X-ray machines passing radiation safety examinations" and "presence of certified radiologist" are examples. Some are productivity measures, such as "percentage of examinations by appropriately trained technician." Although structural measures do not guarantee quality, the difficulties of obtaining process and outcomes measures lead most institutions to use all forms.

Customer satisfaction

Satisfaction emphasizes the user viewpoint, rather than the professional one that prevails with clinical outcomes.

- *Patient satisfaction.* Patient satisfaction is a form of outcomes measure. Data on whether the patient was pleased with the care received are normally collected by careful random survey of treated patients and their families.[10] It is routine to use an outside agency, working with a well-developed, standard protocol that permits comparison to other institutions.[11] Topics surveyed include access, amenities, patient information and education, respect for patients' values and emotional needs, and continuity of care. Surveys are often tailored to specific patient groups.[12] Picker Institute, a leading nonprofit survey organization, provides statistical analysis including correlation of items, benchmarks and peer group comparisons, identification of problem areas, and priorities for improvement.[13]

Less rigorous methods, including internally developed protocols and sampling, can be biased, and they cannot be compared to other institutions. The goal of patient satisfaction is to "delight" the patient, achieving a rating of "very satisfied" and a positive response to questions about returning or recommending the organization to friends and acquaintances. Satisfaction data can also be collected from the community population rather than the patient population. Such data are important for marketing.

- *Referring physician satisfaction.* Referring physicians act as agents for their patients and are concerned with clinical outcomes, patient satisfaction, and cost. If they are dissatisfied, they may divert market share. Their opinion is routinely assessed informally. Formal surveys are an important adjunct in larger institutions.

- *Access.* Access measures reveal whether resources are available to meet demand. They are frequently developed from demand and human resources data. "Imaging facilities in primary care locations," "breast screening sites per 1,000 women over 50," and "percentage of population within 30 minutes of a birthing facility" are examples. The standards for access are set by the marketplace. Logistics management measures can also be used access measures. Delays for routine mammography or diagnosis of a breast lump are examples.

- *Other customer satisfaction.* Some customers of work groups are neither doctors nor patients. The technical support units have other organizational units as customers. Development offices have donors and potential donors as customers. The satisfaction of these groups can be measured by survey.

Examples of performance measures

The performance measurement dimensions are applicable to any level of aggregation, from individual task to healthcare organization as a whole. Figure 5.3 gives three examples, a single home health visit by a trained health aide (an intermediate product), an inpatient episode for hip replacement (a final product), and a comprehensive HMO provider (an organization). As the dimensions are applied to more aggregate situations, they fit closely with the balanced scorecard approaches being used to report governing board performance.

Performance Constraint

Continuous improvement requires that a **constraint**, or acceptable level of performance, be established for all measures in all six dimensions. The kinds of constraints include competitive market performance, profit requirements, comparative performance from noncompetitors, and negotiated expectations.

Figure 5.3 Examples of Performance Measurement

Dimension	Home Health Visit	Hip Replacement	HMO
Demand	# visits requested, by type	# patients referred	# members, market share
	% of all home health in community	% of all hip replacements to citizens of community	% of all insured persons, or total population, by age
	% appropriate home visits	% appropriate surgeries	% of all costs appropriate
	time schedule for visits	delay for surgery	telephone answer delay
Cost/Resources	nurse hours, supply counts, vehicles, etc.	OR time, hospital days, PT visits, number of prostheses, etc.	hospital days, physicians paid, etc.
	costs of physical resources	costs of physical resources	costs of physical resources
	% equipment defects reported	Age of operating theater and equipment	# accredited hospitals
Human Resources	# RNs, aides, etc.	# orthopedic surgeons	# primary care practitioners
	% workers "recommend to others"	% workers "recommend to others"	% workers "recommend to others"
	% aides trained in CPR	% aides trained in exercise	% workers trained in two functions
Outputs/ Productivity	# visits completed visits/employee day	# procedures cases/surgeon	# member months FTE/member month
	$ per visit	$ per case	$ per member month
Quality	% sustain activity level	% walking at 6 weeks	% immunized at 2 years
	% visit protocol met	% care protocol met	patients with appropriate preventive care
	Ratio RNs/aides	Accredited hospital facility	State insurance approval
Satisfaction	% patients "recommend to others"	% patients "recommend to others"	% members "recommend to others"
	% referring physicians "recommend to others"	% referring physicians "recommend to others"	% primary physicians "recommend to others"
	# of insurer panel contracts	# of insurer panel contracts	# of employers offering to employees
	Communities covered	Delay for new patient evaluation	# primary physicians in panel

Market performance

The performance actually accepted by the customer in competitive settings is the clearest and most rigorous constraint known. It creates the acid test of operations wherever it can be applied. If others operate at a certain net revenue, or price paid, any activity that exceeds that price is suspect. (Gross revenue—the price the institution charged or would like to receive— is irrelevant to performance measurement.) Similarly, if competitors can convince patients that their quality, access, or amenities are superior, their achievements must be matched.

Many measures of market performance are simply unavailable, and substitutes must be found. Global payment mechanisms, such as payment per day of care, or per hospitalization, or capitation (payment per member month), are excellent market statements in themselves, but they severely limit the use of price or net revenue as a measure of performance in components below the pricing level. Under these payment mechanisms, for example, no revenue is assigned to any functional unit contributing to the care. As a result, price and profit are not available as indicators of market constraint.

Market performance can be evaluated at a function or final product level if a vendor is willing to accept a contract specifying the six dimensions. Many functional services can be purchased as an alternative to producing them within the organization. When performance is fully specified, the possibility of **outsourcing** or purchasing the function becomes realistic. Many organizations outsource portions of their technical and logistic support services, for example. At least conceptually, a market exists for alternative sources of clinical functions such as imaging, laboratory, home care, and specialist physician services. Specialized independent functional services can sell to integrated organizations. Healthcare organizations can also be vendors, selling services to other organizations. Commercial vendors offer outsourcing for most learning services and for the executive function (contract management). The bids offered by external sources are useful comparisons. If equivalent service can be purchased for a certain price, quality, and satisfaction, the internal function must operate at the same level. If the external vendor offers to meet all imaging demand for $2.5 million per year, the internal department should operate at that cost or less. If equivalent breast screening examinations are offered to the organization for $150 each by an independent imaging company, the internal cost should not exceed $150. (Equivalency is often difficult to judge, but the concept should be clear.)

Profit

With rare exceptions, any organization that expects to survive and grow must earn a profit overall. Profit can be calculated only where net revenue is actually

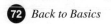

available. Many functional units sell some portions of their service for net prices and can make profit calculations if they can isolate the costs of those services.

Benchmarks

Data on performance of other, similar aggregates are used to establish acceptable performance ranges, in place of or in supplement to direct market tests. Such data usually come from noncompetitors. Healthcare organizations in other communities are happy to exchange comparative information. Organized efforts are necessary to establish definitions and make adjustments necessary to ensure comparability, and alliances have been established for the exchange of comparative data on many performance elements. Competitors protect their performance data, so they are not often known. Various governmental requirements and voluntary agreements open specific measures to comparison.[14] California and Pennsylvania require extensive disclosure, for example. Much data about Medicare are available, and commercial consultants organize them for convenient access.[15]

Benchmarks, or best practices from such comparisons, are used as a guide and long-range target; it is often wise to identify how the organization compares with nonbenchmark organizations as well. The benchmark establishes the long-term goal; the relative rank determines the priority of reaching it. A certain standing in a frequency distribution can be a short term goal or can justify a lower goal while higher priority needs are pursued.

Negotiated constraints

Even in the absence of competitive and comparative data, organizations negotiate performance expectations. Once agreed upon, these are important constraints, with significant rewards and penalties for individual managers. Historical values are important in the negotiations. Improvement can be negotiated; it would be unwise to accept last year's performance as satisfactory for next year. Market price, comparative data, and competitor data are ways to improve the negotiation.

Figure 5.4 shows the kinds of constraint measurement and examples of their application drawn from the three applications shown in Figure 5.3.

Using Performance Management Data

Performance measures are generated as a part of the work itself. Each activity is recorded, either electronically or on paper, in specified forms that generate the data. With six dimensions for each responsibility center (RC) and final product, multiple measures for most dimensions, several dozen important

Figure 5.4 Kinds of Constraint Measurement and Examples

Performance Constraint	*Home Health Visit*	*Hip Replacement*	*HMO*
Competitive	Competitor price, quality, access to patient	Medicare price per case, quality standards	Competitor premium, patient satisfaction
Competitive	Competitor outsourcing bid to insurer or owner	Competitor outsourcing bid to insurer or referring physicians	Offer for merger or acquisition
Profit Requirement	% profit margin	% profit margin on cases paid directly	% profit margin
Benchmark	Best known price/visit, quality, satisfaction	Best known price per case, quality, satisfaction	Lowest comparable premium, highest satisfaction
Negotiated	Historic trend in demand	"Halfway to benchmark"	Planned physician panel expansion

final products, and 50 to 100 work groups, the volume of data that must be processed is very large, running thousands of items per day. To fulfill its purposes, information must be accurate. But there is obviously a limit to the amount of resources that can be expended on data collection. The issue is to design ways of collecting data that are accurate, convenient, and cheap, and the answer is the computer.

Advantages of automation

Computers contribute to efficient data collection in several ways. These advantages are summarized in Figure 5.5.

- Input can be speeded and controlled by programs that prompt for completeness and audit for consistency. Omissions, spelling, and inconsistencies can be corrected immediately, eliminating errors and confusion. For example, the entry "William Smith, Social Security # 187-27-0887, admitted for pediatric asthma" looks reasonable, but checked against an electronic database several questions would arise:
  - Is this William G. Smithe, aged 40, Soc. Sec. # 187-27-0877?
  - If yes, is pediatric asthma the correct diagnosis, or is it adult asthma?
  - If no, what are the middle initial and age?
- Automation makes it possible to eliminate repeated entry. For example, most patient orders must have at least two means of identifying the

Figure 5.5   Contributions of Automated Data Systems

Contribution	*Example*
1. Rapid, audited input	Automatic check for name, identity, spelling, vital statistics
2. No repeat input	All users access central registration file for patient ID and medical condition
3. Recognition for clinical tasks	Protocol suggests normally indicated treatment, prompts for order or explanation before proceeding
4. Verification and cross check of orders	Drugs checked for patient sensitivity, interactions
5. Prompt result reporting	Instantaneous transmission of diagnostic test findings
6. Statistical and accounting calculations	Charges to date, variance, or range of history of laboratory values
7. Accessible archive	Comparison to similar patients or protocol

patient. Electronic identification substitutes an audit of the request for laborious copying of names and numbers. The laboratory will not receive Smithe's specimen and report it as Smith's.

• Automation can change many patient care decisions from recall to recognition by prompting for the clinically indicated next step. Recognition is faster and more accurate than recall. Expectations translate to checklists and prompts that, in themselves, improve performance. If a specific test or procedure is mandatory for a certain condition, a prompt will appear in the automated ordering sequence whenever the doctor identifies the condition.

• By using agreed on care plans, a variety of clinical situations can be programmed to prevent accidental error. For example, the following can be prevented by expanding the audit functions to include clinical guidelines:
  • some accidental misstatements and omissions;
  • inappropriate therapy selections (as with drugs of similar name but different uses);
  • conflicts with prior orders;
  • absence of supporting diagnostic tests or values;
  • interactions between drugs; and
  • failure to obtain consultation or supervision.

• Output can be speeded and organized. When the laboratory does Smithe's tests, the report will be available to the physician immediately, together with the history of Smithe's prior tests. The precision of the laboratory test value and the range of values in a comparable normal population can be added to assist in interpreting the tests.

- Calculations can be made rapidly and cheaply. Smithe's laboratory results can instantaneously update the mean and standard deviation of each test. They can be cross-referenced by his final product, adult asthma. The tests can be entered on his patient ledger, priced, and added to the laboratory daily output statistics.

- An accessible archive is created. The data can be retrieved for Smithe, for the test, for the laboratory, for the insurance intermediary, and for adult asthma. Statistical databases combine Smithe's data with other in each class.

Major data systems

The principal data systems that generate the six dimensions of information are shown in Figure 5.6. Although the groupings can be revised, about 12 systems are necessary to support the information needs of a modern healthcare organization. The systems can be conveniently grouped into those that emphasize capture of data, those that support the background record keeping and analysis, and those that directly support decisions by caregivers and others in the provider organization. Although considerable amounts of data are still processed manually at some stages of their collection, enormous strides have been made in automation in recent years, and even larger ones are likely for the near future. The drawback to computerization is that the systems to do it cost tens or hundreds of millions of dollars and take years to develop. The payback is considerably larger than the investment, however. Even the smallest healthcare organizations are developing computer capability, and it is unlikely that organizations that do not automate most of each of the 12 principal data systems will survive. The activities and status of each system are as follows.

I. **Systems Designed to Capture Data**

   A. *Population assessment systems.* These capture the underlying demographic, economic, and epidemiologic character of the organization's potential market. Current data and trends of geographic distributions, age, child-bearing habits, employment, health insurance, disease patterns, and risk factors are used to evaluate population needs, market share, and market opportunities. The data for these systems come from a variety of sources, but purchase of electronic census and related data is spreading rapidly.

   B. *Membership systems.* These record details of health insurance coverage, including dependents, and utilization for individual subscribers,

Figure 5.6 Relationship of Major Data-Processing Systems

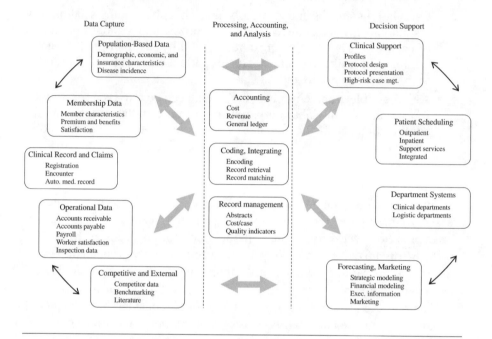

and group, benefits, premium, and account status for groups. The records are essential for insurance operations, but also supply data for clinical support activities. The systems are almost completely automated.

C. *Clinical transaction and claims systems.* These record the name, vital statistics, and details of care for each patient. They also capture records used for payment of providers. Each patient is assigned a unique lifetime number and the systems include elaborate mechanisms to identify patients quickly and correctly. The data from the systems drive much of the processing and accounting activity and are essential for all the decision support systems on the right side of Figure 5.6. Patient registration, order entry, and results reporting are highly automated, and automation is increasing rapidly.

D. *Operational systems.* These record the day-to-day business of the providers, including initial accounting transactions such as payables and payroll. They also record process quality data and worker satisfaction data. The system is essential for provider operation, but it also supports analysis of work processes and worker morale. Many of the accounting transactions are automated, but much of the quality and satisfaction data is manually collected and entered for automated storage and retrieval.

E. *Competitor analysis systems.* These capture data about local competitors and also benchmark and best practice data about similar operations elsewhere. The data come from a wide variety of sources and are frequently estimated or inferred. They are essential for forecasting and marketing activities. The systems are rarely automated.

II. **Processing, Accounting, and Analysis**

A. *Accounting systems.* These tally individual transactions from clinical and operational systems and produce detailed reports of receivables, payables, payrolls, employment benefits, inventories, and equipment depreciation. They generate cost and constraint reports at all levels of aggregation, and much of the general financial reports for the firm as a whole. They perform a variety of cost accounting and financial analyses used by all the operating core, technological, and logistics support activities. They model the long-range financial plan, allowing evaluation of alternative planning scenarios. The systems are highly automated.

B. *Coding and integrating systems.* These systems allow aggregation of accounting and medical record data by disease, patient characteristic, or site of care. They include the various patient classification systems. They are essential to translate individual patient and provider records to aggregates useful for decision support. The systems are almost completely automated.

C. *Record management systems.* These aggregate individual patient care transactions by patient to form the medical record or history. The medical record itself is a critical part of care management. Aggregated by various patient characteristics of interest through the coding system, the information generated is used in all decision support systems. Record systems are partly automated, and major investments are being made to complete automation. It is likely that for inpatient care and major ambulatory treatment, all but a few relatively rare transactions will be automated within the next few years. Office care will be more difficult.

III. **Systems Supporting Decisions**

A. *Clinical support systems.* These generate statistical analyses and profiles that are used to identify patient care improvement opportunities. They also include care protocols and other agreements on clinical procedures and expectations. The systems are largely manual at the present time, but automation will spread with automation of medical record systems.

B. *Patient scheduling systems.* These use historic data on demand and accounting data on availability and cost to schedule patient care transactions. They are partially automated and are growing more sophisticated.

C. *Departmental service and reporting systems.* These govern the internal activities of departments, including many aspects of detailed productivity and quality control. They include personnel scheduling, materials management, work processes, quality inspections, and a variety of internal records. Automation varies by department, but specially designed systems are available for the larger clinical departments and most technical and logistic support activities.

D. *Planning and marketing data systems.* These translate data from all other systems to scenarios and forecasts of future events and are used to evaluate strategies and record strategic decisions. They include financial planning models, models of market development and competitor analysis, and planning databases for facilities, human resources, and information development. Data capture and reporting are increasingly automated through executive information systems. Major strides have been made in the automation of modeling, although the decision processes are supported, rather than directed by the models.

In addition to these sources for routine, ongoing data collection, special nonrecurring studies are also useful. Using research techniques, measurements can be as reliable and valid as desired, within the limits of current technology. Special studies are useful for a variety of purposes, including verifying assumptions about improvement in performance, evaluating new methods or new measures, or collecting very expensive performance measures. Surveys of doctor, patient, and community attitudes, now routine, can be expanded to address particular issues in depth. Processes can be studied in detail, and proposed improvements can be evaluated by special analyses or field trials. Marginal and variable costs can be evaluated in depth. Proposals for new routine measures can be pretested. Investigations of medical and nursing care for specific kinds of cases can be conducted, including formal trials of new methods.

APPROACHES TO QUANTIFICATION

Measuring health and healthcare is a science in itself. Many elements are simply counted by the accounting system. Patients, workers, visits, tests, surgeries, and dollars are examples. Gender, age, address, insurance coverage, worker training, and other characteristics are relatively easy to quantify. The only issues are completeness and uniformity of recording. But to use the six dimensions for continuous improvement, one must address three separate but equally serious problems:

1. *The need to scale performance*—that is, to capture characteristics that otherwise would be only descriptive and subjective. While some important elements are easily counted or measured, others present challenges. Unmet demand, for example, is far more difficult to measure than demand translated to output. Pain is as serious a measurement problem as it is a medical one.

2. *The need for reliability and validity.* It is not enough to measure blood pressure; the value reported must be both reproducible and reflective of the patient's true condition. When these criteria are applied to complex phenomena, multiple dimensions must be considered. The concept of a satisfactory surgery is represented by a checklist of measures, and so is that of a healthy baby.

3. *The need to gain uniformity for fair comparison.* No two patients or treatments are ever alike, but inescapably comparisons must be made between similar groups. What patients are acceptably "similar"? "Healthy newborns" certainly, but identifying comparable groups of impaired newborns is not so obvious. What time period is reasonable? An episode of pregnancy is clear enough, but when is a fracture healed? Many diseases continue over long periods of time without discrete stopping points.

Quantifying the six dimensions is a matter of continually searching for measures that evolve from subjective, almost intuitive beginnings. The measures themselves can be understood as estimations that improve in precision as they evolve. Similarly, the measurement systems grow and mature. Design and improvement of measures involves scaling, specification of populations, and adjustments to compare diverse populations.

Scaling

The process for translating real activities and characteristics to numbers is called scaling. There are four measurement categories, or scales. Which category is used in a given situation will depend on cost and value, and scaling may evolve through several levels over time. Figure 5.7 summarizes scaling.

1. *Nominal scales.* These identify categories that are useful in accommodating the differences in patients, such as gender, race, or specific diagnoses. Classifications for diseases, procedures, and prescription drugs are all nominal scales underpinning healthcare measurement. The International Classification of Diseases is a nominal scale now used almost universally to describe the illnesses leading to hospitalization. It became the foundation for another famous nominal scale,

Figure 5.7 Scales for Quantifying Information

Scale	Description	Examples	Uses	Limitations
Nominal	Scale without rank or comparability	Men/women; DRGs	Identifying different populations	No comparison between groups
Ordinal	Ordered scale, intervals not even in size or importance	Patient satisfaction scores, infant Apgar scores	Classifying complex events by desirability or action required	Improvement moving between intervals differs
Interval	Even, uniform intervals,but no absolute end point	Temperature, blood pressure	Finer classification by desirability or action required	Improvement moving between intervals is constant, but relative improvement is unknown
Ratio	Ordered scale with even or predictable categories and an absolute end point	Height, percentile standing, dollars	Comparison between and within group, calculation of variance and means	Strongest scale; relative change in scale is equal to relative change in objective achievement

DRGs. Other nominal scales are useful in differentiating personnel and activities.

Nominal scales generate **attributes measures**, that is, a binary (yes or no) value for each case. The principal statistic for an attributes measure is the portion passing a certain threshold:

portion passing = number yesses/total number examined

The hip replacement walking measure is a nominal scale, number walking/number of procedures.

2. *Ordinal scales.* These identify categories that move reliably in a uniform direction, so higher numbers represent consistently different situations from lower ones. (Nominal scales are assigned arbitrarily so that high numbers have no intrinsic meaning.) The five numerical classes of Pap smears, for example, indicate progressively more serious disease as the numbers get higher. Burns, cancers, respiratory distress, infant distress, and several other clinical characteristics are

quantified by ordinal scales. For example, intensive care units use an ordinal scale to determine patient condition and necessity for admission.[16] Individual patients' daily nursing requirements are often assessed with ordinal scales.[17] Satisfaction questionnaires use ordinal scales. Ordinal scales are usually treated as attributes measures. Often two or more ordinal categories are grouped together to form the portion passing.

3. *Interval scales.* These are ordinal scales that have uniform values between entries, but an arbitrary end point or starting point. Temperature is an easily recognized interval scale, because two popular scales, Celsius and Fahrenheit, both have uniform ordinal steps (degrees), but they have two different, equally arbitrary zero points. As a result, it is impossible to make relative comparisons. A fever of 100° F is not 1.4 percent worse than normal; the same condition expressed in Celsius is 37.78° C, 2 percent worse than the Celsius normal of 37.0°. Blood pressure is an interval scale. The starting point, atmospheric pressure, is not only variable, it bears no intrinsic relation to the disease of hypertension. A diastolic pressure of 100 mm mercury is not 25 percent worse than 80 mm mercury.

    Interval scales generate **variables measures**; that is, a continuous measure that can take any value over a range.

4. *Ratio scales.* A ratio scale fulfills all the requirements of interval measures but has, in addition, a non-arbitrary zero value. This permits the use of percentages. Height, weight, and percentile standing on comparative distributions are all ratio scales. In accounting, dollars are a ratio scale. Ratios of actual to expected values, such as used in spider diagrams, are ratio scales, even if the underlying measure is not. Percentage of patients walking after hip replacement is a nominal scale, but the actual percentage divided by the expected percentage is a ratio scale. Ratio scales generate variables measures.

Healthcare organizations routinely use all four scaling approaches. While ratio scales have certain advantages, the other approaches are useful in continuous improvement programs as well. Improvement of measures and measurement systems may involve moving from nominal to ordinal or ratio scales.

EVALUATING AND IMPROVING MEASURES

Measures are judged by the extent to which their use allows the organization to improve mission achievement. To be valuable, measures must be valid, reliable and timely.

Validity

A performance measure is valid if the reported values of cases are associated with the exchange objectives (e.g., if patients with higher scores are healthier, if cases with lower values cost less). If an invalid measure is used, energy can be directed toward achieving high scores on that measure rather than achieving the true goals. The result may be a disabling distortion of intended activity. An anecdote may be the best way to illustrate the importance of validity. A factory produced nails, and someone wished to improve performance by setting output goals for the employees. So a goal was set at a certain *number* of nails per hour. After a short time, the goal was exceeded, but the factory was producing mostly tacks. So the goal was changed to a certain number of *pounds* of nails per hour. Again the goal was exceeded, but this time the factory was producing spikes. The moral is that validity of measurements depends on what the goals are. If one wants a variety of nails, one's measures and expectations must reflect that.

Often an elaborate, expensive measurement system is used to establish the validity of a much cheaper one. The ultimate standard for length is an optical measurement system used by the National Bureau of Standards. The validity of the common desk ruler is traceable through several substitutes that are progressively cheaper and less accurate. A measure can be perfectly reliable, but still invalid. Using a ruler that is too short, everyone can agree the distance between two points is almost exactly ten centimeters. A valid ruler would show that it is almost exactly nine centimeters.

In healthcare, validity is usually associated with an objective of health. Thus, if the objective of hip replacement surgery is the full recovery of functioning, an independent panel examining the patient's functioning in his or her life setting several months after surgery would be the ultimate validity, comparable to the optical standard for length. It might be applied in selected situations, to evaluate a less expensive measure, or when new hip replacement processes are considered. Self-reported functioning would be one substitute for the ultimate, much cheaper but potentially subject to bias, like the too-short ruler. The ability to walk a specified distance at a specified postsurgical time would be a second substitute. One or both substitutes might be used to evaluate the annual results for a hip replacement program.

Reliability

A measure is reliable if repeated application to an identical situation yields the same value. The standard deviation of the reported values is the measure of reliability. Lack of reliability impairs precision of measurement. If the average of several measurements is ten centimeters, but the standard deviation of individual measures is one millimeter, the measure is reliable to plus or minus three standard deviations 99 percent of the time, and four standard deviations roughly all but once in a thousand trials.

Reliability is frequently assessed across differing measurement conditions. Time trends in the measure and its standard deviation are common. Testing and retesting against the same population, comparison of different observers, and split sample calculations are common. Reliability is enhanced by clear definitions, good measuring tools, audits, and training of observers. The hip replacement program might check the reliability of its self-assessed function measure over time, by patient categories such as age and the presence of other disease, and against the percentage of nonrespondents. It might review trends, individual observer values, and values by day of the week to identify reliability issues.

Timeliness

There are two important criteria of timeliness: frequency and delay. Delay is the interval between measurement and report. The measurement system that reports too late for the monitor to respond is useless. (In the worst case, efforts to correct a reported problem that no longer exists may destabilize the system.) Reports that are too infrequent allow correctable conditions to exist longer than necessary. Reports that come too often waste the monitor's time. There is a response cycle, a finite time required to respond to a measure. Reporting more frequently than once per response cycle is not useful. In some of the complex issues of quality and productivity, the response cycles are quite long. It may take months to evaluate and redesign the hip replacement process, for example. Weekly reports of outcomes make no contribution; quarterly ones would be more appropriate.

Specification and Adjustment

Most performance measures are dependent both upon the process being measured and the characteristics of the population involved. It is important to separate the two; serious errors result if a difference attributable to a population is taken as reflecting a process. Any comparison of performance measures requires understanding of the difference in population; comparing across similar populations. Two approaches are used: specification and adjustment.

Specification

Specification defines subpopulations with similar characteristics within a larger, more heterogeneous population. Specification is necessary whenever a difference in performance exists between two population subgroups. The characteristic used for specification can be nominal or ordinal. Ratio or interval scales can be converted to specification by grouping them into categories. One might identify similar patient populations by gender, education, an interval scaled condition such as blood pressure, or a ratio scale such as age. If necessary, one could develop specified subpopulations for combinations of characteristics, such as women, over age 50, college graduates, with previous history of diastolic blood pressure over 90 mm mercury. Hip replacement recovery rates might be specified by the degree of loss of function prior to surgery and age. Common taxonomies for patient care performance are shown in Figure 5.8.

Adjustment

Adjusted rates recalculate the whole population rate from the specific rates, standardizing heterogeneous populations to a uniform structure. They are most useful when comparing several different populations, such as the mortality rates for states, which are usually adjusted for age to the age distribution of the United States as a whole. The age-adjusted rate for each state is the mortality rate it would have if its population had the same age distribution as the nation.

Figure 5.8   Common Patient-Specification Taxonomies

Category	*Classifications*
Demographic	Age
	Sex
	Race
	Education
Economic	Income
	Employment
	Social class
Geographic	Zip code of residence
	Census tract
	Political subdivision
Healthcare Finance	Managed versus traditional insurance
	Private versus government insurance
Diagnosis	Disease classification
	Procedure
	Diagnosis-related group (DRG)
	Ambulatory visit group
Risk	Health behavior attribute
	Preexisting condition
	Chronic or high-cost disease

Figure 5.9 Age-Specific, Crude, and Adjusted Rates, Utah versus Florida

Age Category	Utah			Florida		
	Deaths	Population	Death Rate	Deaths	Population	Death Rate
0–14	450	538	8.4	2,742	2,412	11.4
15–44	804	789	10.2	11,822	5,595	21.1
45–64	1,446	245	56.0	19,367	2,548	76.0
65–75	2,894	90	321.6	30,618	1,369	223.7
> 75	4,624	62	754.8	68,168	1,059	643.7
All ages	10,218	1,742	56.3	122,077	12,983	94.0
Crude death rate			56.3			94.0
Utah death rate standardized to Florida population						113.0

Figure 5.9 shows the crude, specific, and age-adjusted death rates for Utah and Florida. Are Floridians more likely to die than Utahns, as the crude rates suggest? Yes, they are if they are under 65, but not among Florida's large retired population. And overall, an age-adjusted comparison shows the Florida rate to be 20 percent lower than Utah, not 73 percent higher as the crude rates indicate. Each adjustment requires additional data and calculations, but the misleading character of the crude rate is clearly shown.

Population characteristics, including mortality and morbidity rates, are often adjusted for age, sex, race, and socioeconomic status, and specific rates are frequently used for specific diseases. Fertility rates are specific to the number of fertile women, and rates of diseases such as cancers and heart disease are expressed for the population over 45.

Severity adjustment

Healthcare organizations frequently adjust performance measures for the severity of illness of their patients. There are two basic approaches. One uses the Medicare DRG payment system as a basis. DRGs are assigned based on discharge diagnosis, grouping clinically similar diagnoses that are also similar in cost. Every Medicare inpatient must be assigned a DRG, and HCFA has assigned a weight to each DRG based on national surveys of the cost of care of those patients. Then for each of the i patient groups:

$$\Sigma(\text{patient}_i * \text{DRG weight}_I)/\Sigma(\text{patient}_i) = \text{average DRG weight, or severity index}$$

and

$$\Sigma(\text{cost/patient}_i)/\Sigma(\text{DRG weight}_I) = \text{weighted cost/patient}$$

The weighted cost/patient (or other performance measure, such as length of stay or clinical outcomes) can more accurately be compared between institutions.

Although the DRG weight is universal and cheap, it has several limitations. The weight explains less than half the variation between cases. The unexplained variation tends to occur among very high cost patients, but these patients are in several DRGs. The assignment process and the weights are focused on the Medicare recipients, almost all over 65 years of age. Younger users of the hospital can be assigned DRGs, but the values are not necessarily correct. One large category of hospitalization, obstetrics, occurs very rarely in the Medicare population, so the basis for assigning the weight is particularly suspect.

Some commercial systems improve on the DRG algorithm. They either create new groups and calculate new weights for them, or expand the existing groups to identify the sicker patients in them. Similar approaches have been developed for outpatient care, but their use is not widespread. Many use the diagnoses and the reported care given, which is reported to insurers using **current procedural terminology (CPT)** groups.[18]

The second severity-weighting approach uses patient conditions other than diagnosis.

Acuity approaches use binary or simple ordinal scales indicating departure from normal function in several physiological and psychological factors known to influence resource use.[19] They are popular for estimating nursing time.[20] Items evaluated include therapeutic and diagnostic needs as well as those involving eating, dressing, and elimination; the emotional state; and the amount of observation ordered by the doctor. Scales are now tailored to the clinical area. Representative acuity variations for obstetrical labor and delivery care are shown in Figure 5.10. For nurse staffing, values for each patient are reported by the head nurse. Computerized systems calculate acuity, assign staffing requirements to individual patients, and add up the nursing personnel required on each floor.

RUGS, a severity grouping system based on functional capability, is widely used in nursing homes.[21] Patients are assigned to category by their ability to eat, dress, toilet, walk, and similar activities, and the weights are established by studies of the nursing time they require.

APACHE is a physiologically-based acuity system, using laboratory values for critical blood chemistry. It was developed in intensive care units and is particularly useful with very ill patients.[22] However, larger scale studies indicate that the contribution of the APACHE approach may be insufficient.[23]

Although severity adjustments are popular, their real value is questionable. An adjustment is useful when it successfully isolates factors approached

Figure 5.10 Patient Acuity Variation

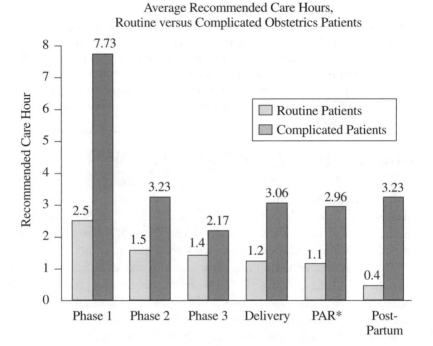

Average Recommended Care Hours,
Routine versus Complicated Obstetrics Patients

---

by radically different mechanisms, such as preventive activity as opposed to care. Formal studies evaluating this capability suggest that most currently available adjustments are of limited value.[24,25] A better approach to the underlying problem of heterogeneity in patient mix is summarized in the following steps:

1. *Finely subdividing the complaints, diagnoses, and procedures* improves the homogeneity of groups. Often a combination of demographic and clinical characteristics identifies acceptably homogeneous groups. Segregating births by mother's age, presence of prenatal care, and Apgar score is an example. Regression analysis helps identify the important variables to use.

2. *Comparing over time, rather than between institutions.* While patient characteristics certainly change over time, the differences at a single institution are much less than those between institutions operating in radically different environments, such as inner city or suburban.

3. *Selecting external comparisons from similar sites.* Results for suburban institutions can be compared to other suburban institutions.

4. *Conducting special studies of situations that still show important variations after the first three steps.* This is a normal part of the Shewhart cycle, but the improvement team can be alert to the possibility that some exogenous factor is causing the problem they address.

5. *Emphasizing continuous improvement rather than identification of error.* It is fear of blame, in the form of reduced reputation, loss of income, or potential tort liability that underlies much concern with acuity adjustment. These elements are deliberately de-emphasized in continuous improvement approaches. Many forms of incentive payment actually exaggerate the problem; that is one reason why they are avoided.

A STRATEGY FOR IMPROVING MEASUREMENT

A strategy for designing measures attempts not only to maximize the value of the measures in improving control, but also to minimize the cost of measurement itself. Rather than addressing specific measures, successful strategies set out classes of measures like Figure 5.2 and address how to obtain large numbers of measures in a coordinated program. Sound strategy also incorporates information improvement into process improvement; each major change in the process should generate better information as well as better results. A change in the protocols for hip replacement should search for new performance measures as well as better clinical results.

Generally, although not universally, the processes that improve measures increase the cost of measurement. Information investments are conceptually weighed in terms of their contribution to value and their cost, assigning priority to those with the highest value/cost ratio. In reality, the data for the comparisons are difficult to obtain, and a number of simplifying assumptions are often necessary. Many healthcare organizations have designated a portion of their investments to information improvement on the belief that a general campaign will pay off. Then information requests are prioritized against each other, but not in competition with other investments.

Cost

The cost of a measurement system is a combination of two elements: first, the resources consumed in obtaining, processing, reporting, and setting expectations for it and second, the costs of incorrect reports. It is convenient to label the first group accounting costs and the second hidden costs. Thoughtful measurement design must always address both.

Accounting costs are frequently buried in other activities. The cost of the data entry to order a test, administer a drug, or take an x-ray are lumped together with other parts of the activity. They can only be identified by special study. Marginal costs of individual new measures are low, but a systematic expansion of data processing capability may cost tens of millions. It may permit hundreds of additional measurements, making the true cost of each unmeasurable. Not only hardware and software is involved in the expansion cost; measurement definitions, scaling, tests of validity, and training of personnel are all initial investment costs.

Accounting costs tend to increase with improvements in reliability, validity, and timeliness, but automation has greatly reduced accounting costs and simultaneously increased the accuracy and timeliness of cost, revenue, output, and productivity information. The same basic data collection and processing system can be used to generate a large number of accurate measures. Careful attention to system design allows improvements in accuracy and timeliness of the information at modest increase in cost.

Hidden costs occur because of two possible incorrect interpretations of the data. *False negatives* occur when a correctable condition is not reported to the monitors, and, therefore, the monitors achieve less performance than they might. *False positives* occur when the measurement system reports a correctable situation when in fact none exists. Both are costly. The first results in suboptimal performance, and the second leads to costly, disruptive, and futile investigations. Hidden costs decrease with improved reliability, validity, and timeliness.

Value

The value of information is measured by the improvement in mission achievement. If a measure contributes cost saving of $5,000, that is its value. A measure that is viewed as essential by a stakeholder is enormously valuable for that reason. A measure that avoids serious error—the compass or the altimeter on an airplane—is essential. A measure nobody refers to is valueless. A measure that misleads has negative value.

While the concept is clear, its assessment is usually a matter of judgment. It is rarely possible to isolate the contribution of a specific measure or even a measurement system. The value of information is frequently confounded by other forces causing behavioral change. For example, market pressures may have pushed the organization to redesign the payroll process. The new process costs less to collect more detailed data. Its reports are expanded and more reliable. They give summary indicators both clearer and faster. And in designing the new process, the group saw some minor changes in other processes that they implemented. When the new process is installed, costs are $5,000 lower, and satisfaction and quality measures are the same to slightly higher. What caused the change? Was it (a) the market pressure that initiated the activity? or (b) the new payroll process? or (c) the improved understanding the work group gained from the study? Isolating the contribution of the new measures from the market pressures and the redesigned process is impossible.

The association between value and reliability, validity, and timeliness is similarly complex. Generally speaking, the more reliable, valid, and timely the measure is, the greater its value will be, but there are two important exceptions. First, when a crude measure is introduced it may cause dramatic changes in performance, the so-called sentinel effect. Second, improvements in measures are only useful up to the point at which the monitor can no longer change actual performance.

In a world where neither costs nor values can be easily assessed, it is difficult to justify expenditure on programs to improve measurement. There does seem to be a clear association between good measurement and success, however. Most well-managed organizations inside and outside of healthcare use measures heavily and are increasing their investment in them. The theory that good management depends on precise, quantitative understanding is compelling and has a number of articulate advocates. (It is inseparable from continuous improvement approaches.) And the performance of companies outside the healthcare field that have pursued information aggressively has substantially exceeded the performance of companies in general.[26]

Well-managed organizations solve the problem by developing a specific information strategy. The strategy has two important elements: a commitment to a continuing investment in information improvement and a plan to move in the directions with the greatest apparent value first. The commitment of leading organizations is quite strong and specific. It extends over a minimum of five years and amounts to 0.25 to 0.5 percent of their net revenue, or 5 to 10 percent of their net profit.[27] Funds are earmarked in the capital budget for information services and are thus protected from the general competitive review.

USING MEASURES TO IMPROVE PERFORMANCE

Information is data processed in ways that help people make decisions. The effective translation of data to information is as important as the quality of the data themselves. It occurs in three different but related ways: analysis of the past to help identify opportunities for improvement, forecasting to the future to help evaluate competing opportunities, and reporting of current performance to help control.

Analyzing Historic Data

Even a partially automated information system quickly builds up a large archive of data that can be systematically mined to understand processes better. The archive, a critical resource for the organization, is carefully managed as part of Information Services.

An issue is identified, questions are posed of the archive, and the answers to the question suggest the directions fruitful for improvement. Figure 5.11 provides a simple illustration; one way to discover improvement opportunities is to search for specific correctable weaknesses, a "special cause" as opposed to a "common cause" in continuous improvement jargon.[28] A series of statistical tests is necessary to rule out various special causes. Any special causes that are found are pursued with their own Shewhart "Plan Do Check

---

Figure 5.11   Investigating a Satisfaction Shortfall: Searching for Improvement by Identifying Correctable Weaknesses

I.   The issue: Patient satisfaction scores have dropped substantially below expectation.

II. The analysis: Search for specialized responses.

Responses	*Analysis*	*Result*
1. Statistically significant?	test mean and variance of most recent sample against previous samples	yes—proceed with analysis no—reevaluate need to proceed
2. Related to certain market segments?	test means of segments	yes—pursue segment specific strategy no—pursue general strategy
3. Related to certain treatment teams?	test means of teams	yes—review with team no—pursue general strategy
4. Related to certain diagnoses?	test means of diagnoses	yes—study those diagnoses no—pursue general strategy
5. Related to certain staffing levels?	test association of source with average staffing level at time of treatment	yes—consider additional staffing no—pursue general strategy

III. General Strategy:

Plan: Develop focus groups of patients and caregivers to identify correctable reasons for low scores.

Do: Devise process changes to address these.

Check: Test changes.

Act: Adopt permanently if improvement results and other dimensions are within acceptable limits.

Act" cycle.[29] An ongoing dialogue between the operators and the database, identifying special causes, is part of the improvement process.

Seven tools of continuous quality improvement

Advocates of continuous improvement have emphasized a set of seven tools for analyzing problems like the satisfaction shortfall.[30] These can be taught directly to operating teams to assist them in improving processes.

1. **Flow process charts** show the steps in a process in the order in which they must be performed, with the criteria and results for various alternatives, or branches. Figure 5.12 shows a simple example. Several flow process charts appear elsewhere in the book. Various kinds of actions, such as evaluations, inspections, and direct services are often shown in different shapes to help follow the process.

2. **Fishbone,** or **cause and effect, diagrams** show relationships between complex flows and allow the team to identify components, test them as specific causes, and focus their investigation. Figure 5.13 illustrates a fishbone diagram that might analyze causes of low staffing, if the test of patient satisfaction scores showed it to be important.

3. The **scatter diagram** is a graphic device for showing association between two measures. Figure 5.14 shows occupancy, a productivity measure, versus bed size for hospitals in southeast Michigan. The relationship indicated by the diagram can be tested using regression analysis. In the case of Figure 5.14, the apparent relationship is significant.

4. The **bar chart** is a display of differing values by some useful dimension, such as day of week, operator, site, or patient group. It is useful for revealing special causes that are related to resources, and correctable by process changes, equipment replacement, and personnel training. For example, the bar chart shown in Figure 5.15 shows varying lengths of stay for surgeons doing cholecystectomies. It reflects considerable variation.

   Pareto analysis simply examines the components of a problem in terms of their contribution to it. It is a bar chart format, with the items rank ordered on a dependent variable such as cost, profit, or satisfaction. The "Pareto Rule" is that in general a few components will include a large part of the problem. Focusing on the biggest contributors allows the team to find solutions that may not work for every case, but that work well enough overall to be valuable. Figure 5.16 is the same subject as Figure 5.15. The expected length of stay from Medicare data has been subtracted from the actual lengths of stay for each patient and the difference has been totaled to create an excess days per physician statistic. The values are ranked in the table and, predictably, a few physicians contribute to the increased stay.

Figure 5.12 Flow Process Chart

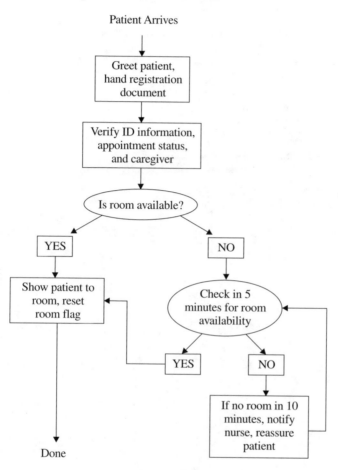

Registration in a Doctor's Office

Patient Arrives

Greet patient, hand registration document

Verify ID information, appointment status, and caregiver

Is room available?

YES

NO

Show patient to room, reset room flag

Check in 5 minutes for room availability

YES

NO

If no room in 10 minutes, notify nurse, reassure patient

Done

5. The **histogram** is built from the bar chart data. It groups individual values and shows the relative frequency of each group. An example is shown in Figure 5.17, again using the cholecystectomy length of stay. This time, individual patient values were grouped by frequency, yielding the display shown in the figure. The few patients who stay a long time contribute to the long tail to the right.

6. The **run chart** displays data over time and allows a visual perception of trends. Figure 5.18 shows a run chart with decreasing demand over several months.

Figure 5.13   Fishbone Diagram

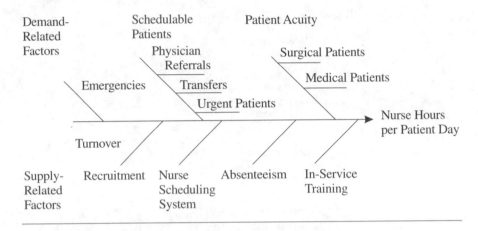

Figure 5.14   Scatter Diagram: Hospital Occupancy by Bed Size (Data from Southeast Michigan, 1990)

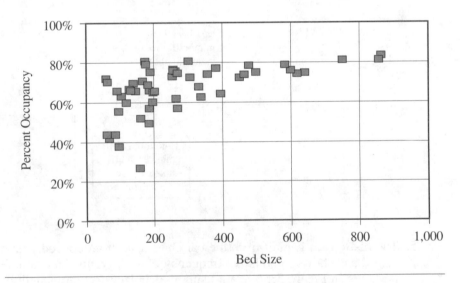

7. The **control chart** is a run chart with the addition of statistical quality control limits. One form of control chart is shown in Figure 5.19. Figure 5.19 shows a success story, a reduction in Caesarean section deliveries that occurred around month 21. It also shows the control limits that would trigger a reinvestigation of Caesarean sections. More complex examples are shown in Figure 5.25.

Figure 5.15 Bar Chart: Average Length of Stay by Attending Physician, Uncomplicated Cholecystectomy

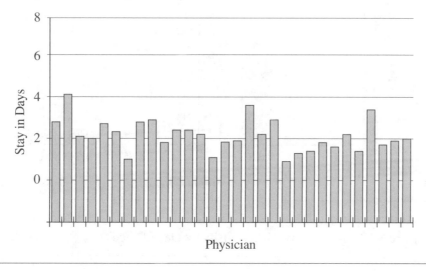

Figure 5.16 Pareto Diagram: Contribution of Days Over Medicare Average, by Physician

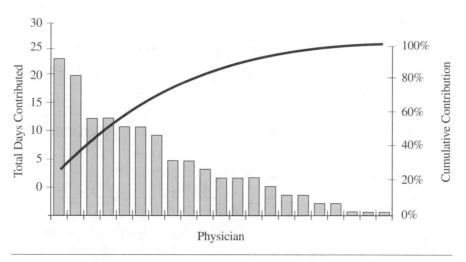

The seven tools can be taught successfully to healthcare workers and are included in elementary continuous improvement training programs. The statistical analyses and graphics can be prepared with common spreadsheet software.[31] Thus a team pursuing the general strategy to overcome the patient

Figure 5.17   Histogram

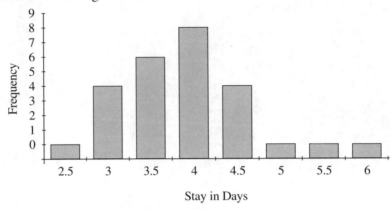

Figure 5.18   Run Chart (Office Visits by Day of Week)

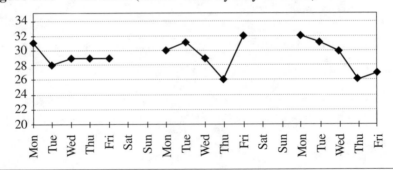

Figure 5.19   Attributes Control Chart (Caesarean Section Percentage by Month)

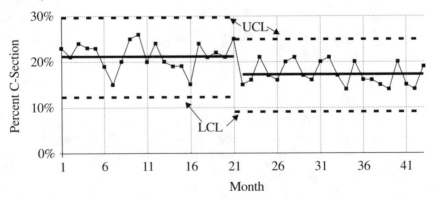

satisfaction shortfall of Figure 5.11 could easily prepare the examples shown here, and the tools would probably help them understand how to improve the care processes and patient satisfaction.

Advanced analytic tools

The seven tools may have their greatest value in teaching people how to think analytically. As tools, their utility is soon exhausted. Notably, they do not allow an untrained team to complete any of the statistical analyses listed in Figure 5.11. An analyst with a knowledge of the data and a graduate degree could answer the questions faster and more reliably. Similarly, they do not address the intricacies of cost analysis. Well-managed institutions provide internal consultants who can support and go beyond the seven tools. The work groups and final product teams at any level can call upon skilled planners, marketers, cost analysts, and management engineers to assist a team at any stage of its efforts. The kinds of analysis they can add include:

- *Advanced graphic displays.* These are often helpful in conveying quantitative information and appear constantly in analyses and proposals. A wide variety of graphs are available on common spreadsheet packages. Selection of the proper graph is important, and an experienced analyst can improve the accuracy and efficiency of information transfer.[32]
- *Univariate statistical analysis.* Arithmetic means, standard deviations, and standard errors are applicable to a great many situations, guiding the team to select topics that are likely to be fruitful. Some statistics—for example, low frequency events—require other tests that are more efficient.
- *Multivariate statistical analysis.* Regression and analysis of variance techniques have expanded dramatically over the past 20 years. A statistician familiar with the different approaches can develop answers faster, and can guard against dangers of using the wrong test or violating conditions for interpreting results.
- *Cost analysis.* Most economic decisions hinge on unit costs and accurate estimates are often problematic. A cost analyst familiar with available data and its limitations can produce the most accurate estimate possible in each specific situation.

Regression Forecasts

Forecasts predict future operating environments. Demand for service and prices of purchased resources are routinely forecast as part of the budget process. The budget office collaborates with planning and marketing to develop forecasts for the most global demand events, such as new patients, hospital admissions, and outpatient visits, broken down into major market segments. Price forecasting is usually developed by market survey or from commercial forecasters who sell opinions.

Global demand and demand for many specific care episodes such as DRGs can be forecast from institutional history, usually by regression analysis.[33] Regression based forecasts are often called *ceteris paribus* forecasts, because they assume that "all other things are equal," particularly that the expressed relationship will continue in the future. Several regression-based techniques are available to develop forecasts from internal historical data. In addition, commercial databases allow forecast of demand by disease episode based on national statistics and population characteristics. Population itself is measured and forecast for political units by a system of federal and state cooperation.[34] Some data are available from commercial sources for small geographic areas, such as zip codes. Thus, most final product teams have two forecasts for future demand:

1. Time series regression analysis of the form
   Demand $= \beta$ (year) $\pm\varepsilon$
2. Epidemiologic analysis of the form
   Demand $= \beta_1$ (population) $+\beta_2$ (age) $+\beta_3$ (sex) $+\beta_4$ (income) $+$ C $\pm\varepsilon$

Demand for specific intermediate products is forecast from regression analysis of the historic relation of the service to more global measures. For example, several recent years' data on the number of laboratory tests is regressed against the number of inpatient admissions, clinic visits, and year. A regression model such as:

$$\text{Lab tests} = \beta_1 \text{ (admissions)} +\beta_2 \text{ (visits)} +\beta_3 \text{ (year)} + \text{C} \pm\varepsilon$$

can be used for the initial forecast, where the forecast year and values for admissions and visits are inserted into the regression equation.

Further refinements can be introduced. Cyclic variation for seasons or days of the week can be accommodated. The demand can be segmented and forecast by segment at whatever level the data and statistical significance will support. The *ceteris paribus* forecasts can be almost fully automated. Well-managed organizations have sophisticated forecasting systems including several forecasting models and a database of agreed-upon forecasts of major measures.

Ceteris paribus forecasts are rarely adequate in themselves. Historically based forecasts are impossible when new services are developed because there is no history to use. "Other things being equal" rarely prevails even in existing services. The opinions and evidence from planning and marketing are used to refine the global forecasts. Line operators can adjust forecasts for areas under their authority, based on their judgment. Line operators are recognized to have excellent judgment about short-term forecasts. Planning and marketing personnel can spot variations from the *ceteris paribus* assumption and make adjustments not possible from computerized models.

Benchmarking Forecasts

Benchmarking is a form of quantitative goal identification establishing the desired forecast, as opposed to the most likely one developed by regression forecasting. A benchmark is the best known value for a specific measure, from any source. Benchmarks are obtained by constructing comparative data sets and ranking them. The benchmark can be a powerful tool to guide process improvement. Related to the benchmark is the process used to generate it, called **best practice**. If both are available, a team might decide to emulate best practice (explicitly abandoning the *ceteris paribus* assumption) and, allowing for implementation delays and learning time, achieve best practice over a few budget cycles. Its forecasts for each cycle would be based on performance relative to the benchmark.

An example of benchmarking and its use is in infant mortality, a complex problem where American healthcare does not do well. Nations with better maternal and infant healthcare are generally below ten deaths per 1,000 births. The best nations achieve less than five, although they are often small, economically advanced, well-educated and ethnically homogeneous populations. Healthcare organizations in American inner cities have a hard time matching these numbers, and it is known that the problems involved include reducing unwanted pregnancies, eliminating mothers' substance abuse and improving their nutrition, providing early prenatal care, and improving care at birth. Not all of these problems are under the control of the healthcare system. Collaboration with other social agencies would be required. Additional funding will be necessary, even though the outcome could reduce overall expenditures. An improved process is thus a multiyear project. A typical inner-city hospital might face forecasts and benchmarks like the ones shown in Figure 5.20. A deliberate program to improve performance might identify an interim goal of nine, and start programs to achieve it in three years.

Performance Modeling

Models are simplified representations of reality that can be manipulated to test various hypotheses about the future. Real-world trials are rarely the best way to begin to evaluate a complex proposal. Models are easier to adjust and less costly if something goes wrong. Modeling recognizes that performance depends on both **exogenous events**, those largely outside the control of the line operator, and **endogenous events**, those largely within the control of the operator. Models require an **objective function**, that is, a

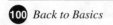

Figure 5.20   Forecasts and Benchmarks Compared to Create a Process-Improvement Strategy

Problem:
High-risk mothers and babies drive infant mortality rates up.

Benchmarks:

World	Japan	4.6/1,000 births
United States	Maine	6.9/1,000 births
Comparable cities		14.2/1,000 births

Strategies	*Time to Visible Result*	*Anticipated change in mortality*
Encourage prenatal care Within three months, open new care center with focus on teen activities, healthcare for teen girls.	 12 months	Year 1: 0% Year 2: 10% Year 3: 20%
Expand use of contraceptives Offer contraceptives and counseling to teen girls and boys.	 12 months	Year 1: 0% Year 2: 05% Year 3: 10%
Drug use prevention and education Work with high schools, police, and social services on drug abatement.	 24 months	Year 1: 0% Year 2: 0% Year 3: 05%

Budget Expectations

Calculation	*Value*
Year 1: No change	21/1,000 births
Year 2: Initial value decreased by 5% for reduced pregnancies 10% for prenatal care	 18/1,000 births
Year 3: Initial value decreased by 10% for reduced pregnancies, 20% for prenatal care, 5% for drug abatement	 14.4/1,000 births

quantitative statement of the relationship between events and desired results, and constraints, limits on the range of acceptable operating conditions.

The modeler can then modify the endogenous assumptions and test the relationship between them and performance, eventually finding an optimal performance within the constraints. Next, in a process called **sensitivity analysis**, the modeler modifies the exogenous events, usually developing most favorable, expected, and least favorable scenarios. These show the robustness of the proposal and indicate the degree of risk involved. Several forms of models are used by well-managed healthcare organizations to evaluate proposals.

The planning department routinely produces short-run and long-run forecasts for a number of important demand measures. It maintains a database that allows generations of forecasts for almost any service demand on request. These are used in strategic positioning, the development of facility and service plans, and the construction of expectations for the next budget year. The reliability of the forecasts, the advice available from the planning department, and the speed with which the request can be serviced are critical elements in long-term success of the organization. The data for incidence rates, advice on segmentation of the population, and ranges of current practice on use are frequently available from national consulting services. Calculation and presentation software are also available to make construction of forecasts, sensitivity analysis, and exploration of alternative scenarios quickly and easy.

Business plans

Models that deal with future events as fixed numbers, rather than as random events subject to a predictable variance, are called **deterministic models**. The most common are business plans, but several others are useful in specific situations.

Business plans are the most universally used model. They describe an operating proposal, identify exogenous and endogenous conditions, and forecast demand, output, revenue, costs, and profit or cost savings over several years. They may use regression or benchmark modeling to forecast components. Demand and prices are usually taken as exogenous, and quality concerns are handled as a constraint. (For example, examining only alternatives that appear likely to give the same or better quality scores.) Business plans are used to justify new programs and capital expenditure, evaluate make-or-buy alternatives, show returns on improved processes, and estimate break-even conditions and earnings associated with increasing demand. The long-range financial plan used by the board is a sophisticated business plan. Scenarios evaluating alternative exogenous and endogenous assumptions are frequently useful for strategy selection.[35]

Business plans assume deterministic conditions, that is, they accept the forecasts without error terms or allowance for random variation. They examine alternative exogenous scenarios using sensitivity analysis. Although they are conceptually algebraic models, they are prepared on computer spreadsheets and presented as year-by-year forecasts. The algebra is buried in the spreadsheet design. Spreadsheet capabilities make graphic summaries easy, and they are widely used and expected.

Many line teams will have members who can prepare elementary business plans. Consultation from technical personnel in planning, marketing, and finance is useful both in the model design and in evaluating the assumptions. The neatness and precision of the spreadsheets and graphs and concealment of the underlying algebra can be misleading. The key questions about business plans deal with the assumptions, such as the sources of forecasts, the realism of alternative scenarios, time allowances made for implementation and learning, and the operating conditions necessary to reach the performance level used in the analysis. As more complex problems are addressed, the spreadsheets themselves get quite elaborate, and the model builder must have extensive experience.[36]

Community-based epidemiologic planning

Healthcare systems now identify geographic communities, or markets, whose healthcare needs they will meet. The demographic, economic, and epidemiological characteristics of these communities are a fundamental data set for planning decisions of all kinds. The general model to estimate local demand for a given service is an equation:

$$
\left\{ \begin{array}{c} \text{Demand for} \\ \text{a service} \end{array} \right\} = \left\{ \begin{array}{c} \text{Population} \\ \text{at risk} \end{array} \right\} \times \left\{ \begin{array}{c} \text{Incidence} \\ \text{rate} \end{array} \right\} \times \left\{ \begin{array}{c} \text{Average} \\ \text{use per} \\ \text{incidence} \end{array} \right\} \times \left\{ \begin{array}{c} \text{Market} \\ \text{share} \end{array} \right\}
$$

It can be applied to either intermediate services or final products. It is usually calculated for specific risk groups to accommodate the fact that most conditions for which people seek healthcare differ by age, sex, income, and other factors.[37] The individual terms must themselves be forecast, using regression analysis, benchmarking, or other techniques. State agencies now prepare detailed population forecasts that are more reliable than any other sources, except for very small geographic areas. Sensitivity analyses evaluate alternative forecasts, greatly improving the final decision process.

Examples of the use of the model are shown in Figure 5.21. Obstetrics is the easiest to understand. It also has the best supporting data, allowing great refinement in the estimate. Obstetrical deliveries occur only to young women. The population at risk and the anticipated fertility rates are frequently available for each year of age. The use per incident for deliveries is essentially one. Market share can be measured from history because births are recorded both by the mother's address and the site of delivery. All of these data must be forecast into the future. The fertility rates and market share can be forecast from history or by survey of child-bearing intentions.

The remaining examples of Figure 5.21 show the application of the model in other areas. Post-partum care days in obstetrics resemble the

Figure 5.21 Applications of the Epidemiologic Planning Model

Example	Population at Risk	Incidence Rate	Use per Incident	Market Share
Obstetrics deliveries	Fertile women	Births/fertile woman-year	1 deliveries/ woman	% of all births to women in community
Post-partum care	Delivered women	Births/fertile woman-year	2.0 days/ delivery	% of all births to women in community
Well-baby visits	Infants < 1 year	Births/fertile woman-year	4.0 visits/ year	% of all well-baby visits in community
Emergency department visits	Economic, geographic subsets of population	ED visits/ person for each subset	1.0 visits/ arrival	% of community visits seeking this ED
Hip replacements	Population aged 50–65, over 65	Hip replacement/ person for each subset	1.0 surgeries/ patient	% of candidates seeking this institution

forecast for deliveries, but each mother uses about two days, a number that differs by locale. Well-baby visits are planned events important to provide immunizations, instruction to the mother, and early detection of developmental problems. The population at risk is all babies born in the last year; the incidence and the number of visits per baby are set by policy; and the market share is closely related to the obstetrics share. The forecast would be used not only to estimate demand, but as a quality standard—a well-managed health insurance program will strive to achieve 100 percent of scheduled visits.

Emergency department visits are expensive, and managed care strategies call for minimizing them. They are a function of availability of health insurance, other primary care sources, and lifestyle. As a result, the population at risk would be segregated economically or geographically to identify different incidence rates. For many purposes, it would also be necessary to adjust for time of day and day of week. This would be done by using several different incidence rates. The use term could be set at one, yielding a forecast of visits, or the average number of hours of use, yielding an estimate of use of facilities. Hip replacement surgery occurs almost exclusively among the elderly, and the use term can be adjusted to forecast either procedures or expected days of inpatient stay.

Using the incidence of diseases, the model can forecast many final product episodes. Epidemiologic studies have developed the incidence of most common and expensive illness and analyzed the population characteristics associated with it. Data are available from the Centers for Disease Control and Prevention[38] and commercial sources. Estimates can be compared to actual values for diseases reducible by prevention or management, such as cancer, heart disease, and AIDS, to reveal unique risks or treatment practices in the community. These are useful in identifying cost-improvement possibilities. A simple example is births to very young single mothers. These are associated with high-cost problems in infant care. Programs to reduce these births by discouraging teenaged pregnancy are cost-effective. Programs to reach young mothers early in their pregnancies reduce the risk and cost of problems. Under capitation insurance contracts, these gains work directly to reduce overall cost of care.

Other deterministic models

Other algebraic models can be developed as needed. They show the relationship between exogenous characteristics and desired endogenous ones, such as the relation between demand and staffing, and are useful for illustrating assumptions and gaining improved understanding of operating possibilities.[39]

PERT (project evaluation and review technique) charts are programs for analyzing construction projects and similar sets of complex, time-dependent, interrelated activities. The value of PERT charts lies in their ability to identify critical paths, the sequences and timetables of events that will delay the overall project if they are not met. PERT charting is routine for major construction projects and renovations. It is also useful for complex new program development. Commercial software supports the analysis, but the inputs require substantial knowledge of change processes. PERT charting is generally done by one or two people in the organization who are experienced with it.

A variety of programming models are used in commercial applications, including linear programming and forms of dynamic programming. These models differ from the business plan in their ability to find the optimum set of endogenous conditions. They have found limited use in healthcare, although linear programming is theoretically applicable to personnel staffing and inventory management. The few applications that have occurred have been incorporated in specific software for departmental operation. A technique called data envelopment analysis allows estimation of optimal operational efficiency in certain multidimensional problems.[40] Development of programming models is demanding. Special coursework is essential, along with extensive experience in other modeling forms.

Stochastic models

Some situations cannot be effectively modeled by deterministic techniques. They are usually those where the exogenous conditions cannot be predicted easily in advance, but still have an important effect on the outcomes. Stochastic means subject to chance variation. **Stochastic models** incorporate chance variation in the analysis and evaluation of the solutions. The traditional example of a stochastic problem is the arrival of women for obstetric delivery. Each event is unpredictable even a few hours in advance, yet it is so important that the healthcare organization must have adequate staff and facilities to serve the patient when she arrives. A model will be constructed showing how often the staff and facilities will be overtaxed for a given level of average demand. Because the demand is random with wide variation from hour to hour, a deterministic model based on the average demand would be disastrously unsatisfactory.

Figure 5.22 shows the results of a model to determine obstetric birthing rooms and staffing. (The model is simplified to illustrate the issues involved.) On the average, women arriving for delivery will require two rooms and staff groups. Just under 2,200 women deliver each year, and they require on the average about eight hours of service. But because of the stochastic demand, they will keep two rooms and staff occupied most of the time, need a third about 20 percent of the time, a fourth about 10 percent, a fifth less than 5 percent. Only about once a year will six units be required. Quality and patient satisfaction require that some provision be made for the five-unit and six-unit situations, but because of the cost, the solution will not be to routinely staff for five units, nor to build six units.[41]

Stochastic models are usually constructed around **Monte Carlo simulation**, a computerized test of a model situation by repeated trial. Although advanced spreadsheet software has the capability of doing Monte Carlo simulation, the most important parts of the model are its design and the measurement of the parameters. The birthing room example in Figure 5.22 requires not only forecasts of mean values but reliable distributions of arrival times, service times, and staffing requirements. The final evaluation will weigh probabilities of rare events and the extent to which they violate constraints against the cost of meeting them.

Simulation can also be adapted to expand sensitivity analysis of deterministic models. Exogenous variables must be given realistic distributions

Figure 5.22   Stochastic Analysis of Birthing Room Requirements (% of time rooms in use)

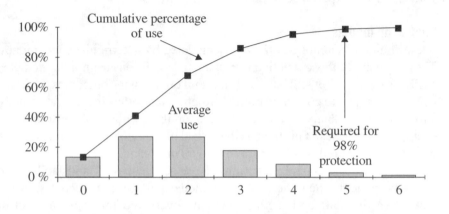

of possible values, and the impact of variation can be explored to reveal changes required in endogenous variables and resulting values of the objective function. A range of scenarios, rather than just a few extremes, can be evaluated.[42] Advanced software is usually necessary to do this and is offered by several vendors. These systems allow financial planning in a stochastic mode and are called **decision support systems** (DSS). To date, they have found limited application in healthcare, probably because they require very large, reliable databases.[43] New program analysis has been reported in a proposed health promotion center[44] and a pharmacy.[45] As healthcare organizations improve their automated data archives, DSS applications will grow. At least theoretically, a sophisticated DSS model could be used with a process improvement team in real time, allowing the team to experiment with various changes to endogenous events and see the impact on constraints and objective function almost immediately.[46]

Experimentation

Many improvement possibilities require more than an abstract model evaluation. Relationships between exogenous and endogenous events and final objectives are not always easy to state or even understand. All models are simplifications of reality; one of the most common simplifications is omission of interactions between various events. As a result, real world trials do not always behave as the model indicated. In addition, trials offer opportunities to demonstrate, convince, and teach. The model site can be the teaching site to roll out the results to the larger organization. For these reasons, the "check" step of PDCA frequently includes a field trial.[47]

Quantitative information contributes to the field trial in several ways. It allows the improvement team to analyze relationships between various events and design the improvement itself. It supports simple models that rule out unpromising experiments and reveal correctable weaknesses in promising ones. Models also show the kinds of data required for evaluation and the length of trial necessary to achieve reliable results. They often suggest potential difficulties with the trial or its interpretation that can be accommodated in design or analysis to strengthen the conclusions.

The most rigorous form of experiments are random controlled trials carefully designed and controlled to yield results appropriate to a large, uncontrolled population or market, such as the United States or all developed countries. They are supported by research funds from large corporations or government. Design and publication are both subject to rigorous critical review. Many healthcare organizations participate in alliances or networks formed for the purpose of research. Most clinical research developing and testing new methods of diagnosis and treatment is done this way.

Experiments on operations are difficult to do at the same level of rigor. Trials are often pre/post, using historical data as a control, or pre/post with a control. The results are superior to no trial at all and are usually strong enough to support decisions. Technically, a single organization can represent only itself. Transferability from one organization to another may be limited; indeed the objective may be to develop a unique competitive advantage for a single firm.

The level of rigor is only one of the considerations in the trial design. The cost of the trial, including potential dangers to patients or employees, and other benefits such as building consensus or serving as a training site must also be considered. A good field trial is one that:

- presents no increased danger to patients or staff;
- is free of avoidable distortion or bias;
- is conducted over enough patients or events to yield statistically significant results;
- evaluates an improvement worth several times the accounting cost of conducting the trial; and
- can be modified in course to yield the greatest possible overall improvement.

These standards are considerably less rigorous than those for formal research. The loss of rigor increases the chance that the result may be caused by something other than the experimental modification, and the chance that a second trial will not yield the same results. The so-called **Hawthorne effect** is a frequent issue. A famous series of experiments showed that the fact of experimentation and the attention it drew could improve performance, independent of the experiment itself.[48] Organization field trials often approach the problem of rigor by making allowance for the Hawthorne effect and related risks in judging the results, and by approaching the experiment sequentially. Thus, very strong initial results lead to continuation of the trial; weaker ones to consideration of improvements in the proposal; and disappointing ones to discontinuation. If feasible, the continuation can be undertaken on a second site, where pride of authorship is less likely to enhance the results.

A field trial should have the following components:

1. A hypothesis or proposal expressing the relationship between an endogenous event, process, or method, and an objective function, such as "If we change Process A in a certain defined way, we will achieve better outcomes as measured by cost, profit, and quality."

2. Justification from literature or analysis of operational data suggesting that the hypothesis is plausible, that the answer is not obvious, and that a trial is likely to yield improvements worth many times its cost.

3. A method of implementing the change in a real field setting, including site, initial investment in equipment and training, safety factors, and time schedules.

4. A method of measuring the changes in outcomes and any other variables important to the decision.

5. An estimation of the length or size of the trial necessary to demonstrate the improvement.

6. A review of the moral and practical implications for patients and employees involved in the trial.

7. A critical analysis of the reliability, validity, and value of the expected results, including a review of confounding factors that should be considered.

While the steps seem onerous, a field trial involves a disruption of an ongoing process and the danger of doing harm is always present. The steps can be simplified in undemanding situations; operating teams try new approaches constantly as part of their learning. But a trial involving more than a few people in direct personal communication deserves at least a review of all seven items.

Well-managed institutions establish mechanisms facilitating review of field trials. The support includes consultants trained in experimental design and analysis and ad hoc work groups to gain consensus on methods, explore implications, and provide a critical analysis. A **human subjects committee** can contribute unbiased review of potential dangers to patients and employees. It is required by most funding bodies for formal research, but it clearly has a role whenever a process change involves patient care or risks to employees. Similarly, large-scale trials can be given critical review by formal committees from outside the area in question, emulating the research review process.

MONITORING AND CONTROLLING

Control, the ability to achieve desired future events, is the essence of all economic activity and the central justification for the organization.[49] Control implies both predictability and uniformity. Variation is a measure of the lack of control, and monitoring is the measurement of variation. Control is actually achieved by individuals and organizations through a series of human interactions where the quantitative measurement of relevant factors is only a supplement to more powerful and less precise processes. As activities and organizations grow more complex, the role of quantification becomes more central, but it never replaces the underlying human factors.

Continuous improvement theory emphasizes that control is built in, not monitored, and certainly not imposed. Control begins with the design of service and process. The right process, training, tools and supplies, and demand levels lead to control; failures in these cannot be replaced by incentives or statistical systems. A monitoring process, statistical systems, and incentives are necessary to maintain the system after it is designed. Even if it was perfectly designed at the outset, an unmonitored system will deteriorate as a function of environmental changes, wear, and fatigue. Monitoring detects the need for maintenance and the opportunity for improvement.

Cybernetic Systems

The concept of monitoring begins with a cybernetic system, the addition of a separate, new activity to a process. A process translates inputs—including demand and resources—to outputs—goods or services sold for revenue and profit. It can be represented as shown in Figure 5.23A. The monitor shown in Figure 5.23B is added to evaluate the performance, identify necessary corrections, and make them. The monitor relies on the same measures of performance that were shown in Figure 5.2. The word **cybernetic** comes from the ancient Greek *cybernos*, or helmsman, the monitor who kept the ship on course. Monitors of some systems are purely mechanical; the thermostat on the heating system is an example. Most human activities are monitored by the person doing them.

Figure 5.23 Cybernetic System

A. Activity Converting Inputs to Outputs

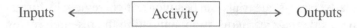

B. Cybernetic System with Monitor

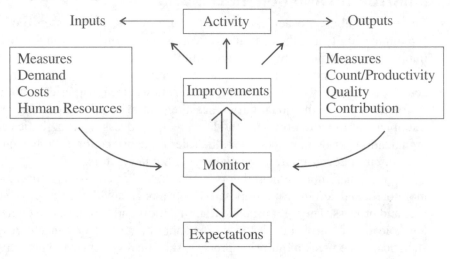

Figure 5.23B applies to any process, from a nurse giving patient care to a complete healthcare organization. The monitor in direct contact with the process is called the primary monitor. It is possible to monitor monitors, thus establishing a nest of sequential monitoring functions. The accountability hierarchy is such a nest; each level monitors not the underlying activities, but the performance of the level immediately below it. The governing board can be understood as the primary monitor for the organization as a whole.

The monitor, whether it is the nurse, the governing board, or anyone in between, proceeds by comparing the performance information (technically the signal) against the expectation. If the two are not identical, an error signal is generated and the monitor acts upon it. This does not automatically require quantification; the nurse will be working with a wide variety of verbal, visual, and sensory data that is not quantified at all. Quantification is necessary when the direct contact is lost.

As an example of an activity beyond the individual worker, consider a nursing station shown in Figure 5.24. The head nurse is the monitor; nurses and other nursing personnel are the major resources; arriving patients are the demands; and treated patients are the outputs. The budget for a nursing unit will specify quantitative expectations for all six performance dimensions, and measures of achievement will reach the head nurse regularly on these and many other indicators. (Some will be by direct observation and will not be quantitative.) The head nurse will compare signals to expectations. He or she will expect no error signals, and in a well-managed institution will rarely see them. The failures that do occur should always be studied for ways to eliminate them in the future, by changing the process. The head nurse's main effort will turn to possibilities for further improvement, which can be evaluated and implemented in future years' expectations.

Spider Charts

Ratio-scaled performance can be reported on spider charts at any level of the organization from the work group up. The Henry Ford Health System does

Figure 5.24   Examples of Monitor Function on a Nursing RC

Dimension	*Measures*	*Possible Improvements*
Demand	Number of patients	Patient satisfaction, physician satisfaction, scheduling, case management
Costs	Labor costs	Personnel scheduling, cross-training, new processes
	Supplies costs	New processes, clinical protocols
Human Resources	Employee satisfaction	Personnel scheduling, supervisory training, new job requirements
Output/ Productivity	Cost per visit or per day	Change processes to reduce variable costs, increase demand to reduce fixed costs
	Cost per member month	Change processes to reduce variable costs, decrease demand, reduce fixed costs by elimination
Quality	Recovery rates	Personnel training, clinical protocols, new processes
	Patient satisfaction	Personnel training, clinical protocols, new processes
	Procedure	Personnel training, clinical protocols, new processes
Contribution	Profit or cost target	Search for improvable inputs, outputs, and processes

this, interlocking the performance measures and representing all the quadrants (cost, quality, satisfaction, and market share). The charts themselves are easily created from spreadsheet software, but careful attention must be paid to defining the performance measures, expectations, and data collection processes to insure reliable and valid reports. The charts provide a quick, graphic summary of performance on up to 16 variables.

Statistical Quality Control

Statistical quality control will be necessary to identify variations that are significant or likely to be correctable.[50] Significant variations can be called special cause variation or error signals. Nonsignificant variations can be called random variation, common cause variation, or noise. Significance can be tested by standard statistical techniques, and statistical quality control is now frequently automated and graphically reported.[51] Measures for a specific time period are taken for a sample or for all activity during the period. Each measurement is called a lot, and lots are collected sequentially. Values and control limits for both the mean and the variance covering sequential time periods can be plotted for variables statistics (those arising from interval and ratio scales), as shown in Figure 5.25. The more common attributes measures can be expressed as a percentage passing (or failing) the threshold for each time period and plotted over time as shown in Figure 5.19. All three of these graphs are control charts. They can be reviewed over time for trends or changes, using statistical techniques to identify the special cause or statistically significant variation.

Several alternatives and improvements can make the statistical tests more sensitive in specific situations. For further discussion at an elementary level, see Gitlow, *Planning for Quality, Productivity, and Competitive Position,* and at an advanced level Feigenbaum's *Total Quality Control* (see Suggested Readings).

Control charts allow monitors to scan large numbers of measures and quickly identify where further improvements are likely.[52] However, there are a number of ways in which the analysis can be misused. Misuse will waste resources, and it may be destructive because it diverts us from important alternatives or results in insupportable accusations and loss of morale. Here are some of the principal problems:

1. The lots must be from the same process. Many uncontrollable events change medical care processes over time, such as changes in the condition of arriving patients. Runs of uncommon patients and other factors affecting the lots must always be ruled out before "outliers" are acknowledged.

Figure 5.25 Process Control Charts for Variables Measures

A. Control Chart for the Mean

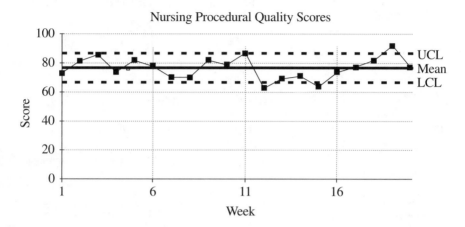

B. Control Chart for Variation

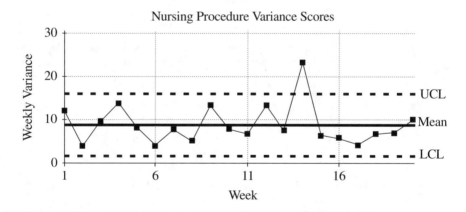

2. No inference of good or poor quality can ever be made about a lot until special causes have been identified or ruled out. It is useful to use 99 percent confidence limits (three times the standard deviation) to identify outliers. This reduces the number of outliers identified and raises the probability that a correctable cause can be found.

3. No inference of good or poor quality can ever be made about individual cases in the lot using this approach (or about the practitioners treating the patients in the lot). Many outliers are actually random events.

SUGGESTED READINGS

Austin, C. J., and S. B. Boxerman. 1995. *Quantitative Analysis for Health Services Administration.* Chicago: Health Administration Press.

Deming, W. E. 1986. *Out of the Crisis.* Boston: Massachusetts Institute of Technology Center for Advanced Engineering Study.

Feigenbaum, A. V. 1991. *Total Quality Control,* 3rd ed. (rev.). New York: McGraw-Hill.

Flood, A. B., S. M. Shortell, and W. R. Scott. 1997. "Organizational Performance: Managing for Efficiency and Effectiveness." In *Essentials of Health Care Management,* edited by S. Shortell and A. D. Kaluzny, 381–429. New York: Delmar.

Krowinski, W. J., and S. R. Steiber. 1996. *Measuring and Managing Patient Satisfaction,* 2nd ed. Chicago: American Hospital Publishing.

Mendenhall, W., and R. J. Beaver. 1994. *Introduction to Probability and Statistics*, 9th ed. Belmont, CA: Duxbury Press.

Montgomery, D. C., L. A. Johnson, and J. S. Gardiner. 1990. *Forecasting and Time Series Analysis,* 2nd ed. New York: McGraw-Hill.

NOTES

1. K. Castaneda-Mendez, K. Mangan, and A. M. Lavery, "The Role and Application of the Balanced Scorecard in Healthcare Quality Management." *Journal for Healthcare Quality* 20(1), pp. 10–13 (January–February, 1998).

2. P. Eastman, "NCI Adopts New Mammography Screening Guidelines for Women." *Journal of the National Cancer Institute* 89(8), pp. 538–39 (April 16, 1997); Anonymous, "NIH Consensus Statement. Breast Cancer Screening for Women Ages 40–49." *NIH Consensus Statement* 15(1), pp. 1–35 (January 21–23, 1997).

3. R. S. Kaplan and R. Cooper, *Cost & Effect: Using Integrated Cost Systems to Drive Profitability and Performance.* Boston: Harvard Business School Press (1998).

4. J. J. Baker, "Activity-Based Costing for Integrated Delivery Systems." *Journal of Health Care Finance* 22(2), pp. 57–61 (Winter, 1995).

5. D. J. Brailer, E. Kroch, M. V. Pauly, and J. Huang, "Comorbidity-Adjusted Complication Risk: A New Outcome Quality Measure." *Medical Care* 34(5), pp. 490–505 (May, 1996).

6. T. P. Hofer, S. J. Bernstein, R. A. Hayward, and S. DeMonner, "Validating Quality Indicators for Hospital Care." *Joint Commission Journal on Quality Improvement* 23(9), pp. 455–67 (September, 1997).

7. M. L. Millenson, *Demanding Medical Excellence: Doctors and Accountability in the Information Age.* Chicago: University of Chicago Press (1997).

8. ———, "Perspective on Measurement." *Health Affairs* 17(4): 7–41.

9. M. Johantgen, A. Elixhauser, J. K. Bali, M. Goldfarb, and D. R. Harris, "Quality Indicators Using Hospital Discharge Data: State and National Applications." *Joint Commission Journal on Quality Improvement* 24(2), pp. 88–105 (February, 1998).

10. J. H. Seibert, J. M. Strohmeyer and R. G. Carey, "Evaluating the Physician Office Visit: In Pursuit of a Valid and Reliable Measure of Quality Improvement Efforts." *Journal of Ambulatory Care Management* 19(1), pp. 17–37 (January, 1996).

11. R. C. Ford, S. A. Bach and M. D. Fottler, "Methods of Measuring Patient Satisfaction in Health Care Organizations." *Health Care Management Review* 22(2), pp. 74–89 (Spring, 1997).

12. W. J. Krowinski, S. R. Steiber, *Measuring and Managing Patient Satisfaction*, 2nd Ed. Chicago: American Hospital Publishing (1996).

13. Pickert Institute home page: www.pickert.org (October 28, 1998 version).

14. R. Hodges, L. Kelley, and A. Wilkes, "Benchmarking and Networking Through Collaborative Groups." *Journal for Healthcare Quality* 18(1), pp. 26–31 (January–February, 1996).

15. See, for example, publications and services of the Medstat Corporation: www.medstat.com; Sachs Group: www.sach.com; and HCIA, Inc.: www.hcia.com (October 27, 1998).

16. W. A. Knause, E. A. Draper, and D. P. Wagner, "The Use of Intensive Care: New Research Initiatives and Their Application for National Health Policy," *Milbank Memorial Fund Quarterly* 61, pp. 561–583 (Fall, 1983).

17. R. C. Jelinek, "An Operational Analysis of the Patient Care Function," *Inquiry* 6(2), pp. 53–58 (June, 1969).

18. J. P. Weiner, B. H. Starfield, D. M. Steinwachs, and L. M. Mumford, "Development and Application of a Population-Oriented Measure of Ambulatory Care Case-Mix." *Medical Care* 29(5), pp. 452–72 (May, 1991); B. Starfield, J. Weiner, L. Mumford, and D. Steinwachs, "Ambulatory Care Groups: A Categorization of Diagnoses for Research and Management." *Health Services Research* 26(1), pp. 53–74 (April, 1991).

19. P. A. Gross, "Practical Healthcare Epidemiology: Basics of Stratifying for Severity of Illness." *Infection Control & Hospital Epidemiology* 17(10), pp. 675–86 (1996).

20. C. Y. Phillips, A. Castorr, P. A. Prescott, and K, Soeken, "Nursing Intensity: Going Beyond Patient Classification." *Journal of Nursing Administration* 22(4), pp. 46–52 (April, 1992).

21. B. E. Fries, D. P. Schneider, W. J. Foley, and M, Dowling, "Case-Mix Classification of Medicare Residents in Skilled Nursing Facilities: Resource Utilization Groups (RUG-T18)." *Medical Care* 27(9), pp. 843–58 (September, 1989).

22. V. J. Gooder, B. R. Farr, and M. P. Young, "Accuracy and Efficiency of an Automated System for Calculating APACHE II Scores in an Intensive Care Unit." *Proceedings/AMIA Annual Fall Symposium*, pp. 131–5 (1997); T. A. Mackenzie, A. Greenaway-Coates, M. S. Djurfeldt, and W. M. Hopman, "Use of Severity of Illness to Evaluate Quality of Care." *International Journal for Quality in Health Care* 8(2), pp. 125–30 (April, 1996).

23. L. I. Iezzoni, A. S. Ash, M. Shwartz, J. Daley, J. S. Hughes, and Y. D. Mackiernan, "Judging Hospitals by Severity-Adjusted Mortality Rates: The Influence of the Severity-Adjustment Method." *American Journal of Public Health* 86(10), pp. 1379–87 (October, 1996).

24. L. I. Iezzoni, "The Risks of Risk Adjustment." *Journal of the American Medical Association* 278(19), pp. 1600–7 (November, 19 1997); L. I. Iezzoni, A. S. Ash, M. Shwartz, J. Daley, J. S. Hughes, and Y. D. Mackiernan, "Judging Hospitals by Severity-Adjusted Mortality Rates: The Influence of the Severity-Adjustment Method." *American Journal of Public Health* 86(10), pp.1379–87 (October, 1996).

25. J. W. Thomas and M. L. Ashcraft, "Measuring Severity of Illness: Six Severity Systems and Their Ability to Explain Cost Variations." *Inquiry* 28(1), pp. 39–55 (1991).

26. The Malcom Baldrige National Quality Award home page: www.quality.nist.gov (October 27, 1998).

27. J. R. Griffith, V. K. Sahney, and R. A. Mohr, *Reengineering Healthcare: Building on Continuous Quality Improvement.* Chicago: Health Administration Press (1995).

28. W. E. Deming, *Out of the Crisis.* Boston: Massachusetts Institute of Technology, Center for Advanced Engineering Study, pp. 309–371 (1986).

29. *Ibid*, p. 39 (1986).

30. Joint Commission on Accreditation of Healthcare Organizations, *Six Hospitals in Search of Quality, Striving Towards Improvement.* Oakbrook Terrace, IL: JCAHO, pp. 255–259 (1992).

31. D. C. Kibbe and R. P. Scoville, "Computer Software for Healthcare CQI," and "Tutorial: Using Microsoft Excel for Healthcare CQI." *Quality Management In Healthcare* 1(4), pp. 50–58 (Summer, 1993) and 2(1), pp. 63–71 (Fall, 1993).

32. S. L. Jarvenpaa and G. W. Dickson, "Graphics and Managerial Decision Making: Research Based Guidelines." *Communications of the ACM* 31(6), pp. 764–74 (1988).

33. T. W. Weiss, C. M. Ashton, and N. P. Wray, "Forecasting Areawide Hospital Utilization: A Comparison of Five Univariate Time Series Techniques." *Health Services Management Research* 6(3), pp. 178–190 (August, 1993).

34. U.S. Bureau of the Census, *Current Population Reports: Cooperative Program for Federal-State Population Estimates*, Series P-26. Washington DC: U.S. Department of Commerce, Bureau of the Census.

35. R. D. Zentner and B. D. Gelb, "Scenarios: A Planning Tool for Healthcare Organizations." *Hospital & Health Services Administration* 36(2), pp. 211–22 (Summer 1991).

36. P. Kokol, "Structured Spreadsheet Modeling in Medical Decision Making and Research." *Journal of Medical Systems* 14(3), pp. 107–17 (1990).

37. J. R. Griffith, W. M. Hancock, and F. C. Munson, *Cost Control in Hospitals.* Chicago: Health Administration Press, pp. 23–89 (1976).

38. Centers for Disease Control, US Dept. of Health and Human Services, home page: www.cdc.gov (October 27, 1998).

39. M. Kim and W. M. Hancock, "Applications of Staffing, Scheduling and Budgeting Methods to Hospital Ancillary Units." *Journal of Medical Systems* 13(1), pp. 37–47 (1989).

40. Y. L. Huang, "An Application of Data Envelopment Analysis: Measuring the Relative Performance of Florida General Hospitals." *Journal of Medical Systems* 14(4), pp. 191–6 (1990).

41. J. D. Thompson, "Predicting Requirements for Maternity Facilities." *Hospitals* (Feb. 16, 1963).

42. L. C. Gapenski, "Using Monte Carlo Simulation to Make Better Capital Investment Decisions." *Hospital & Health Services Administration* 35(2), pp. 207–19 (Summer, 1990).

43. M. E. Hatcher and C. Connelly, "A Case Mix Simulation Decision Support System Model for Negotiating Hospital Rates." *Journal of Medical Systems* 12(6), pp. 341–63 (1988).

44. M. E. Hatcher and N. Rao, " A Simulation Based Decision Support System for a Health Promotion Center." *Journal of Medical Systems* 12(1), pp. 11–29 (1988).

45. A. S. Zaki, "Developing a DSS for a Distribution Facility: An Application in the Healthcare Industry." *Journal of Medical Systems* 13(6), pp. 331–46 (1989).

46. M. E. Hatcher, "Uniqueness of Group Decision Support Systems (GDSS) in Medical and Health Applications," *Journal of Medical Systems* 14(6), pp. 351–34 (1990).

47. C. H. Moore, "Experimental Design in Healthcare." *Quality Management in Healthcare* 2(2), pp. 13–26 (Winter, 1994).

48. F. J. Roethlisberger and W. J. Dickson, *Management and the Worker: An Account of a Research Program Conducted by the Western Electric Company, Hawthorne Works, Chicago*. Cambridge, MA: Harvard University Press (1939).

49. A. D. Chandler, *The Visible Hand: The Managerial Revolution in American Business*. Cambridge, MA: Belknap Press (1977).

50. P. E. Pisek, "Tutorial: Introduction to Control Charts." *Quality Management in Healthcare* 1(1), pp. 65–74 (Fall, 1992).

51. H. Gitlow, S. Gitlow, A. Oppenheim, and R. Oppenheim, *Tools and Methods for the Improvement of Quality*. Homewood, IL: Irwin, pp. 78–110 (1989).

52. L. J. Finison, K. S. Finison, "Applying Control Charts to Quality Improvement." *Journal for Healthcare Quality* 18(6): 32–41 (Nov–Dec, 1996).

Planning and Budgeting

Louis C. Gapenski, Ph.D.

Planning and budgeting play a critical role in the finance function of all
health services organizations. In fact, one could argue—and usually
win—that planning and budgeting are the most important of all finance
related tasks. *Planning* encompasses the overall process of preparing for
the future. Because of its importance to organizational success, most health
services managers, especially at large organizations, spend a great deal of
time on activities related to planning.

Budgeting is an offshoot of the planning process. A set of *budgets* is the
basic accounting tool used to tie together managerial planning and control
functions. In general, organizational plans focus on the long-term big picture,
whereas budgets address the details of both planning for the immediate future
and, through the control mechanism, ensuring that current performance is
consistent with organizational plans and goals.

This chapter includes an introduction to the planning process and a
discussion of how budgets are used within health services organizations.
In particular, the chapter focuses on how managers can use flexible budgets
and variance analysis to help exercise control over current operations. Unfortunately, in this chapter, only the surface of these very important topics
can be scratched.[1]

THE PLANNING PROCESS

The *strategic plan* is the foundation of any organization's planning process.
It begins with the organization's mission statement, scope, and objectives.

Editor's Note: This chapter is from Chapter 8 of *Healthcare Finance* by Louis C. Gapenski,
1999, HAP

The strategic plan then outlines the broad strategies to be followed to achieve the plan's stated objectives. Although the strategic plan is the lynchpin of the planning and budgeting process, it does not provide managers with detailed operational guidance. The "how to" or perhaps "how we expect to" portion of the planning process is contained in the *operating plan.*

Operating plans can be developed for any time horizon, but most organizations use a five-year horizon. Thus, the term *five-year plan* is often used in place of *operating plan.* In a five-year plan, the plans are most detailed for the first year, with each succeeding year's plan becoming less specific. Unlike the strategic plan, which is short on specifics, the five-year plan contains considerable detail concerning who is responsible for what particular function and when specific tasks are to be accomplished.

Table 6.1 contains Bayside Memorial Hospital's annual planning schedule. This schedule illustrates the fact that for most organizations, the planning process is essentially continuous. Next, Table 6.2 outlines the key elements of the hospital's five-year plan with an expanded section for the financial plan (Part 7 of the operating plan). A full outline would require several pages, but Table 6.2 at least provides insights into the format and contents of a five-year plan. Note that the first two chapters of the operating plan are drawn from the organization's strategic plan.

For Bayside, much of the planning function takes place at the department level, with technical assistance from the marketing, planning, and financial staffs. Larger firms with divisions would begin the planning process at the divisional level. Each division would have its own mission and goals as well as objectives and budgets designed to support its goals; these plans are then consolidated to form the overall corporate plan.

Section A of the financial plan (Part 7 of the operating plan) focuses on long-term financial planning at the organizational level. Its first component is a review of the business' current financial condition, which provides the basis or starting point for the remainder of the financial plan. Next, the capital budget, which outlines future capital acquisitions (i.e., long-term asset purchases), is presented. This information feeds into the pro-forma financial statements, which are projected for the next five years.[2] Finally, the organization's external financing requirements are listed, along with a plan for obtaining these funds. As can be seen from its content, Section A of the financial plan provides an overview of the financial future of the organization.

Section B of the financial plan concerns current asset and current liability management, which often is called *working capital management.* Here, the financial staff receives overall guidance regarding day-to-day, short-term financial operations. Section C of the financial plan provides short-term operating benchmarks for all levels of management. For example, the

Table 6.1   Bayside Memorial Hospital: Annual Planning Schedule

Months	*Action*
April–May	Marketing department analyzes national and local economic factors likely to influence Bayside's patient volume and reimbursement rates. At this time, a preliminary volume forecast is prepared for each service line.
June–July	Operating departments prepare new project (long-term asset) requirements, as well as operating cost estimates based on the preliminary volume forecast.
August–September	Financial analysts evaluate proposed capital expenditures and department operating plans. Preliminary forecasted financial statements are prepared with emphasis on Bayside's overall sources and uses of funds and forecasted financial condition.
October–November	All previous input is reviewed and the hospital's five-year plan is drafted by the planning, financial, and departmental staffs. At this stage, the operating and cash budgets are finalized. Any changes that have occurred since the beginning of the planning process are incorporated into the plan.
December	The five-year plan, including all budgets for the coming year, is approved by the hospital's executive committee, and then submitted to the board of directors for final approval.

accounting plan provides financial goals at the micro level by division, contract, or diagnosis, and is used to control operations through frequent comparisons with actual results.

If financial planning were compared to planning a cross-country road trip, Section A could be thought of as a roadmap of the United States, which provides the overview, while Section C could be thought of as the state maps, which provide the details. The bulk of this chapter is devoted to a discussion of Section C, specifically, the preparation and use of budgets.

INTRODUCTION TO BUDGETING

Budgeting involves detailed plans, expressed quantitatively in dollar terms, that specify how resources will be obtained and used during a specified period of time. In general, budgets rely heavily on revenue and cost estimates.

To be of greatest usefulness, managers must think of budgets not as accounting tools, but as managerial tools. Budgets are more important to

---

Table 6.2   Bayside Memorial Hospital: Five-Year Plan Outline

Part 1   Corporate mission, scope, and objectives
Part 2   Corporate strategies
Part 3   Projected business environment
Part 4   Summary of projected business results
Part 5   Marketing plan
Part 6   Operating plan
Part 7   Financial plan
     A.   Long-term plan
        1. Financial condition analysis
        2. Capital budget
        3. Pro-forma financial statements
        4. External financing requirements
     B.   Working capital management plan
        1. Overall working capital policy
        2. Cash budget
        3. Cash and marketable securities management
        4. Inventory management
        5. Credit policy and receivables management
        6. Short-term financing
     C.   Accounting plan (first year only)
        1. Revenue budget
        2. Expense budget
        3. Operating budget
        4. Control procedures
Part 8   Administration and human resources plan

---

managers than to accountants because budgets provide the means to plan and communicate operational expectations within an organization. Every manager within an organization must be aware of the plans made by other managers and by the organization as a whole, and budgets provide the means of communication. In addition, the budgeting process and the resultant final budget provide the means for senior managers to allocate limited resources among competing demands within an organization.

Although planning, communication, and allocation are important purposes of the budgeting process, perhaps the greatest value of budgeting is that it establishes financial benchmarks for control. When compared to actual results, budgets provide managers with feedback about the relative financial performance of the enterprise, whether it is a department, diagnosis, contract, or the organization as a whole. Such comparisons help managers evaluate the performance of individuals, departments, product lines, reimbursement contracts, and so on.

Furthermore, budgets provide managers with information about what needs to be done to improve performance. When actual results are not as good as those specified in the budget, managers use *variance analysis* to identify the areas causing the sub-par performance. In this way, managerial resources can be brought to bear on those areas of operations that offer the most promise for financial improvement. Finally, the information developed by comparing actual results with planned results (i.e., the control process) is useful in improving the overall accuracy of the planning process. Managers want to meet budget targets, and hence most managers will think long and hard when those targets are being developed.

BUDGET TYPES

Although an organization's immediate financial expectations are expressed in a document called *the budget*, typically the document is composed of several different budgets. Unlike financial statements, budget formats are not controlled by external requirements, so a great deal of room exists in the budgeting process for managerial innovation and creativity. The specific types and contents of the budget are dictated by the organization's mission, structure, and managerial preferences. Nevertheless, several primary types of budgets are used, either formally or informally, at virtually all health services organizations.

Statistics Budget

The *statistics budget* is the foundation budget in that it develops the data used in the other budgets. In general, the statistics budget identifies the volume of services to be provided and the resources necessary to provide those services. Because the statistics budget feeds into all other budgets, accuracy is particularly important. The statistics budget does not provide detailed data on required resources such as staffing or short-term operating asset requirements, but rather it provides general guidance.

Some organizations, especially smaller ones, may not have a separate statistics budget, but instead may incorporate its data directly into the revenue and expense budgets, or perhaps into a single operating budget. The advantage of having a separate statistics budget is that it forces all forecasting within the organization to begin with the same set of volume and resource assumptions. Unfortunately, volume estimates, which are the heart of the statistics budget and which drive all other forecasts, are among the most difficult to make.

To illustrate the complexities of volume forecasting, consider the volume forecast procedures followed by Bayside Memorial Hospital. To begin, the demand for services is divided into four major groups: inpatient, outpatient, ancillary, and other services. Volume trends in each of these areas over the past five years are plotted and a first approximation forecast is made, assuming a continuation of past trends. Next, the level of population growth and disease trends are forecasted. For example, what will be the growth in the over-65 population in the hospital's service area? These forecasts are used to develop volume by major diagnoses and to differentiate between normal services and critical care services.

Bayside's managers then analyze the competitive environment. Consideration is given to such factors as the hospital's inpatient and outpatient capacities, its competitors' capacities, and new services or service improvements that either Bayside or its competitors may institute. Next, Bayside's managers consider the effect of the hospital's planned pricing actions on volume. For example, does the hospital have plans to raise outpatient charges to boost profit margins or to lower charges to gain market share and utilize excess capacity? If such actions are expected to affect volume forecasts, these estimates must be revised.

Marketing campaigns and contracts or loss of contracts with managed care plans also affect volume, so probable developments in these areas must be considered. This facet of the forecast is particularly important to Bayside, which is in the process of buying physician group practices and creating an integrated delivery system. The success or failure of this venture could have a significant impact on future volume estimates.

If the hospital's volume forecast is off the mark, the consequences can be serious. First, if the market for any particular service expands more than Bayside has expected and planned for, the hospital will not be able to meet its patients' needs. Potential patients will end up going to competitors, and Bayside will lose market share and perhaps miss a major opportunity. However, if its projections are overly optimistic, Bayside could end up with too much capacity, which means higher than necessary costs because of excess equipment, inventory, and staff. All this would result in low profitability, which could degrade the hospital's ability to compete in the future.

Revenue Budget

Detailed information from the statistics budget feeds into the *revenue budget*, which combines volume data with reimbursement data to develop revenue forecasts. Bayside's managers consider the hospital's pricing strategy for managed care plans, conventional fee-for-service contracts, and private-pay patients, as well as trends in inflation and third-party payor reimbursement, all of which affect operating revenues. Also, price changes related to other income, such as lease rates to tenant physicians, must be considered.

The end result is a compilation of revenue forecasts by service, both in the aggregate—for example, inpatient operating revenue—and on an individual diagnosis basis. The individual diagnosis forecasts are summed and then compared with the aggregate service group forecasts. Differences are reconciled and the result is a revenue forecast for the hospital as a whole, but with breakdowns by service categories and by individual diagnoses. Finally, both the amount and the **timing** of future revenues are important. Thus, the revenue budget must forecast not only the amount of revenue expected, but also when it is likely to be received, typically by month.

Expense Budget

Like the revenue budget, the *expense budget* is derived from data in the statistics budget. The focus here is on the costs of providing services, rather than the resulting revenues. The expense budget typically is divided into labor (salaries, wages, and fringe benefits) and nonlabor components. The nonlabor components include expenses associated with such items as depreciation, leases, administrative and medical supplies, and medical training and education. Expenses normally will be broken down into fixed and variable components. (As discussed later in this chapter, cost structure information is required if an organization uses flexible budgeting techniques.) Finally, at larger organizations, the expense budget may be composed of several component budgets, each one focusing on a single category of expense such as labor, supplies, or utilities.

Operating Budget

For larger organizations, the *operating budget* is a combination of the revenue and expense budgets. For smaller businesses, the statistics, revenue, and expense budgets often are combined into a single operating budget. Because the operating budget (and, by definition, the revenue and expense budgets) is prepared using accrual accounting methods, it can be roughly thought of as a pro-forma (or forecasted) income statement. However, unlike the income statement, which is typically prepared at the organizational level, operating budgets are prepared at the unit level, say, a department or product line. Because of its overall importance to the budgeting process, especially for managers, most of this chapter focuses on the operating budget.

Cash Budget

Finally, the *cash budget* focuses on the organization's cash position. Because the operating budget and its component budgets use accrual accounting, they do not provide cash flow information. Like the statement of cash flows, which recasts the income statement to focus on cash, the cash budget recasts the operating budget to focus on the actual flow of cash into and out of a business. Thus, the cash budget tells managers whether the business will be generating excess cash, which will have to be invested, or experiencing a cash shortfall, which will have to be covered in some way.

The primary difference between a cash budget and the statement of cash flows is time period. The statement of cash flows generally is prepared on an annual (and perhaps quarterly) basis, and is used for long-term cash planning. The cash budget is prepared on a monthly, weekly, or daily basis, and is used for short-term cash management.

BUDGET DECISIONS

In addition to the types of budgets used within an organization, managers must make several other decisions regarding the budget process.

Timing

Virtually all health services organizations have annual budgets, which set the standards for the coming year. However, it would take too long for managers to detect adverse trends if budget feedback were solely on an annual basis, so most organizations also have quarterly budgets, while some even have monthly, weekly, or daily budgets. Not all budget types have to use the same timing pattern. Additionally, many organizations prepare budgets for one or more *out years*, or years beyond the next budget year. Out year budgets are more closely aligned to financial planning than to operational control.

Conventional Versus Zero-Based Budgeting

Traditionally, health services organizations have used the *incremental/dec-remental,* or *conventional, approach* to budgeting. In this approach, the previous budget is used as the starting point for creating the new budget. Each line on the old budget is examined, and typically, minor changes are made to reflect changes in circumstances. Also, in the conventional approach, it is common for most budget changes to be applied more or less equally across departments and programs. For example, labor costs may be assumed to increase at the same inflation rate for all departments within an organization. In essence, the traditional approach to budgeting assumes that prior budgets are based on operational rationality, so the main issue is determining what changes (typically minor) must be made to the previous budget to account for changes in the operating environment.

As its name implies, *zero-based budgeting* starts with a clean slate.[3] For example, departments begin with a budget of zero. Department heads, then, must fully justify every line item in their budgets. In effect, departments and programs must justify their very existence each budget period. Often, budgets must be created that show the type and amount of department or program services that could be offered at alternative funding levels. Senior management, then, can use this information to make rational decisions about what budgets should be cut in the event of funding constraints.

Conceptually, zero-based budgeting is superior to incremental/decremental budgeting. Indeed, when zero-based budgeting was first introduced in the 1970s, it was widely embraced. However, what should be obvious is that the managerial resources required for zero-based budgeting far exceed those required for conventional budgeting. Therefore, many organizations that initially adopted zero-based budgeting soon concluded that its benefits were not as great as its costs. There is evidence, however, that zero-based budgeting is making a comeback among health services organizations because of the fact that market forces now require providers to continually apply cost-control efforts.

Top-Down Versus Bottom-Up Budgeting

There is no other area of accounting in which behavioral implications are more important than in budgeting. A budget affects virtually everyone in the organization, and individuals' reactions to the budgeting process can have considerable influence on an organization's overall effectiveness. One of the most important decisions regarding budget preparation is whether the budget should be created top down or bottom up.

In the *bottom-up*, or *participatory*, *approach*, budgets are developed by department or program managers first. Presumably, such individuals are most knowledgeable regarding their departments' or programs' financial needs. These budgets, then, are submitted to the finance department for review and compilation into the organizational budget, which must be approved by top management. Unfortunately, the aggregation of department or program budgets often results in an organizational budget that is not financially feasible. In such cases, the component budgets must be sent back to the original preparers for revision, which starts a negotiation process aimed at creating a budget acceptable to all parties or at least to as many parties as possible.

A more authoritarian approach to budgeting is the *top-down approach* in which little negotiation takes place between junior and senior managers. This approach has the advantages of being relatively expeditious and reflecting top management's perspective from the start. However, by limiting involvement and communication, the top-down approach often results in less commitment among junior managers and employees than does the participatory approach. Most people will perform better and make greater attempts to achieve budgetary goals if they have been consulted in setting those goals. The idea of participatory budgeting is to involve as many managers, and even employees, as possible in the budgetary process.

Fixed Versus Flexible Budgeting

As its name implies, the dollar amounts in a *fixed budget* are set in stone. A fixed budget, once it is approved, ignores the fact that revenues and expenses are tied to volume. One can think of a fixed budget as assuming no uncertainty in the volume forecast. Conversely, a *flexible budget* explicitly recognizes that rarely will the forecasted volume be realized. In essence, the flexible budget assumes perfect foresight **after the fact** because it adjusts the initial budget to recognize the actual volume of services provided. Flexible budgeting is discussed in detail in later sections of this chapter.

CONSTRUCTING A SIMPLE OPERATING BUDGET

Table 6.3 contains the 1998 operating budget for Carroll Clinic, a large inner-city primary care facility. As with most financial forecasts, the starting point for the operating budget, which was developed in October of 1997, is volume. A *volume projection* gives managers a sense of the extent of business to be performed, and hence a starting point for making revenue and cost estimates. As shown in Part I of Table 6.3, Carroll Clinic's expected patient volume for 1998 comes from two sources: a fee-for-service (FFS) population expected to generate 36,000 visits and a capitated population expected to average 30,000 members. Historically, annual utilization by the capitated population has averaged 0.15 visits per member-month, so this population is expected to generate $30,000 \times 12 \times 0.15 = 54,000$ visits in 1998. Therefore, in total, Carroll's patient base is expected to produce $36,000 + 54,000 = 90,000$ visits. Armed with this Part I volume projection, Carroll's managers can proceed with revenue and cost projections.

Part II contains revenue data. The clinic's net collection for each FFS visit averages $25. Some visits will generate greater revenues and some will generate less. On average, though, expected revenue is $25 per visit. Thus, 36,000 visits would produce $25 \times 36,000 = \$900,000$ in FFS revenues. Additionally, the capitated population will produce a revenue of $3 PMPM, for total revenues of $3 \times 30,000 \times 12 = \$3 \times 360,000$ member months $= \$1,080,000$. Considering both patient sources, total revenues for the clinic are forecasted to be $900,000 + \$1,080,000 = \$1,980,000$ in 1998.

Because of the uncertainty inherent in the clinic's volume estimates, it is useful to recognize that total revenues will be $1,980,000 only if the volume forecast holds. In reality, Total revenues = ($25 \times$ Number of FFS visits) + ($3 \times$ Number of capitated member-months). If the actual number of FFS

Table 6.3   Carroll Clinic: 1998 Operating Budget

I.   *Volume Assumptions:*
A.	FFS	36,000	visits
B.	Capitated lives	30,000	members
	Number of member months	360,000	
	Expected utilization per member-month	0.15	
	Number of visits	54,000	visits
C.	Total expected visits	90,000	visits

II.   *Revenue Assumptions:*
A.	FFS	$ 25	per visit
		× 36,000	expected visits
		$ 900,000	
B.	Capitated lives	$ 3	per member-month
		× 360,000	actual member months
		$ 1,080,000	
C.	Total expected revenues	$ 1,980,000	

III.   *Cost Assumptions:*
A.	Variable Costs:		
	Medical staffing	$ 1,200,000	(48,000 hours at $25/hour)
	Supplies	150,000	(100,000 units at $1.50/unit)
	Total variable costs	$ 1,350,000	
	Variable cost per visit	$ 15	($1,350,000/90,000)
B.	Fixed Costs:		
	Overhead, plant, and equipment	$ 500,000	
C.	Total expected costs	$ 1,850,000	

IV.   *Pro-Forma Profit and Loss (P&L) Statement:*
Revenues:	
FFS	$ 900,000
Capitated	1,080,000
Total	$ 1,980,000
Costs:	
Variable:	
FFS	$ 540,000
Capitated	810,000
Total	$ 1,350,000
Contribution margin	$ 630,000
Fixed costs	500,000
Projected profit	$ 130,000

visits is more or less than 90,000 in 1998 or the number of capitated lives is something other than 30,000, the resulting revenues will be different from the $1,980,000 forecast.

Part III of Table 6.3 focuses on expenses. To provide the quantity and quality of care to support the forecasted 90,000 visits, the clinic is expected to use 48,000 hours of medical labor, at an average cost of $25 per hour, for a total medical staffing expense of $48,000 \times \$25 = \$1,200,000$. Thus, medical staffing costs are expected to average $\$1,200,000 / 90,000 = \$13.33$ per visit in 1998. In reality, all medical staffing costs are not variable, but there are a sufficient number of part-time clinical workers such that medical labor hours are closely related to the number of visits.

Supplies expense, the bulk of which is inherently variable in nature, historically has averaged about $1.50 per bundle (unit) of supplies, with 100,000 units expected to be used to support 90,000 visits. (A unit of supplies is a more or less standard package that contains both administrative and clinical supplies.) Thus, supplies expense is expected to total $150,000, or $\$150,000 / 90,000 = \$1.67$ per visit. Taken together, Carroll's variable costs are forecasted to be $\$133.33 + \$1.67 = \$15$ per visit in 1998. The same amount can be calculated by dividing total variable costs by the number of visits: $\$1,350,000 / 90,000 = \$15$.

Finally, the clinic is expected to incur $500,000 of fixed costs for 1998, primarily administrative overhead labor costs, depreciation, and lease expense. Therefore, to serve the anticipated 90,000 visits in 1998, costs are expected to consist of $1,350,000 in variable costs plus $500,000 in fixed costs, for a total of $1,850,000. Again, it is important to recognize that some costs (in Carroll's case, a majority of costs) are tied to volume. Thus, total costs can be expressed as ($15 \times$ Number of visits) + $500,000. If the actual number of visits in 1998 comes in at more or less than 90,000 in total, then total costs will differ from the $1,850,000 budget estimate.

The final section (Part IV) of Table 6.3 contains Carroll Clinic's budgeted 1998 *profit and loss (P&L) statement*, the heart of the operating budget. A P&L statement is, in reality, a simplified pro-forma income statement. The difference between the projected revenues of $1,980,000 and the projected variable costs of $1,350,000 produces a contribution margin of $630,000, which when compared to forecasted fixed costs of $500,000 produces a budgeted profit of $130,000. The amount of data (the number of lines) shown in an operating budget varies considerably. Most budgets are more complex than the Carroll Clinic example shown in Table 6.3. The illustration has purposely been kept simple for ease of discussion.

Although the format of the P&L statement encourages sensitivity analysis (i.e., "what if" scenarios), the purpose of an operating budget is not so much to forecast profits as it is to set financial goals for the clinic. Although this first step in the operating budget very much resembles a typical pro-forma analysis, the significance of the budgeted bottom line number of $130,000 and its underlying volume, revenue, and expense assumptions become much more important in terms of managerial accountability. In effect, the operating budget can be thought of as a psychological contract between the organization and its managers. Thus, the $130,000 profit forecast becomes the overall financial benchmark for the clinic in 1998, and individual managers will be held accountable for the revenues and expenditures needed to meet the budget.

VARIANCE ANALYSIS

Variance analysis is an important technique for controlling financial performance. This section includes a discussion of the basics of variance analysis, including flexible budgeting, as well as an illustration of the process.

Variance Analysis Basics

In accounting, a *variance* is the difference between a budgeted value, often called a *standard*, and the actual value. Thus, *variance analysis* is an examination and interpretation of differences between what has actually happened and what was planned. If the budget is based on realistic expectations, variance analysis can provide managers with very useful information. Variance analysis does not provide all the answers, but it does help managers ask the right questions. (Note that the accounting definition of variance is different from the statistical definition, although both meanings connote a difference from some base value.)

Variance analysis is essential to the managerial control process. Actions taken in response to variance analysis often have the potential to dramatically improve the operations and financial performance of the organization. For example, many variances are controllable, so managers can take actions to avoid unfavorable variances in the future. The primary focus of variance analysis should not be to assign blame for unfavorable results. Rather, the goal of variance analysis is to uncover the cause of operational problems so that these problems can be avoided, or at least minimized, in the future. Unfortunately, not all variances are controllable by management. Nevertheless, knowledge of such variances is essential to the overall management and well-being of the organization. It may be necessary to revise plans, for example, to tighten controllable costs in an attempt to offset unfavorable cost variances in areas that are beyond managerial control.

Static Versus Flexible Budgets

To be of maximum value to managers, variance analysis must be approached systematically. The starting point for such analysis is the *static budget,* which is the original approved budget unadjusted for differences between planned and actual (i.e., realized) volumes. However, at the end of a budget period, it is not likely that realized volume will equal budgeted volume, so any resulting variances will be based on an apples-to-oranges comparison.

To illustrate the comparison problems that arise with static budgets, consider Carroll Clinic's 1998 operating budget contained in Table 6.3. The profit projection, $130,000, is predicated upon specific volume assumptions: 36,000 visits for the FFS population and 360,000 member months, which results in 54,000 visits for the capitated population. At the end of 1998, the clinic's managers will compare actual profits with budgeted profits. The problem, of course, is that it is highly unlikely that actual profits will be based upon 36,000 fee-for-service visits and 360,000 member months (with 54,000 visits) for the capitated population. Thus, if Carroll's managers were to merely compare the realized profit with the $130,000 in the budget, they would not know whether any profit difference is caused by volume differences or underlying operational differences.

To provide an explanation of what is driving the profit variance, managers must adopt a flexible budget. A *flexible budget* is one in which the static budget has been adjusted to reflect the actual volume achieved in the budget period. Essentially, flexible budgets are an after-the-fact device to tell managers what the results would have been under the volume level actually attained, **assuming all other budgeting assumptions held**. The flexible budget permits a much more in-depth variance analysis than is possible with a static budget. However, a flexible budget requires the identification of variable and fixed costs, and hence places a larger burden on the organization's managerial accounting system.

Variance Analysis Illustration

To illustrate variance analysis, consider Carroll's static budget for 1998 (Table 6.3), which projects a profit of $130,000. Data used for variance analysis is tracked in various parts of Carroll's managerial accounting information system throughout the year, and variance analyses are performed monthly. This allows managers to take necessary actions during the year to positively influence annual results. For purposes of this illustration, however, the monthly feedback is not shown. Rather, the focus is on the year-end results, which are contained in Table 6.4.

Total Variance, Volume Variance, and Management Variance

The variance analysis begins with a calculation of Carroll's *total variance*. Total variance is merely the difference between the realized profit (Table 6.4)

Table 6.4 Carroll Clinic: 1998 Results

I. *Volume:*
    A. FFS   40,000   visits
    B. Capitated lives   30,000   members
        Number of member months   360,000
        Actual utilization per   0.20
        member-month
            Number of visits   72,000   visits

    C. Total actual visits   112,000   visits

II. *Revenues:*
    A. FFS $ 25   per visit
                                          × 40,000   actual visits
                                          $ 1,000,000
    B. Capitated lives $ 3   per member-month
                                          × 360,000   actual member months
                                          $ 1,080,000

    C. Total actual revenues $ 2,080,000

III. *Costs:*
    A. Variable Costs:
            Medical staffing $ 1,557,400   (59,900 hours at $26/hour)
            Supplies   234,600   (124,800 units at $1.88/unit)
                Total variable costs $ 1,792,000

            Variable cost per visit $ 16   ($1,792,000/112,000)

    B. Fixed Costs:
            Overhead, plant,
            and equipment $ 500,000

    C. Total actual costs $ 2,292,000

IV. *Profit and Loss Statement:*
            Revenues:
                FFS $ 1,000,000
                Capitated   1,080,000
                Total $ 2,080,000

            Costs:
                Variable:
                    FFS $ 640,000
                    Capitated   1,152,000
                    Total $ 1,792,000

            Contribution margin $ 288,000
            Fixed costs   500,000
            Actual profit   ($ 212,000)

and the static profit (Table 6.3): Total variance = Actual profit − Static profit, or −$212,000 − $130,000 = −$342,000. Although this large negative value should generate considerable concern among Carroll's managers, a variance analysis based on the static budget is not capable of providing any insights into why profit expectations were not met. For this, a flexible budget variance analysis is required.

Table 6.5 contains three profit and loss statements (budgets) for 1998. The static budget taken from Table 6.3 is the forecast made at the beginning of 1998, while the actual budget taken from Table 6.4 reflects after-the-fact results. The flexible budget in the center column of Table 6.5 reflects projected revenues and costs at the realized (actual) volume as opposed to the projected volume, but incorporating all other assumptions that went into the static budget in Table 6.3. By analyzing differences in these three budgets, Carroll's managers can gain insights into why the clinic ended the year with a profit shortfall (from budget) of $342,000.

Before the total variance is decomposed for analysis, it is useful to examine the flexible budget in more detail. The flexible budget maintains

Table 6.5   Carroll Clinic: Static, Flexible, and Actual Budgets for 1998

	Static Budget	Flexible Budget	Actual Budget
Assumptions:			
FFS visits	36,000	40,000	40,000
Capitated visits	54,000	72,000	72,000
Total	90,000	112,000	112,000
Revenues:			
FFS	$ 900,000	$1,000,000	$1,000,000
Capitated	1,080,000	1,080,000	1,080,000
Total	$1,980,000	$2,080,000	$2,080,000
Costs:			
Variable:			
FFS	$ 540,000	$ 600,000	$ 640,000
Capitated	810,000	1,080,000	1,152,000
Total	$1,350,000	$1,680,000	$1,792,000
Contribution margin	$ 630,000	$ 400,000	$ 288,000
Fixed costs	500,000	500,000	500,000
Profit	$ 130,000	($ 100,000)	($ 212,000)

the original budget parameters of Revenues = ($25 × Number of FFS visits) + ($3 × Number of capitated member-months), and Expenses = ($15 × Number of FFS visits) + ($15 × Number of capitated visits) + $500,000. However, the flexible budget *flexes* (adjusts) revenue and costs to reflect actual volume levels. Thus, in the flexible budget column, Revenues = ($25 × 40,000) + ($3 × 360,000) = $1,000,000 + $1,080,000 = $2,080,000, and Expenses = ($15 × 40,000) + ($15 × 72,000) + $500,000 = $600,000 + $1,080,000 + $500,000 = $2,180,000.

The flexible budget can be described as follows. The $2,080,000 in total revenues is what the clinic **would have expected** for 40,000 FFS visits and a capitated membership of 30,000. The total variable costs of $1,680,000 are the costs that Carroll **would have expected** for 40,000 FFS visits and 72,000 capitated visits (based on a membership of 30,000). By definition, the fixed costs should be the same, within a reasonable range, no matter what the volume level. Thus, the $100,000 loss shown on the flexible budget represents the profit expected given the initial assumed revenue, cost, and volume relationships coupled with a forecasted volume equal to the realized volume.

Table 6.6 breaks down the total variance of −$342,000 into its two component variances. The total variance is the difference between actual profit and static profit, so it represents changes caused by all factors including volume differences and management factors. But, the flexible budget profit is the profit expected under the realized volume, assuming all other budget assumptions hold. Thus, the difference between the flexible budget profit and the original static budget profit, which is called the *volume variance*, is solely caused by volume differences. Carroll's 1998 volume variance is −$100,000 − $130,000 = −$230,000.

Any profit differences not caused by volume must be caused by factors that are controllable management, and the *management variance* is defined as the actual profit less the flexible profit. In Carroll's case, Management variance = −$212,000 − (−$100,000) = −$112,000. Because all differences are classified as either volume differences or management differences, the sum of the volume variance and the management variance must equal the total variance: −$230,000 + (−$112,000) = −$342,000.

Variance analysis, along with the flexible budget, has helped Carroll's managers better understand the clinic's 1998 operating results. If they did not have a budget process, they simply would have received a year-end profit and loss statement that would have told them that they lost $212,000. The budget data and variance analysis contained in Tables 6.5 and 6.6 disclose several important operational issues. First, the overall situation is **worse** than the $212,000 loss reported for 1998 because Carroll's managers had reason to believe that the clinic would realize a profit of $130,000 in 1998. The

Table 6.6 Variance Summary Under Flexible Budgeting

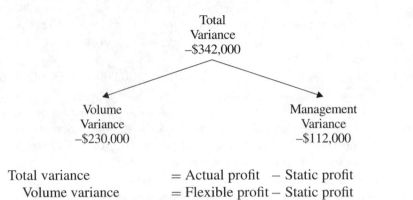

Total variance	= Actual profit − Static profit
Volume variance	= Flexible profit − Static profit
Management variance	= Actual profit − Flexible profit

total variance of −$342,000 shows the true magnitude of the problem and provides a starting point for further analysis.

Carroll's managers also know that the total variance of −$342,000 consists of a $230,000 shortfall caused by volume differences and a $112,000 shortfall caused by managerial control problems. About 67 percent of the total variance ($230,000 / $342,000) is caused by volume differences, over which Carroll's managers have limited control. Of course, volume is an issue of management concern at the clinic. Carroll's managers want more capitated lives with a utilization rate that is the same or less than the current rate, as well as more FFS visits. The bad news, however, is that their ability to influence volume is limited.

The good news is that Carroll's managers have a much better chance of attacking that portion of the total variance (33 percent) caused by management variables. With improved efficiency of operations at least up to the standards assumed in the static budget, the clinic would have suffered a shortfall from projections in 1998 of only $230,000, rather than the actual total variance of $342,000. Put another way, operating at standard efficiency would have resulted in a loss on the actual budget of only $100,000, not the $212,000 that actually occurred. Further variance analysis is needed to determine precisely where the managerial efficiency problem lies.

Volume Variance Breakdown
As shown in Table 6.7, volume variance typically has two components. Although the Carroll Clinic example contains a mix of FFS and capitated

Table 6.7   Volume Variance Components

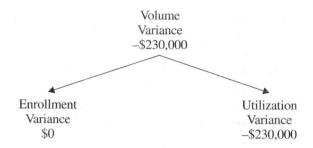

Volume variance   = Flexible profit – Static profit
   Enrollment variance   = Static profit   – Static profit
   Utilization variance   = Flexible profit – Static profit

Note: In our example, there were no enrollment differences. However, if some patients are capitated, and there are enrollment differences between expected and realized budgets, the situation becomes more complex. Then, it is necessary to create two flexible budgets: one flexed for both enrollment and utilization, and one flexed only for enrollment. With two flexible budgets, the volume variances are calculated as follows:

Volume variance   = Flexible (enrollment and utilization) profit — Static profit.
   Enrollment variance   = Flexible (enrollment) profit   — Static profit.
   Utilization variance = Flexible (enrollment and utilization) profit — Flexible (enrollment) profit.

patients, planned capitated enrollment is equal to actual enrollment (360,000 member months), so there is no enrollment component to the volume variance. In general, with a capitated population, the volume variance breakdown shows both the difference from budget caused by utilization rate changes and the difference caused by changes in the size of the population served.[4]

In general, the utilization variance (−$230,000) is the difference in the volume (i.e., the number of visits) multiplied by the contribution margin on each visit. Because Carroll Clinic has two different patient populations (FFS and capitated), there are two different contribution margins. For the capitated population, there were 18,000 more visits realized in 1998 than were planned (72,000 actual visits versus 54,000 budgeted). The contribution margin for this population using budgeted rather than actual costs is −$15 per visit. This is the budgeted variable cost per visit because there are no incremental revenues associated with visits by capitated patients. Thus, the 18,000 additional visits for this population resulted in a reduction in profits of $-\$15 \times 18,000 = -\$270,000$, which, of course, is only one component of the utilization variance of $-\$230,000$.

The overall effect of this $-\$270,000$ can be understood by examining the static and flexible budget columns in Table 6.5. Moving from the static to the flexible budget, essentially adjusting for volume differences, shows no change on the capitated revenue line; revenue remains at $\$1,080,000$. However, variable costs for the capitated population increased from $\$810,000$ to $\$1,080,000$, or by $\$270,000$. This amount is the expected budgeted cost increase caused by the additional 18,000 visits. The fact that variable costs for the capitated population increased to $\$1,152,000$ in the actual budget is caused by reasons other than utilization changes.

The other subcomponent of the utilization variance is related to the FFS population. There were 4,000 FFS visits above the static budget, each with a budgeted contribution margin of $\$25$ revenue $- \$15$ variable cost $= \$10$. Thus, the volume variance for the FFS population is $\$10 \times 4,000 = \$40,000$, a positive number. The $+\$40,000$ reflects the fact that the clinic's profitability is positively related to the number of FFS visits. Again, the $+\$40,000$ can be understood by examining the static and flexible budget columns of Table 6.5. Moving from the static budget to the flexible budget, FFS revenues increase by $\$100,000$. At the same time, FFS variable costs increase by only $\$60,000$, which results in a profit increase of $\$40,000$. The positive $\$40,000$ utilization variance caused by FFS patients partially offsets the negative $\$270,000$ utilization variance caused by the capitated population. Combining the utilization variances of the two populations gives $+\$40,000 - \$270,000 = -\$230,00$, which is the overall utilization variance and, with no enrollment variance, the overall volume variance.

What did Carroll's managers learn from the volume variance analysis? A major portion, $\$230,000$, of the overall profit shortfall from standard of $\$342,000$ can be explained by volume discrepancies. Within the volume variance, the problem is actually a little worse within the capitated population than the aggregate variance data reveal. That is, there was a $\$270,000$ shortfall caused by utilization control problems within the capitated population, which was partially offset (i.e., disguised) by the benefits ($+\$40,000$) of increased FFS utilization. Thus, the breakdown of volume variance reveals a major issue that Carroll's managers must address—its utilization management of the capitated population. Either utilization management must be tightened or utilization forecasts need to be revised (i.e., increased), which may cause Carroll to reconsider its pricing on this managed care contract.

Management Variance Breakdown

Now consider the management variance of $-\$112,000$.[5] This value represents the profit shortfall from standard that results not from volume assumption errors, but from cost factors that presumably are more controllable by management.

For Carroll, the realized cost per visit was $16, while the standard budgeted cost was only $15. Thus, total costs in 1998 to handle 112,000 visits (40,000 FFS plus 72,000 capitated) amounted to $1 × 112,000 = $112,000 more than budgeted. Table 6.5 shows the $112,000 cost overrun as the difference between actual total costs of $1,792,000 and flexible budget costs of $1,680,000.[6] This management variance, which results from production (i.e., cost) inefficiencies, can be broken down according to population served. However, in Carroll's situation, it costs the same on a per visit basis to treat both FFS and capitated patients, so the cost overruns are the same proportionally for each population: $40,000 on FFS and $72,000 on capitated patients.

As previously stated, the management variance of −$112,000 indicates that Carroll has cost-control problems. Furthermore, the major resources involved in operating costs are medical staffing and supplies, so it would be valuable to Carroll's managers to learn which of the two areas contributed most to the management variance. Perhaps an even deeper investigation can be made within staffing and supplies: Is too much of each resource being used or is too much money being paid for what is being used? Table 6.8 examines the components of the management variance. Most of the budget data required to calculate the component variances are contained in Part III of Table 6.3 (the static budget) and Table 6.4 (the actual results).

First, consider medical staffing, which represents labor utilization. The original static budget of $1,200,000 was based on the expectation that it would require 48,000 hours of work at $25 per hour to treat 90,000 visits. However, actual staffing amounted to 59,900 hours at $26 per hour to treat 112,000 visits, for a total cost of $1,557,400. If 48,000 hours are expected to be sufficient to provide for 90,000 visits, a labor efficiency ratio of 90,000 / 48,000 = 1.875 visits per hour results. In effect, for every hour of labor expended, the expectation is that the clinic can serve 1.875 patients. With this productivity assumption, the clinic would expect a staffing requirement of 112,000 / 1.875 = 59,733 hours to provide for the 112,000 visits realized in 1998. The flexed value for labor hours when combined with the standard labor cost of $25 per hour produced a flexible, volume adjusted labor cost of $25 × 59,733 = $1,493,325. The difference between the flexible and actual budget staffing costs produces a medical staffing variance of $1,493,325 − $1,557,400 = −$64,075.

Of the management variance of −$112,000, −$64,075 is caused by medical staffing and the remainder is caused by supplies; there is no fixed cost variance. The $64,075 medical staffing variance can be decomposed into

Table 6.8   Detailed Analysis of the Management Variance

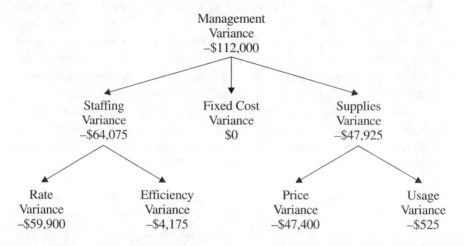

Management variance = Actual profit − Flexible (enrollment and utilization) profit
Fixed cost variance = Flexible fixed costs − Actual fixed costs
Staffing variance = Flexible staffing costs − Actual staffing costs
Rate variance = (Static rate − Actual rate) × Actual labor hours
Efficiency variance = (Flexible hours − Actual hours) × Static rate
Supplies variance = Flexible supplies costs − Actual supplies costs
Price variance = (Static price − Actual price) × Actual units
Usage variance = (Flexible units − Actual units) × Static price

that portion caused by productivity (the efficiency variance) and that portion caused by wage rates (the rate variance). As suggested previously, the flexible hours allowed based upon the initial productivity assumption were 59,733. However, the actual hours required were 59,900. The difference between the number of hours suggested by the flexible budget and the actual number needed is 59,733 − 59,900 = −167. An overage of 167 hours, coupled with a budgeted hourly rate of $25, produces a staffing efficiency variance of −167 × $25 = −$4,175. Thus, of the $64,075 overrun in medical staffing costs, $4,175 is caused by productivity inefficiencies and the remainder ($59,900) must be caused by paying more for labor than the clinic had originally planned (rate variance). The rate variance can be calculated directly by first comparing the actual labor rate of $26 per hour to the budgeted rate of $25 per hour, for a cost rate of $1 per hour above standard. When this additional cost is multiplied by the actual number of hours worked in 1998 (59,900), the rate variance of −$59,900 is obtained.

What can Carroll's managers learn from the medical staffing variance data? The numbers indicate that only a very small portion of the cost overrun was caused by productivity problems; the vast majority of the overrun was caused by higher-than-expected wages. This suggests that Carroll's managers have to take a close look at the clinic's wage rates to ensure that they are not paying more than the local market for labor dictates. Of course, Carroll wants to have quality employees, but at the same time, management needs to be concerned about labor costs.

How did Carroll do in 1998 regarding supplies costs? At the beginning of the year, Carroll estimated supplies costs of $150,000, based on the assumption that 100,000 units at $1.50 per unit would be needed for 90,000 visits. However, actual usage was 124,800 units that cost a total of $234,600, or about $1.88 per unit, to accommodate 112,000 visits. If 100,000 units were budgeted for 90,000 visits, then supplies usage was forecasted to be $100,000 / 90,000 = 1.11$ units per visit. Thus, with an actual number of visits of 112,000 in 1998, Carroll should have used $1.11 \times 112,000 = 124,450$ units according to standard usage. (There are some rounding differences in these calculations.) At a budgeted cost of $1.50 per unit, total supplies costs should have been $1.50 \times 124,450 = \$186,675$ for the 112,000 visits that occurred in 1998. However, $234,600 was actually spent on supplies, for a variance of $186,675 - \$234,600 = -\$47,925$.

If $-$47,925$ of the management variance of $-$112,000$ is caused by supplies, the remainder, as discovered previously, must be caused by staffing. Within the $-$47,925$ supplies variance, the amount caused by excess utilization (the usage variance) and the amount caused by price differentials (the price variance) can be determined. The flexible budget suggests that the appropriate usage was 124,450 units. However, in 1998, 124,800 units were actually consumed. The difference between the flexed usage and the actual usage produces a usage overage of $124,450 - 124,800 = -350$ units. At a budgeted cost of $1.50 per unit, the usage variance is $-350 \times \$1.50 = -\$525$.

If $-$525$ of the supplies variance of $-$47,925$ is caused by usage differences, the remainder ($-$47,400$) must be caused by price differences. To find the price variance directly, Carroll paid $1.50 - \$1.88 = -\$0.38$ above budget for each of the 124,800 units actually consumed, for a price variance of $-$0.38 \times 124,800 = -\$47,400$, with a small rounding error.

What did Carroll's managers learn from the supplies variance analysis? They know that the supplies cost overrun was caused almost totally by price increases; supplies usage was almost on target when volume differences are accounted for. Thus, it would be prudent for management to investigate the clinic's purchasing policy to see if prices can be lowered through such actions

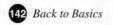

as changing vendors, making larger purchases at a single time, or joining a purchasing alliance.

Final Comments on Variance Analysis

In summary, variance analysis, combined with flexible budgeting, helps managers identify the factors that cause realized profits to be different from those expected. If profits are higher than expected, managers can see why and then try to exploit those factors even further in the future. If profits are lower than expected, managers can identify the causes and then embark on a plan to correct the deficiencies. Larger health services organizations have made significant improvements in their use of flexible budgeting and variance analysis. The benefit from expanding the level of information detail is that it is easier for managers to isolate and presumably rectify problem areas. Fortunately, the marginal cost of obtaining such detailed information is lower now than ever before because detailed managerial accounting information is being generated both to support cost-control efforts and to aid in pricing and service decisions.

THE CASH BUDGET

Thus far, our discussion of budgeting has focused on the operating budget. As shown in the Carroll Clinic illustration, the operating budget, along with the budgetary control process, provides managers with numerous insights into the efficiency of an organization's operations. However, the operating budget is based on accrual accounting principles, and hence does not provide managers with much information about a business' cash position. This situation is corrected by the *cash budget*.

To create a cash budget, managers forecast both fixed asset and inventory requirements, along with the times when such payments must be made. This information is combined with projections about the delay in collecting accounts receivable, wage payment dates, interest payment dates, and so on. All this information is then combined to show the organization's projected cash inflows and outflows over some specified period. Generally, businesses use a monthly cash budget forecasted over the next year, plus a more detailed daily or weekly cash budget for the coming month. The monthly cash budget is used for liquidity planning purposes and the daily or weekly budget for actual cash control.

Creating a cash budget does not require the application of a complex set of accounting rules. Rather, all the entries in a cash budget represent the actual movement of cash into or out of the organization. Table 6.9 contains a monthly cash budget that covers six months of 1999 for Madison Homecare,

Table 6.9   Madison Homecare: May through October Cash Budget

	Mar	Apr	May	June	July	Aug	Sept	Oct
Collections Worksheet:								
1. Billed charges	$50,000	$50,000	$100,000	$150,000	$200,000	$100,000	$100,000	$ 50,000
2. Collections:								
a. Within 30 days			19,600	29,400	39,200	19,600	19,600	9,800
b. 30–60 days			35,000	70,000	105,000	140,000	70,000	70,000
c. 60–90 days			5,000	5,000	10,000	15,000	20,000	10,000
3. Total collections			$ 59,600	$104,400	$154,200	$174,600	$109,600	$ 89,800
Supplies Worksheet:								
4. Amount of supplies ordered	$10,000	$ 15,000	$ 20,000	$ 10,000	$ 10,000	$ 5,000		
5. Payments made for supplies		$ 10,000	$ 15,000	$ 20,000	$ 10,000	$ 10,000	$ 5,000	
Net Cash Gain (Loss):								
6. Total collections (from Line 3)			$ 59,600	$104,400	$154,200	$174,600	$109,600	$ 89,800
7. Total purchases (from Line 5)			$ 10,000	$ 15,000	$ 20,000	$ 10,000	$ 10,000	$ 5,000
8. Wages and salaries			60,000	70,000	80,000	60,000	60,000	60,000
9. Rent			2,500	2,500	2,500	2,500	2,500	2,500
10. Other expenses			1,000	1,500	2,000	1,000	1,000	500
11. Taxes				20,000			20,000	
12. Payment for capital assets						50,000		
13. Total payments			$ 73,500	$109,000	$104,500	$123,500	$ 93,500	$ 68,000
14. Net cash gain (loss)			($ 13,900)	($ 4,600)	$ 49,700	$ 51,100	$ 16,100	$ 21,800
Borrowing/Surplus Summary:								
15. Cash at beginning with no borrowing			$ 15,000	$ 1,100	($ 3,500)	$ 46,200	$ 97,300	$113,400
16. Cash at end with no borrowing			$ 1,100	($ 3,500)	$ 46,200	$ 97,300	$113,400	$135,200
17. Target cash balance			10,000	10,000	10,000	10,000	10,000	10,000
18. Cumulative surplus cash (loan balance)			($ 8,900)	($ 13,500)	$ 36,200	$ 87,300	$103,400	$125,200

a small, for-profit home health care company. Madison's cash budget, which is broken down into three sections, is typical, although there is a great deal of variation in formats used by different organizations.

The first section of the cash budget contains the *collections worksheet*, which translates the billing for services provided into cash revenues. Because of its location in a summer resort area, Madison's patient volume, and hence billings, peak in July. However, like most health services organizations, Madison rarely collects when services are provided. What is relevant from a cash budget perspective is not when services are provided or when billings occur, but rather when cash is collected. Based on previous experience, Madison's managers know that most collections occur 30 to 60 days after billing. In fact, Madison's managers have a collections table that allows them to forecast, with some precision, the timing of collections. This table was used to convert the billings shown on Line 1 of Table 6.9 into the collection amounts shown on Lines 2 and 3.

The next section of Madison's cash budget is the *supplies worksheet*, which accounts for timing differences between when supplies are ordered and when they are paid for. Madison's patient volume forecasts, which are used to predict the billing amounts shown on Line 1, are also used to forecast the supplies (primarily medical) needed to support patient services. These supplies are ordered and received one month prior to expected usage, as shown on Line 4. However, Madison's suppliers do not demand immediate payment. Rather, Madison has, on average, 30 days to pay for supplies after they are received. Thus, the actual payment occurs one month after purchase, as shown on Line 5.

The next section combines data from the collections and supplies worksheets with other projected cash outflows to show the *net cash gain (loss)* for each month. Cash from collections is shown on Line 6. Lines 7 through 12 list cash payments that are expected to be made during each month including payments for supplies. Then, all payments are summed, with the total shown on Line 13. The difference between expected cash receipts and cash payments, Line 6 minus Line 13, is the net cash gain or loss during the month, which is shown on Line 14. For May, there is a forecasted net cash flow of −$13,900, where the parentheses indicate a negative cash flow (loss).

Although Line 14 contains the meat of the cash budget, Lines 15 through 18 (the *borrowing/surplus summary*) extend the basic budget data to show Madison's forecasted cash position for each month. Line 15 shows the forecasted cash on hand at the beginning of each month, assuming that no borrowing takes place. Madison is expected to enter the budget period, the beginning of May, with $15,000 of cash on hand. For each succeeding month, Line 15 is merely the value shown on Line 16 for the previous month. The values on Line 16, which are obtained by adding Lines 14 and 15, show the cash on hand at the end of each month assuming no borrowing takes place. For May, Madison expects a cash loss of $13,900 on top of a starting balance of $15,000, for an ending cash balance of $1,100 in the absence of any borrowing. This amount is the cash at beginning with no borrowing amount for June, which is shown on Line 15.

To continue, Madison's target cash balance (i.e., the amount that it wants on hand at the beginning of each month), which is shown on Line 17, is $10,000. The target cash balance is subtracted from the forecasted ending cash with no borrowing amount to determine the firm's borrowing requirements (shown in parentheses) or surplus cash (shown without parentheses). Because Madison expects to have ending cash, as shown on Line 16, of only $1,100 in May, it will have to borrow $1,100 − $10,000 = −$8,900 to bring the cash account up to the target balance of $10,000. Assuming that this amount is indeed borrowed, the total loan outstanding will be $8,900 at the end of May. (The assumption is that Madison will not have any loans outstanding on May 1 because the beginning cash balance exceeds the firm's target balance.)

The cumulative cash surplus or required loan balance is shown on Line 18; a positive value indicates a cash surplus, while a negative value indicates a loan requirement. The surplus cash or loan requirement shown on Line 18 is a **cumulative amount**. Thus, Madison is projected to borrow $8,900 in May; it has a cash shortfall during June of $4,600, as reported on Line 14, so its total loan requirement projected for the end of June is $8,900 + $4,600 = $13,500, as shown on Line 18.

The same procedures are followed in subsequent months. Patient volume and billings are projected to peak in July, accompanied by increased payments for supplies, wages, and other items. However, collections are projected to increase by a greater amount than costs and Madison expects a $49,700 net cash inflow during July. This amount is sufficient to pay off the cumulative loan of $13,500 and have a $36,200 cash surplus on hand at the end of the month.

Patient volume and the resulting operating costs are expected to fall sharply in August, but collections will be the highest of any month because they will reflect the high June and July billings. As a result, Madison would normally be forecasting a healthy $101,100 net cash gain during the month. However, the company expects to make a cash payment of $50,000 to purchase a new computer system during August, so the forecasted net cash gain is reduced to $51,100. This net gain adds to the surplus, so August is projected to end with $87,300 in surplus cash. If all goes according to the forecast, later cash surpluses will enable Madison to end this budget period with a surplus of $125,200.

The cash budget is used by Madison's managers for liquidity planning purposes. For example, the Table 6.9 cash budget indicates that Madison will need to obtain $13,500 in total to get through May and June. Thus, if the firm does not have any marketable securities to convert to cash, it will have to arrange a loan, typically a line of credit, to cover this period. Furthermore, the budget indicates a $125,200 cash surplus at the end of October. Madison's managers will have to consider how these funds can best be utilized. Perhaps the money should be paid out to shareholders as dividends, or be used for fixed asset acquisitions or be temporarily invested in marketable securities for later use within the business. This decision will be made on the basis of Madison's overall financial plan.

This brief illustration shows the mechanics and managerial value of the cash budget. However, before concluding this discussion of the cash budget, several additional points need to be made. First, if cash inflows and outflows are not uniform during the month, a monthly cash budget could seriously understate a business' peak financing requirements. The data in Table 6.9 show the situation expected on the last day of each month, but on any given day during the month it could be quite different. If all payments had to be made on the fifth of each month, but collections came in uniformly throughout the month, Madison would need to borrow cash to cover within-month shortages. For example, August's $123,500 of cash payments may occur before the full amount of the $174,600 in collections have been made. In this situation, some amount of cash would have to be obtained to cover shortfalls in August, even though the end of month cash flow after all collections have been made is positive. In this case, Madison would have to prepare a weekly or daily cash budget to indicate such borrowing needs.

Also, because the cash budget represents a forecast, all the values in the table are **expected** values. If actual patient volume, collection times, supplies purchases, wage rates, and so on, differ from forecasted levels, the projected cash deficits and surpluses will be incorrect. Thus, there is a reasonable chance that Madison may end up needing to obtain a larger amount of funds than is indicated on Line 18. Because of the uncertainty of the forecasts, spreadsheet programs are particularly well-suited for constructing and analyzing cash budgets. For example, Madison's managers could change any assumption, say, projected monthly volume or the time third-party payors take to pay, and the cash budget would automatically and instantly be recalculated. This would show Madison's managers exactly how the firm's cash position would change under alternative operating assumptions. Typically, such an analysis is used to determine how large a credit line to establish to cover temporary cash shortages.[7] In Madison's case, such an analysis indicated that a $20,000 line is sufficient.

KEY CONCEPTS

Planning and budgeting are important managerial activities. In particular, budgets allow health services managers to assess financial performance and to ensure that operations are carried out in a manner consistent with expectations. The key concepts of this chapter are:

- *Planning* encompasses the overall process of preparing for the future, while *budgeting* is the accounting process that ties together planning and control functions.
- The *strategic plan*, which provides broad guidance for the future, is the foundation of any organization's planning process. More detailed managerial guidance is contained in the *operating plan*, often called the *five-year plan*.

- The *financial plan*, which is the financial portion of the operating plan, contains a *long-term plan*, *working capital management plan*, and *accounting plan.*
- *Budgeting* provides a means for communication and coordination of organizational expectations and allocation of scarce resources. In addition, budgeting establishes benchmarks for control.
- There are several types of budgets including the *statistics budget*, *revenue budget, expense budget, operating budget,* and *cash budget.*
- The *conventional*, or *incremental/decremental, approach* to budgeting uses the previous budget as the basis for constructing the new budget. *Zero-based budgeting* begins each budget as a clean slate, and hence all entries have to be justified each budget period.
- *Bottom-up budgeting*, which begins at the unit level, encourages maximum involvement by junior managers. Conversely, *top-down budgeting*, which is less participatory in nature, is a more efficient way to communicate senior management's views.
- The *operating budget* is the basic budget of an organization, in that it sets the profit expectations for the budget period. A critical element of the operating budget is the *profit and loss (P&L) statement*, which is a simplified income statement.
- A *variance* is the difference between a budgeted (planned) value, or *standard*, and the actual (realized) value. *Variance analysis* examines differences between budgeted and realized amounts, with the goal of finding out why things went either badly or well.
- A budget that fully reflects realized results is called the *actual budget.* When the original budget, or *static budget*, is recast to reflect the actual volume of patients treated, but with all other static budget assumptions unchanged, the result is called a *flexible budget.* To be most useful, variance analysis examines differences between the actual, flexible, and static budgets.

NOTES

1. For an in-depth treatment of budgeting within health services organizations, see A. G. Herkimer, Jr., *Understanding Health Care Budgeting* (Rockville, MD: Aspen, 1988).
2. Financial statement forecasting is an important function of any business' financial staff. However, this discussion will be left to other texts. For more information, see L. C. Gapenski, *Understanding Health Care Financial Management* (Chicago: AUPHA Press/Health Administration Press, 1996).
3. For an extensive discussion on zero-based budgeting within hospitals, see M. M. Person, III, *The Zero-Base Hospital* (Chicago: Health Administration Press, 1997).
4. By assuming no change in enrollment, the example has been simplified to make variance analysis easier to understand at the introductory level. In essence, the Carroll Clinic analysis

is similar to a variance analysis in which all patients are under FFS. Without enrollment variance, only one flexible budget is required. However, had enrollment differences been built into the illustration, two different flexible budgets would have been required. See the note to Table 6.7.

5. Variances can be defined such that the resulting value is either a positive or a negative number. For example, when cost variances are calculated, they can be defined so that a negative variance implies costs less than standard, which is good, or costs greater than standard, which is bad, depending on which budget value is subtracted from the other. In this example, all variances have been defined such that a negative number indicates an undesirable variance and not necessarily that the realized value is less than the standard. For example, a higher-than-standard wage rate would be a negative variance, even though realized wages were higher than standard.

6. In this illustration, no difference exists in revenues between the flexible and actual budgets, so the management variance is also the difference in profit between these two budgets.

7. A *credit line* is an agreement between a borrower and a financial institution that obligates the institution to furnish credit over a time period, typically a year, up to the agreed-on amount. The borrower may use some, all, or none of the credit line. Usually, credit lines require borrowers to pay an up-front fee for the credit guarantee called a *commitment fee*.

REFERENCES

Gapenski, L. C. 1996. *Understanding Health Care Financial Management*. Chicago: AUPHA Press/Health Administration Press.

Herkimer, A. G., Jr. 1988. *Understanding Health Care Budgeting*. Rockville, MD: Aspen.

Person, M. M., III. 1997. *The Zero-Base Hospital*. Chicago: Health Administration Press.

Information Technology Today

Charles J. Austin, Ph.D., and Stuart B. Boxerman, D.Sc.

T he delivery of health services is an information-intensive process. High-quality patient care relies upon careful documentation of each patient's medical history, health status, current medical conditions, and treatment plans. Administrative and financial information is essential for efficient operational support of the patient care process. A strong argument can be made that the health services industry is one of the most information-intensive sectors of our economy. But health services organizations have been slow to adopt the use of modern information technology in the delivery of care and the management of services. This situation, however, is changing, given rapid advances in technology and the forces of change in the healthcare system itself.

This chapter discusses how the management of health services organizations can be improved by the *intelligent* use of information. Some management theorists discount the value of information in the management process, stating that management is still more of an art than a science. They argue that experience, judgment, intuition, and a good sense of the political environment are the critical skills involved in making administrative decisions. On the other end of the spectrum are the technocrats, who argue that management and information are inseparable, that all management decisions need to be completely rational and based entirely on an analysis of comprehensive information. The focus of this chapter lies between these two extreme views of the managerial world. The use of information has both costs and benefits

Editor's Note: This chapter is from Chapter 1 of *Information Systems for Health Services Administration, Fifth Edition,* by Charles J. Austin and Stuart B. Boxerman, 1997, HAP associated with it. These costs and benefits need to be assessed, and health administrators need to develop their skills in using information intelligently.

The health services industry is in the midst of a period of great change. Pressures for improved management information are growing as health services organizations face ever-increasing demands to lower costs, improve quality, and expand access to care. Market-driven healthcare reform has led to rapid expansion of managed care, development of integrated delivery systems through mergers and acquisitions, and radical changes in systems of payment for services. Health services organizations have grown larger and more complex, and information systems must keep pace with the dual effects of organizational complexity and continued advances in medical technology.

The intelligent use of information in health services management does not just happen. Rather, the administrator must ensure that it occurs in a systematic, formally planned way. This chapter, then, deals with two important matters: the management of information resources in health services organizations and the effective use of information in organizational management.

Careful distinction should be drawn between data and information. As used in this chapter, *data* are raw facts and figures collected by the organization. *Information*, on the other hand, is defined as data that have been processed and analyzed in a formal, intelligent way, so that the results are directly useful to clinicians and managers. All too often, computerized data banks are available, but are little used because of inadequate planning of information content and structure needed to support management planning and control.

An essential element for successful information systems implementation is carefully planned teamwork by clinicians, managers, and technical systems specialists. Information systems developed in isolation by technicians may be "technically pure and elegant in design," but rarely will they pass the test of reality in meeting organizational requirements. On the other hand, very few administrators and clinicians possess the equally important technical knowledge and skills of systems analysis and design, and the amateur analyst cannot hope to avoid the havoc that can result from a poorly designed system. A balanced effort is required: operational personnel contribute ideas on systems requirements and organizational realities, and technical personnel employ their skills in analysis and design.

Computer technology has advanced to a high level of sophistication in recent years. However, computers are only tools to aid in the accomplishment of a wider set of goals. Analysis of information requirements in the broader organizational context always should take precedence over a rush to computerize. Information technology by itself is not the answer to management problems; technology must be part of a broader restructuring of the organization, including reengineering of business processes. Alignment of information systems strategy with business goals of the health care organization is essential (DeFauw and L'Heureux 1995).

CATEGORIES OF INFORMATION SYSTEMS

Computerized information systems in healthcare fall into four categories: clinical, administrative, strategic decision-support, and electronic networking applications (see Figure 7.1.).

Clinical information systems support patient care and provide information for use in strategic planning and management. Applications include computerized patient records systems, automated medical instrumentation, clinical decision-support systems (computer-aided diagnosis and treatment planning), and information systems that support clinical research and education.

Operational administrative systems support nonpatient care activities in the health services organization. Examples include financial information sys-

---

Figure 7.1 Categories of Health Information Systems

Clinical
  1. Computerized Patient Records
  2. Medical Decision Support
  3. Automated Instrumentation
  4. Clinical Research and Education

Administrative
  1. Financial
  2. Scheduling
  3. Human Resources
  4. Materials Management
  5. Office Automation

Strategic Decision Support
  1. Planning and Marketing
  2. Financial Forecasting
  3. Resource Allocation
  4. Performance Assessment
  5. Outcomes Measurement

Electronic Networking
  1. Insurance Billing and Claims Processing
  2. Regional/National Databases
  3. Online Purchasing
  4. Provider Networks

tems, payroll, purchasing and inventory control, outpatient clinic scheduling, office automation, and many others.

Strategic decision-support systems assist the executive management team in strategic planning, managerial control, performance monitoring, and outcomes assessment. Strategic information systems must draw on both internal data from clinical and administrative systems in the organization as well as external data on community health, market-area demography, and activities of competitors. Consequently, information system integration—the ability of organizational information systems to communicate electronically with one another—becomes very important.

Most health services organizations also engage in electronic data interchange with external organizations for such activities as insurance billing and claims processing, accessing clinical information from regional and national databases, and communicating among providers in an integrated delivery system.

HISTORICAL OVERVIEW

The first computer systems in healthcare date to the early 1960s when a small number of hospitals began to automate selected administrative operations, usually beginning with payroll and patient accounting functions. These systems were developed by analysts and computer programmers hired by the hospital and were run on large and expensive centralized computers referred to as "mainframes." Little attention was given to the development of clinical information systems to support patient care. A few systems were developed for the electronic storage and retrieval of abstracts of inpatient medical records. But these systems contained limited information and were operated on a postdischarge, retrospective basis.

Advances in technology during the 1970s expanded the use of information systems in hospitals and marked the beginning of limited applications in other organizational settings, including clinics, physician practices, and long-term care facilities. Computers became smaller and less expensive, and some vendors began to develop "applications software packages," generalized computer programs that could be used by any hospital, clinic, or physician's office that purchased the system. Most of these early software packages supported administrative operations—patient accounting, general accounting, materials management, scheduling, and practice management. Some clinical systems were developed as well, particularly for hospital clinical laboratories, radiology departments, and pharmacies.

A revolution in computing occurred in the 1980s with the development of powerful and inexpensive personal computers (PCs), desktop devices with computing power and storage capacity that equaled or exceeded the large mainframe systems of the 1960s and 1970s. A second major advance in this period was the development of electronic data networks in which personal computers and larger systems could be linked together to share information on a decentralized basis. An increasing number of vendors entered the healthcare software business, and a much larger array of products became available for both administrative and clinical support functions. The use of personal computers in physicians' offices, particularly for practice management, became commonplace.

The early 1990s were marked by dramatic changes in the healthcare environment with the advent of market-driven healthcare reform and rapid expansion of managed care. As a result, much greater attention began to be given to the development of clinical information systems and strategic decision-support systems to assist providers in achieving a critical balance between costs and quality in the delivery of care.

THE CHANGING HEALTHCARE ENVIRONMENT

The rapidly changing healthcare environment of the 1990s has made the employment of information technology more important than ever. Several factors are influencing this change. Most notable is the influence of market-driven healthcare reform, which has resulted in an expansion of managed care, the development of integrated delivery systems by providers of care, and major changes in insurance and payment mechanisms for the delivery of health services. Major forces of change in healthcare are discussed in the sections that follow.

Expansion of Managed Care

Managed care is a new paradigm for the delivery of health services, resulting from concern among large employers, insurance companies, and government agencies about rapid escalation in the costs of healthcare. There is no simple definition of *managed care* since it can assume many different forms. However, Wozmak (1995) provides the following functional definition:

> Managed care is a system of providing and paying for medical care that includes a panel of providers who agree to deliver services at an agreed upon fee. Financial incentives are included for patients to use the identified providers that make up the panel (Wozmak 1995, 12).

Managed care can assume many different forms. Three of the more common arrangements are health maintenance organizations (HMOs); preferred provider organizations (PPOs); and exclusive provider arrangements (EPAs).

HMOs provide coverage of specified health services to plan members for a fixed premium, prepaid in advance (usually on a monthly basis). Physician services may be provided by employing a group of physicians on a salaried basis; contracting with physicians who have organized as a partnership, professional corporation, or association; contracting with multiple physician groups; or contracting with an individual practice association, which in turn contracts with individual physicians and medical groups.

PPOs are insurance programs in which plan members receive better benefits (usually through reduced deductible and copayment amounts) when they use services offered by preferred providers. Patients can use nonparticipating providers, but at a higher cost. Providers are usually paid on a fee-for-service basis, but agree to discounts in order to receive the preferred provider designation.

EPAs have been initiated "by major self-insured employers who decided to cut out the middlemen—health insurers and third party administrators—and make their own deals in the medical marketplace" (Coile 1990, 135). Pricing is established using the company's actual experience with its own employees' utilization of health services. Strong financial incentives are employed to limit or exclude services by providers who are not part of the company's EPA plan.

Membership in managed care plans has increased rapidly. Enrollment in HMOs grew to 59 million covered individuals in 1995 (Kertesz 1996).

Health services organizations operating in this environment must have vastly improved financial and clinical information about their operation in order to monitor the costs and quality of services and negotiate successfully with managed care plans.

Development of Integrated Delivery Systems (IDS)

In responding to the imperatives of managed care, many hospitals, medical group practices, and other health services organizations have come together to form integrated delivery systems. An IDS can be defined as "an organization that is accountable for the costs and clinical outcomes associated with delivery of a continuum of health services to a defined population." An IDS is composed of a network of hospitals, physicians, and other healthcare providers who furnish all needed services to a patient population, in some cases for a fixed annual payment.

Integrated delivery systems build on the HMO concept but are more flexible in the organizational relationships that are established among providers. Most networks will either own or be closely aligned with an insurance product.

Physicians are actively engaged in IDS development activities. Medical group practices may enter directly as partners in a system. Hospitals and physicians are joining together to form physician-hospital organizations (PHOs) in order to compete for managed care business. In some cases, hospitals are buying physician practices in order to be able to employ their own cadre of physicians, particularly those in primary care (family practice, internal medicine, pediatrics, and obstetrics).

Integrated delivery systems are tied together by information about the patients being served. Success will be heavily dependent upon the ability to provide good clinical, financial, and customer service information to those who purchase health services from the IDS.

Changes in Reimbursement

Managed care will result in significant changes in methods of payment for health services. Traditional systems of fee-for-service payment are increasingly being replaced by *contractual discounts* and *capitation*. These systems of reimbursement are designed to reduce costs. Providers are being asked to share in the financial risks traditionally assumed by insurers and purchasers of care.

All managed care plans require that physicians, hospitals, and other healthcare providers accept discounts from their regular prices or fee schedules in order to be included in the plan as participating or preferred providers.

An increasing number of plans are moving toward capitated payment in which a provider agrees to accept a fixed fee (monthly or annual) for all patient care provided to a defined population (the enrollees in the managed care health plan). Results from a recent survey of 19 HMOs revealed that 17 employ capitation in contracting for specialty medical services (Wong 1994).

Capitation requires that providers assume some of the financial risk in providing patient care. Capitated payment systems offer incentives for reducing unnecessary utilization of services, and place a premium on prevention and strategies for keeping people healthy.

Capitated contracting makes it essential that health services organizations have good information about their own service patterns as well as information on the health needs of the population to be covered by the contract. Without such information, it is impossible to determine an acceptable capitation rate for the practice.

Outcomes Assessment

Balancing the costs and quality of patient care is an important requirement in today's healthcare delivery system. Purchasers of care, insurance companies, and managed care plans are placing emphasis on *outcomes assessment* as a method for striking this delicate balance between costs and quality.

Outcomes assessment involves measuring the effectiveness of alternative treatment modalities on clinical outcomes for specific groups of patients and specific medical conditions. Outcomes assessment can be used to compare the quality of care delivered by individual providers. Managed care plans are using outcomes information in seeking out the *lowest cost* treatment protocols that have been shown to have *at least equal medical effectiveness* to other available treatment modalities. Much of the impetus behind outcomes research stems from a desire to use the results of the research for cost-control purposes.

The federal government's Agency for Health Care Policy and Research (now Agency for Health Care Research and Quality) has established a grant program to support outcomes research. The results of these research studies will likely be used in the following ways:

1. Effectiveness results will be used in determining what types of treatments will be eligible for reimbursement under public and private health insurance plans.
2. Large purchasers of care will use effectiveness results in making selections among HMOs and individual providers.
3. Healthcare providers will use effectiveness results in measuring their own performance and implementing programs of continuous quality improvement.
4. Individual physicians will use effectiveness information to explain treatment options to patients and involve them in decision making.
5. At the national level, outcomes information will be use to establish practice guidelines for common and high-cost medical conditions, such as treatment of prostate cancer and hip replacement (Unger 1992).

Health services organizations will need to develop good clinical information systems to monitor their operations and develop their own clinical effectiveness measures. Computerization of patient records will take on increasing importance as we move into the future.

Report Cards

The concept of outcomes measurement is being extended to formal systems of quality reporting. These "report cards" are used by consumers and purchasers to assist in selection of a health plan. Report cards have been developed by individual employers, industry coalitions, some of the larger HMOs, accrediting organizations, and professional associations.

The Cleveland Health Quality Choice Coalition is a voluntary collaborative effort involving hospitals, the medical society, corporate CEOs, human resource and benefits managers, and small businesses in the Cleveland, Ohio, metropolitan area. The purpose of the Coalition is to assess the quality and efficiency of healthcare in the community and distribute the results to Coalition members. Outcomes information has been reported for 31 hospitals, including the following measures:

1. Patient satisfaction
2. In-hospital mortality
3. Length of stay for different procedures
4. Hospital acquired complications
5. Severity adjusted outcomes for medical, surgical, and obstetrical patients (Rosenthal and Harper 1994).

Some of the nation's largest HMOs are developing their own quality report cards as well. Efforts are under way to develop reporting standards in order to minimize variations and facilitate comparisons among plans. The National Committee for Quality Assurance has developed the Health Plan Employer Data and Information Set (HEDIS) to facilitate standardized reporting on a national basis.

INFORMATION TECHNOLOGY IN THIS ENVIRONMENT OF CHANGE

Healthcare organizations operating in this environment of change must develop sophisticated information systems to support clinical operations and strategic management. The major priorities for system development include:

1. development of repositories of computerized patient records;
2. a shift in emphasis from inpatient systems to ambulatory care systems;
3. development of enterprisewide computer networks to support integrated delivery systems;
4. development of strategic decision-support systems for risk analysis, financial forecasting, outcomes assessment, and quality improvement; and
5. development of new applications as some integrated delivery systems take on the dual roles of provider and insurer.

Computerized Patient Records

In 1991, a distinguished committee of the Institute of Medicine, National Academy of Science, issued a report calling for the development of a national system of computer-based patient records (CPRs) (Dick and Steen 1991). Such a system would serve multiple objectives (see Figure 7.2.). The ready availability of complete medical records should improve the quality of patient care to an aging and highly mobile population. The productivity of healthcare workers would be enhanced since essential demographic and medical information would need to be captured and entered into the system only once, avoiding unnecessary duplication of effort. Information on insurance coverage and eligibility would be available electronically to physicians, hospitals, and other providers of health services. Data captured in such a system would be very useful in health services research and policy formulation.

The Institute of Medicine (IOM) Committee envisioned a standardized patient record format that would be available on a national basis through electronic data interchange (EDI) technology. This massive undertaking would ultimately require computerization of all records, from those maintained in large medical centers to those in solo physician practices. Many problems would need to be addressed to bring such a system to reality, including funds for developmental costs and systems to protect the confidentiality of patient information. The Committee recommended that a developmental effort be undertaken by a follow-up organization, the Computer-Based Patient Record Institute (CPRI) which would "promote and facilitate development, implementation, and dissemination of the CPR."

Market-based healthcare reform is providing additional impetus to the development of computerized patient records and clinical information systems. As integrated delivery systems are formed, clinical and financial information must be readily available and shared electronically with all providers in the system—hospitals, physician offices, long-term care facilities, home health agencies, etc. Emphasis seems to be shifting from a single, national system of electronic patient records to systems developed at the local or regional level.

In discussing the major barriers to effective integration of healthcare delivery systems, Shortell, Gillies, and Anderson (1994, 56) state that " . . .

Figure 7.2   Objectives for Computer-Based Records

Institute of Medicine Report

1. Support patient care and improve its quality.
2. Enhance productivity of healthcare professionals.
3. Reduce administrative costs associated with healthcare delivery and financing.
4. Support clinical and health services research.
5. Accommodate future developments in healthcare technology, policy, management, and finance.
6. Protect patient data confidentiality.

systems must expand their information capabilities to link patients and providers across all settings involved in the continuum of care, from acute inpatient care to care provided in the physician's office to care provided in the patient's home."

Barea (1993) describes the development of a clinical information system at Egleston Children's Hospital at Emory University in Atlanta:

> Having measurable outcomes and tracking this information in a clinical database will save the institution money as physicians improve utilization. . . . Proven success will be critical as contracts are negotiated with employers, HMOs and other entities (Barea 1993, 44).

Many healthcare organizations are planning to build "data warehouses" containing complete clinical, financial, and administrative data on every patient. These repositories of patient records can be centralized in one large computer file or they may be "virtual" systems in which the data are distributed across a number of departmental systems. These data warehouses require solid computer architecture in their design and must employ industry-wide standards for data definition and coding. Security is essential to protect privacy and confidentiality of patient information (Talbott 1994).

Ambulatory Care Systems

Managed care and market-based reform have caused a major shift in emphasis from acute inpatient care to services delivered on an outpatient basis (including surgery). As a result, health services organizations are placing increased emphasis on the development of ambulatory care information systems.

Park Nicollet Medical Center in Minneapolis, Minnesota, has developed an advanced ambulatory care information system to support patient care and strategic management in the multiple clinics operated by the Center. All clinic sites are linked electronically to a centralized patient database and accounting system. The system enables physicians and staff members at any clinic to access patient records from other sites, schedule appointments with other physicians, and schedule laboratory and radiology procedures at the central facility.

Data from the information system are used to generate a number of performance reports, including patient satisfaction, ratios of patients to staff, and other key indicators of cost and quality. Outcome reports are generated on the cost-effectiveness of alternative treatment modalities, with data from these assessments used to create practice guidelines for the clinics. The system also generates strategic management reports. Population-based data are used to monitor health status, illness patterns, prevention and wellness practices, and service utilization rates (Kralewski et al. 1994, 22–23).

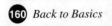

Enterprisewide Systems

As healthcare organizations band together to form integrated delivery systems, development of enterprisewide information and communications networks becomes a high priority. Often this involves the need to integrate diverse information systems developed by individual provider organizations who have come together through mergers, acquisitions, or joint ventures.

An enterprisewide system must include an electronic network infrastructure to facilitate sharing of clinical and financial information among members of the integrated delivery system: physicians, hospitals, ambulatory care centers, home health service agencies, long-term care facilities, and other components of the system.

One approach to establishing an information infrastructure that can support the goals of an integrated delivery system is to participate in or promote the development of a community health information network (CHIN) (Weaver 1993). A CHIN expands the communications network to include employers, insurers, government agencies, and other providers in the community. CHINs provide authorized users access to relevant patient and financial information from multiple sources. There is some skepticism about CHIN development among healthcare executives:

> Executives are coming to realize that they are often ill-positioned—technologically, operationally, and strategically—to move toward a true community information network. Instead, many hospital-based integrated delivery systems are going back a few steps and regrouping, putting in place plans that span the entire system before making the leap to community-wide information management (Appleby 1995, 43).

The Internet provides one option for development of intrasystem communications among components of an integrated delivery system. Applications include intercompany messaging, e-mail, web browsing, and access to knowledge-based resources for physicians.

Strategic Decision-Support Systems

Historically, information systems in hospitals and other health services organizations have focused on day-to-day operations: admitting and discharging patients, ordering lab tests, reporting results from radiology, processing the payroll, preparing bills for insurance payments, and the like. Until recently, very little priority was assigned to the use of information for strategic planning and management in healthcare facilities. Managed care and market-driven reform have quickly changed this situation. Organizations that wish to survive in the current environment must be able to:

1. assess the health risks of the populations they serve or plan to serve in the future;
2. forecast the costs and revenues anticipated from contracts with HMOs and exclusive provider arrangements; and
3. measure the clinical outcomes of services provided and continuously improve service quality in order to compete successfully for business in the medical marketplace.

Meeting these strategic objectives requires development of databases of clinical and financial information plus decision-analysis programs to support executive management.

Some vendors are developing software products for decision-support purposes. Dilts, Kappeler, Durham & Co. established a data repository for health networks used to develop computer models of treatment costs. The software will search the database and build a profile of resource consumption for a typical patient for a given procedure. The profiles are used to forecast the profitability of capitation proposals (Morrissey 1994, 82).

New Types of Applications

With the expansion of managed care and concurrent development of integrated delivery systems, many healthcare organizations are now playing dual roles as providers of care and insurers of populations served by the network. For example, Intermountain Health Care System of Salt Lake City, Utah, includes multiple hospitals, clinics, and other facilities providing health services to patients in its region. In 1992, Intermountain also operated three managed care plans with enrollment of more than 200,000 individuals (Hard 1992).

Systems such as Intermountain must develop a full range of information systems to support patient care (clinical, administrative, and decision support). In addition, integrated delivery systems involved in direct contracting and offering insurance products such as HMOs or PPOs must develop a complete range of insurance products to support sales and marketing; actuarial and underwriting activities; service contracting; eligibility; billing; utilization review; and claims processing, among others (Austin and Sobczak 1993).

Recent surveys of leaders in healthcare confirm these trends. Executives responding to the fifth annual survey of information systems trends sponsored by *Modern Healthcare* indicated that redesigning their computer systems for managed care was their highest information technology priority (Morrissey 1995). These findings are supported by results from the 1996 Leadership Survey conducted by the Healthcare Information and Management Systems Society and Hewlett-Packard Corporation. Respondents indicated that the most significant force driving information technology investments was the need to control costs due to pressures of managed care. The survey also indicated movement of computer technology to outpatient settings, including ambulatory clinics, physicians' offices, and group practices— far out pacing development of applications in traditional inpatient settings (HIMSS/HP 1996).

THE HEALTHCARE INFORMATION PROFESSIONAL

A number of trade and professional organizations support the work of information professionals in the healthcare field.

1. American College of Healthcare Information Administrators (ACHIA). A subunit of the American Academy of Medical Administrators, ACHIA is a personal membership organization for information administrators with special focus on continuing education and research in healthcare information administration.

2. American Health Information Management Association (AHIMA). Formerly the American Medical Record Association, AHIMA is comprised of information professionals who specialize in the utilization and management of clinical data.

3. American Medical Informatics Association (AMIA). "Medical informatics" is a term used to describe the science of storage, retrieval, and optimal use of biomedical information for problem solving and medical decision making. AMIA is a personal membership organization of professionals interested in computer applications in biomedicine.

4. Center for Healthcare Information Management (CHIM). CHIM is a trade association of corporate members representing the leading firms (hardware, software, and consulting) in the healthcare information technology industry.

5. College of Healthcare Information Management Executives (CHIME). CHIME is a personal membership organization of chief information officers (CIOs) in the healthcare field. CHIME provides professional development and networking opportunities for its members.

6. Healthcare Information and Management Systems Society (HIMSS). HIMSS is a personal membership organization representing professionals in four areas: clinical systems, information systems, management engineering, and telecommunications. HIMSS provides professional development opportunities to its members through publications and educational programs.

For more information on these and other related professional organizations, the reader is directed to the Annual Market Directory issue of *Health Management Technology*. The 1996 Directory lists 41 associations and includes addresses and contact information for each organization in the listing.

SUMMARY

Healthcare is an information-intensive process. The management of health services organizations can be improved through intelligent use of information. This requires systematic planning and management of information resources in order to develop information systems that support patient care, administrative operations, and strategic management.

Health information systems fall into four categories: clinical, administrative, strategic decision-support, and electronic network applications. Clinical information systems support patient care and provide information for strategic planning and management. Administrative systems support nonpatient care activities such as financial management, human resource management, materials management, scheduling, and office automation. Strategic decision-support systems assist executives in planning, marketing, management control of operations, performance evaluation, and outcomes assessment. Electronic network applications are used for insurance billing and claims processing, ordering medical supplies, and exchanging information across provider networks.

Change is occurring rapidly in healthcare. Major forces of change include:

1. expansion of managed care;
2. development of integrated delivery systems;
3. changes in reimbursement, including contractual discounts and capitation;
4. outcomes assessment to improve quality and reduce costs; and
5. demand for "report cards" on the performance of health plans and providers of care.

These environmental forces have resulted in reordering of the information system priorities of health services organizations. These new priorities include:

1. development of computerized patient records systems;
2. shift in emphasis from inpatient to ambulatory care systems;
3. development of enterprisewide electronic networks within integrated delivery systems;
4. development of strategic decision-support systems for risk analysis, financial forecasting, outcomes assessment, and quality improvement; and
5. development of new insurance-type applications within integrated delivery systems.

REFERENCES

Appleby, C. 1995. "The Trouble with CHINs." *Hospitals & Health Networks* 69 (9): 42–44.

Austin, C. J., and P. M. Sobczak. 1993. "Information Technology and Managed Care." *Hospital Topics* 71 (3): 33–37.

Barea, A. 1993. "Links to Physicians as Requirements of Reform?" *Healthcare Informatics* (September): 42–44.

Coile, R. C. 1990. *The New Medicine: Reshaping Medical Practice and Health Care Management.* Rockville, MD: Aspen Publishers.

DeFauw, T. D., and D. L'Heureux. 1995. "How to Strategically Align Information Resources with the Goals of an Integrated Delivery System." *Healthcare Information Management* 9 (4): 3–10.

Dick, R. S., and E. B. Steen, eds. 1991. *The Computer-Based Patient Record: An Essential Technology for Health Care.* Washington, DC: National Academy Press.

Hard, R. 1992. "Well-managed Information Vital to Effective Managed Care Contracting." *Hospitals* 66 (11): 50.

Healthcare Information and Management Systems Society and Hewlett-Packard Company (HIMSS/HP). 1996. *Seventh Annual Leadership Survey: Trends in Health Care Computing.* Chicago: Healthcare Information and Management Systems Society.

Kertesz, L. 1996. "HMO Enrollment Soars." *Modern Healthcare* October 28: 10.

Kralewski, J. E., A. deVries, B. Dowd, and S. Potthoff. 1994. *The Development of Integrated Service Networks (ISNs).* A Report for the MinnesotaCare Legislative Oversight Committee. University of Minnesota, School of Public Health, February 21.

Morrissey, J. 1994. "Hunting for Data to Limit Risks of Managed Care." *Modern Healthcare* 24 (46): 80–82.

———. 1995. "Information Systems Refocus Priorities." *Modern Healthcare* (February 13): 65–66.

Rosenthal, G. E., and D. L. Harper. 1994. "Cleveland Health Quality Choice: A Model for Collaborative Community-Based Outcomes Assessment." *Journal on Quality Improvement* 20 (8): 425–42.

Shortell, S. M., R. R. Gillies, and D. A. Anderson. 1994. "The New World of Managed Care: Creating Organized Delivery Systems." *Health Affairs* (Winter): 46–64.

Talbott, N. 1994. "Managing Information: Today's Integrated Healthcare Enterprises." *Healthcare Informatics* (June): 24–28.

Unger, W. J. 1992. "The Interdependence of Outcomes Management." *Decisions in Imaging Economics.* 5 (4): 4–7.

Weaver, C. 1993. "CHINs: Infrastructure for the Future." *Trustee* 46 (12): 12.

Wong, L. K. 1994. "Specialty Services Capitation Contracting by HMOs." *Medical Group Management Journal* (September–October): 96–100.

Wozmak, M. S. 1995. "Managed Care: A Primer." *American Academy of Medical Administrators Executive* (January–February): 12–14.

ADDITIONAL READINGS

American Hospital Association. 1993. *Transforming Health Care Delivery: Toward Community Care Networks.* Chicago: The Association.

Catholic Health Association. 1993. *A Handbook for Planning and Developing Integrated Delivery* St. Louis, MO: The Association.

Coile, R. C. 1995. "Assessing Healthcare Market Trends and Capital Needs: 1996–2000." *Healthcare Financial Management* 49 (8): 60–2, 64–5.

Health Care Advisory Board. 1994. *Report on Capitation.* Washington, DC: The Board.

Health Management Technology. 1996. *Annual Market Directory* Atlanta, GA: Argus, Inc.

Norman, K. C., and J. J. Moynihan. 1994. "Electronic Data Interchange: An Electronic Network Strategy for Managed Care." *Managed Care* 2 (1): 54–61.

Rontal, R. 1993. "Information and Decision Support in Managed Care." *Managed Care* 1 (3): 3–14.

Shortell, S. M., R. R. Gillies, D. A. Anderson, J. B. Mitchell, and K. L. Morgan. 1993. "Creating Organized Delivery Systems: The Barriers and Facilitators." *Hospital & Health Services Administration* (Winter): 447–66.

Evaluation and the Decision-Making Process

James E. Veney, Ph.D., and Arnold D. Kaluzny, Ph.D.

Many, if not most, managers deny—or are at the very least skeptical of—anything as abstract as a "decision model." In reality, however, managers are always being influenced by information, or lack thereof, that implicitly or explicitly forms the basis of their decisions about the nature of a problem and about the effects of some program and/or service actvity implemented to address that problem. The purpose of this chapter is to describe what will be referred to as the *evaluation-based decision model*, a model that formally incorporates information into the decision-making process about the problem being studied and the effects of program and service activity on that problem.

This chapter is presented in four sections, each dealing with an aspect of the decision-making process. The first section describes the evaluation-based decision model and how this model relates to other decision models that may be used to make program decisions or other types of decisions and the criteria appropriate to guide the use of these models. The other three sections of the chapter describe components of the evaluation-based decision model: needs assessment, program implementation, and outcomes assessment.

As shown in Figure 8.1, each phase of program operation is generally associated with particular types of questions in program evaluation and with related evaluation techniques. Needs assessment, for example, is most closely related to the issue of relevance and adequacy; it adopts survey-related

Editor's Note: This chapter is from Chapter 2 of *Evaluation and Decision Making for Health Services, Third Edition,* by James E. Veney and Arnold D. Kaluzny, 1998, HAP

Figure 8.1 Schematic View of Components of Evaluation

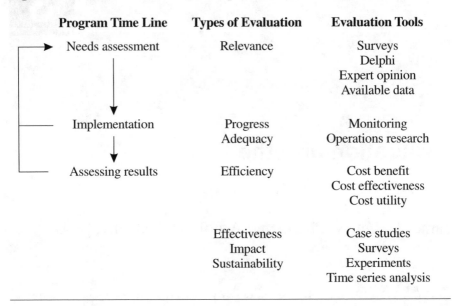

Program Time Line	Types of Evaluation	Evaluation Tools
Needs assessment	Relevance	Surveys Delphi Expert opinion Available data
Implementation	Progress Adequacy	Monitoring Operations research
Assessing results	Efficiency	Cost benefit Cost effectiveness Cost utility
	Effectiveness Impact Sustainability	Case studies Surveys Experiments Time series analysis

techniques such as random sample surveys, Delphi studies and solicitation of expert opinion, and use of available data. Program implementation is most closely related to the issue of progress and adopts techniques like monitoring and related operations research techniques. Results assessment is related to issues of efficiency, effectiveness, outcomes, and sustainability and adopts, again, survey techniques, cost-benefit and cost-effectiveness analysis, time series analysis, and experimentation. The detailed discussion of these methodological techniques is the major focus of the subsequent sections of the book.

THE EVALUATION-BASED DECISION MODEL

Central to the evaluation-based decision model is the idea of "cybernetics" (Weiner 1948). The term cybernetics has become popular as a way of defining a methodological approach to a wide variety of scientific and management endeavors and is closely linked with general systems theory and its applications in the social, organizational (Scott 1998; Senge 1990), and management sciences (Deming 1986, 93). The idea of cybernetics is intuitively simple (Hage 1974) and is characterized by two major components:

- There exists a system of interrelated variables that represent some production process—in the broadest sense, a process for accomplishing an end. These variables include inputs, throughputs, and outputs.
- Some of the variables in the input-throughput-output system are being regulated and controlled by decisions made on the basis of the feedback of information about the state of the system.

The essence of the evaluation-based decision model is shown in Figure 8.2. This figure is a schematic of the input-throughput-output model showing the feedback of information that leads to control where control is based on communication of information in any system, whether complex or simple. This view of cybernetics and its application within the evaluation-based decision model is the fundamental basis of managerial decision making.

The conceptual basis of the model is relatively simple. It begins with the assumption that verifiable ends (outcomes) exist that are expected to result from the activity. The extent to which the activity has been successful in producing these verifiable ends can thus be evaluated at various points in time during the life of the program and at its completion. The information about the gap between the expected outcomes and the actual outcomes is then used to modify either inputs or process, during program operation or before a similar program is launched in the future, to attempt to reduce the gap between the verifiable expected outputs and the actual outputs. If no verifiable outcomes do exist, the very initiation and implementation of such activity can and should be challenged.

ALTERNATE DECISION-MAKING MODELS

The evaluation-based decision model is but one of the four models available to managers and must be viewed in the context of the other three alternatives:

Figure 8.2   The Evaluation-Based Decision Model

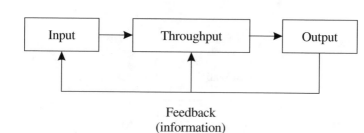

Feedback
(information)

random-walk decision making, traditional decision making, and mechanistic decision making. Figure 8.3 presents the four types of decision making as defined by the four cells of a two-by-two means/ends table. The horizontal axis is defined as a verifiable (i.e., to know when a process has been successful is possible) versus a nonverifiable end and on the vertical axis by whether the means to obtain the end is accepted or not accepted. Accepted or not accepted means that in a given setting a particular decision process and, hence, course of action would generally be expected to produce the desired outcomes in a direct, linear manner with no error along the way. An accepted means is essentially a recipe for moving directly to the desired output with no mistakes.

It should be understood that these decision-making modes are ideal types. By that, we mean that in virtually no real decision-making situation will the ideal type that we described be the only method that is likely to be brought to bear. Further, we do not claim that the ideal-type decision models we are going to suggest are totally exhaustive of all decision models. Nevertheless, it is useful to suggest these types as a point of departure.

To understand this typology, consider the category "accepted means and verifiable end." This is the *mechanistic model* of decision making (Deutsch 1968). Mechanistic decision making occurs when the ends are verifiable and the appropriate decision process (the means) is known and accepted. This is the realm, for example, of linear programming. If a hospital wishes to maximize its dollar profits from a course of action (a verifiable end) subject to a set of constraints, the decision process, and thus the course of action, can be determined by a widely understood and accepted mathematical algorithm. The means is accepted, and at some point the fact that the result of the set of decisions is the optimum result can be verified. Yet trying other alternative decisions in this context is generally not necessary because the linear programming model is the model known to produce the optimum result.

Figure 8.3 Means Ends Decision Table

		Ends	
		Non Verifiable	Verifiable
Means	Not Accepted	Random Walk	Cybernetic
	Accepted	Traditional	Mechanistic

When a nonverifiable end or set of nonverifiable ends is desired, and no accepted means of reaching these ends exists, the decision process is in the realm of the *random walk*. Because the goals or ends are not verifiable and the appropriate decision process, and thus course of action, for reaching the nonverifiable goals are not accepted or specified, any decisions will be as good as any others. In essence, a random decision process is adequate. The random process may ultimately arrive at a desired result, but it will not be verifiable, in any case.

Appropriately, managers are uncomfortable with random decision making. What very often happens during this situation of being uncomfortable is that a particular means is institutionalized even in the absence of verifiable ends or confirmation that the accepted means will produce a verified desired end. This is the mode of *traditional decision making*. In this mode of decision making decisions can be made for long periods of time without ever being subjected to any further scrutiny than that they adhere to a particular institutionalized decision-making process. In effect, the process becomes the product.

If program goals or ends can be stated in ways that achievement of the ends can be verified but no accepted means to obtain the ends exists, the decision-making process may be in the realm of *cybernetic*, or *evaluation-based decision making*. In this form, information about the extent to which a particular decision or set of decisions brings the program closer to the verifiable ends can be used to modify the decisions next taken. By doing this, an effort can be made to assure that the result comes ever closer to the desired ends.

When ends are not verifiable or the necessary effort to verify them is not likely to be made (the realm of random walks or traditional decision making), evaluation cannot proceed because evlauation refers specifically to the assessment of the extent to which ends are reached. Further, no reason to conduct evaluation would exist. In the absence of verifiable ends no information will be produced that can be used for making better decisions than the ones already being made.

DECISION MODE DRIFT

Despite the efforts and good intentions of both managers and evaluators, much of decision making follows closely either the random walk model or the traditional model. Much of what goes by the name of evaluation is actually a process of examining decisions that are made either on the basis of random walks or of tradition. To the extent that this is true, much that goes by the name of program evaluation is wasted effort because in both situations the ends are not verifiable.

A number of reasons can be cited for why decision making tends to drift toward the random walk mode, and particularly toward the traditional mode. The ability to verify that an end has been achieved is the central problem. What may begin as a clear effort to operate within the evaluation-based decision realm (i.e., clearly defined and verifiable ends available to assess results of decisions and courses of action through feedback) may quickly drift to either the random walk mode or to the traditional mode of decision making since verifiable ends are not easily accessible.

Decision mode drift may happen for several reasons. Program managers may decide that the cost of verifying program ends is greater than expected or greater than the value of verification. This perception is usually accompanied by a stated or unstated rationale that is something like "I know that this is the right course of action, so it is not reasonable to spend 25 percent of my program delivery budget on evaluation that will only confirm what I already know." In fact, this is probably often true.

Originally specified and verifiable goals may not express the full range of results expected from a program. It is unfortunate that verifiable goals may often be relatively trivial in the context of a program—the goal of a training program may be to impart the ability to deliver a complex skilled service, but the only verifiable (measurable) goal for the training program may be that a certain number of persons have been subjected to training. As goals become more complex, the decision-making process drifts toward the traditional or random walk modes.

Results that managers see from a program may not be as attractive as they had hoped. In this situation, there is a tendency to kill the messenger by dismantling what might be a fairly serious cybernetic decision effort and falling back into the random walk or traditional modes, in which the lack of attempts to verify achievement of ends will not be a threat to program personnel or continuation of the program itself.

Mechanistic decision making, which is an appropriate realm of evaluation only to the extent that continued verification of the efficacy of a particular decision process is desired, may also drift toward traditional modes of decision making as ends become more complex. What may be a straightforward, mechanistic decision process in the presence of a relatively simple set of goals (e.g., a linear programming model to maximize hospital profits) may revert to traditional decision making as the goals become more difficult to measure (e.g., improved community health status). The ideal situation would be that the mechanistic decision process would retrench at cybernetic decision making, but this will happen only if the necessary steps are taken to specify in measurable terms and to verify the more complex ends.

EVALUATION-BASED VERSUS MECHANISTIC DECISION MAKING

Why is the evaluation-based model—implying feedback of information about the extent to which a given decision results in achievement of a given goal—the proper realm of evaluation, while evaluation is likely to be redundant in a setting in which mechanistic decision making—implying both a verifiable end and an accepted way to reach the end—is used? As a simple example, consider the problem of finding the square root of a number. The square root of a number is defined as that number which when multiplied by itself will give the original number. Today, with the widespread availability of battery-powered calculators that provide square roots to ten decimal places at the push of a button, hardly anyone thinks of finding square roots as a decision problem, except possibly in the most trivial sense (i.e., "to find the square root of a number, enter the number into the hand calculator and push the square root button").

Not too long ago, however, finding a square root for a large number was far from a trivial matter. Tables of square roots were published in mathematics texts, but they always required approximation. People learned to use logarithms to find square roots, but these also usually required approximations. Anyone going to school before the 1960s probably learned a tedious method for extracting square roots, which most have long forgotten. This was a mechanistic method in the sense that if people learned the necessary steps and followed them faithfully without making any mistakes in arithmetic, they could produce the square root of any number to any number of decimal places desired without ever checking to see if the process was producing the right result. The result was assured by the decision-making process.

The square root of a number can also be found by a purely cybernetic decision process (i.e., feedback method) that many of us hit upon independently when we first had access to electrically powered mechanical calculators that would multiply relatively quickly but that would not take square roots directly. With this method, memorizing an accepted decision process was not needed. All that was required was to make a first guess at the square root of the number and then multiply the guess by itself. The result, however wrong it may have been, was compared to the original number for which the square root was desired. If the result was bigger than the original number, then the original guess at the square root was too large and had to be adjusted down. If the result was smaller than the original number, the original guess at the square root was too small and had to be adjusted up. The size of the adjustment in either direction depended on how bad the first guess was. On the basis of this adjustment, a new number to approximate the square root was selected and the process repeated. This could be done as many times as necessary to obtain the accuracy required by the application.

In effect, this method used feedback of information (evaluation) about the difference between what was produced and what was desired to make a decision about what to do next. This was an evaluation-based decision process and was within the appropriate realm of evaluation. To determine which method was best in this situation is unnecessary. Either method produced a usable result. Many situations exist, however, in which no mechanistic method of decision making is available. In such settings, only cybernetic decision making and evaluation are likely to produce the results desired.

USING DECISION-MAKING MODELS

Given the complexity within which evaluation occurs, what criteria are appropriate in the use of each model? Three tests are available for managers and can be applied in a variety of situations: instrumental, efficiency, and social tests (Thompson 1967, 84–87). The appropriateness is a function of the degree of clear formulation or ambiguity of standards of desirability and the completeness or incompleteness of cause-and-effect relationships. Table 8.1 presents the relationship of these tests to our four decision-making models.

Instrumental Tests

As shown in Table 8.1, instrumental tests are primarily appropriate for decision making within the evaluation-based model. Here the standards of desirability are reasonably clear, and the cause-and-effect relationships are uncertain. For example, will national health insurance produce greater access to health services for all people? Will managed care programs contain costs of providing services to various segments of the population, and do consensus conferences as a means of technology assessment change physician practice patterns? These are essentially technical questions in which the major criterion is to ascertain only whether the desired ends were achieved, without considering resource utilization or the exact means by which this was accomplished.

In this area the evaluator can make the most important contributions to program decision making. The tools available to the evaluator—measurement techniques, sampling, survey designs, experimentation—are all techniques that conform to the instrumental approach to information. As long as an issue is basically technical, the evaluator is in the most effective realm, although the evaluator is always at risk of challenge if the results do not conform to the expectations of important constituent groups.

For example, in a randomized clinical trial of coronary care units, an

Table 8.1 Decison Models and Criteria

Criteria	Decision Models			
	Cybernetic	*Mechanistic*	*Traditional*	*Random Walk*
Instrumental	X			
Efficiency		X		
Social			X	X

initial report showing a greater death rate for those treated in hospitals than those treated at home was mistakenly reversed. When these data were presented to a group of cardiologists, they demanded that the trials be declared unethical and the study be stopped immediately because the results did not conform to their expectations. When the mistake was identified and the data presented correctly, the same group could not be persuaded to declare the trials unethical but found all sorts of problems with the study sampling and measurement procedures (Cochrane 1972).

Not all questions can be answered on the basis of instrumental tests. Many questions of belief and values are simply not subject to technical verification or refutation. Even in those areas where technical criteria (empirical verification) can apply, measurement may be so difficult or complex that arriving at even a technical answer is impossible. Furthermore, the myriad of desirable ends that a particular program is to accomplish and the difficulty of objectively measuring all these ends usually make hoping that technical rationality alone can resolve all decision-making problems for program operation impossible.

Efficiency Tests

Where instrumental criteria in the broad sense raise the question of whether demonstrating empirically that the means employed produces the ends desired is possible, efficiency criteria tackles the question of whether the specific means employed is the most efficient means for producing the ends desired. This is critical to the mechanistic model, in which cause-and-effect relationships are well understood. The assumption is that alternative means exist by which a particular end may be reached or, at the very least, that the program has the option of producing a certain amount of a desired end and that the means will be exercised only to the extent that the cost of producing the amount of the end desired is acceptable.

Again, if evaluation is limited to the aspect of technical rationality that may be seen as economic, rationalilty, evaluators are generally on firm ground. Cost-benefit anlaysis, cost-effectiveness analysis, and optimization techniques available from operations research are all capable of producing useful information about the most efficient means of realizing desired ends.

Social Tests

As shown in Table 8.1, social tests are appropriate to random walk and traditional decision-making models, where standards of desirability are ambiguous regardless of cause-and-effect relationships. Under these conditions, criteria are validated by authority or consensus.

Abortion, for example, is technically an effective means of birth control. Yet in many countries both its legal and social acceptability remain in contention. Many genetic defects and genetically transmitted diseases could be effectively controlled from a technical standpoint through programs to control procreation. Again, in most societies these programs would be neither legally nor socially acceptable. Substantial questions could be raised as to whether the notion of primary healthcare as currently promoted by the World Health Organization (WHO) and the United Nations Children's Fund (UNICEF) is technically the most rational way to approach the goal of "health for all by the year 2000." This modality, which relies heavily on local self-help and to a great extent on lay practitioners, has a substantial degree of social rationality for many of the developing nations in which it is to be implemented. On the other hand, because of the continuing restrictions on what non-physicians may legally do in many of these societies, the legal rationality of the primary care programs may still be subject to question.

Similarly, a given program may be more a means of controlling resources, maintaining a particular elite in power, or providing a hope to special interest groups or disgruntled portions of the population than a way of actually eliminating or reducing the problem to which the program is manifestly addressed. Every large-scale program, despite its true relationships to desired ends from the technical standpoint, is likely to have a substantial component of political rationality in its formulation. For example, recent federal and state programs designed to regulate the utilization management practices of managed care plans offer prime illustrations of political rationality in program design. Some of these programs require managed care plans to offer minimum hospital stays for certain medical procedures such as childbirth, while others specify the conditions under which certain medical procedures can be performed on an outpatient basis.

Clearly, to implement governmental programs and regulations that established standards of practice for every possible medical procedure and condition would be impossible. Consequently, the existing piecemeal programs are unlikely to have a significant effect on the quality of care delivered through managed care plans. Nevertheless, these programs serve the political purpose of appeasing the healthcare consumers and providers who express concerns about quality of care within managed care plans.

When the prevailing criteria of program planners and managers are primarily social, the evaluator may have little effect on decision making. In fact, the evalutor's findings will probably be largely irrelevant to decision making because decisions are being made on the basis of criteria that are not essentially technical and that cannot be verified empirically. In this case, the evaluator may provide useful insights to decision makers about the technical characteristics of the program and perhaps clarify political trade-offs but cannot expect the work to have a significant impact on the decision. The evaluator should be aware of the appropriate tests within each decision model. Failure to apply the appropriate tests within each model will limit the ability of the evaluation to influence the decision-making process—as well as elucidate the evaluator's own role in that process.

COMPONENTS OF THE EVALUTION-BASED DECISION MODEL

Needs assessment, implementation, and assessing outcomes are critical elements in the evaluation-based decision model. Following are descriptions of each component, their respective approaches, and their challenges.

Needs Assessment

Needs assessment is the first stage in program implementation and is the process of determining the nature and extent of the problems that a program is designed to address; it is the assessment of the relevance and adequacy of the program. In particular, this means that information about the problem—a gap between the desired state of some verifiable end and the actual state of that verifiable end—is used as the basis on which to structure, direct, and assess the adequacy of a program. This information may include:

- the nature of the problem;
- its extent;
- who or what it affects;
- where and when it occurs;
- its frequency; and
- any other salient information.

But is is information about the problem on which the nature of the program is based, not particularly on guesses about the problem (random walk decision making) or the assumption in the absence of data that the problem fits into a previously defined mold (traditional decision making).

A needs assessment may possibly indicate that the problem is amenable to solution by one or another systematic decision-making technique, such as linear programming. This decision in itself, however, should be made within the context of information about the actual nature of the problem.

At least two reasons exist why evaluation-based decision making may fail to be used in determining the problem that the program is to address and how it will be addressed. The first of these reasons is the problem of institutionalized (previously accepted) means, and the second is expert bias. Institutionalized objectives limit effective needs assessment, particularly as they restrict the range of issues that a program may be permitted to address. Expert bias refers to the basic misconception that many experts may have about what the actual problem may be.

The issue of instutionalized objectives is one in which the problem is stated in such a way that only one or a limited number of program solutions can be adopted. For example, use of family planning services in a country may be a function of the quality and extent of training of service providers. The use will also be a function of the political situation, the degree to which people desire family planning, the availability of supplies and equipment and attractive clinics in which to provide services, and a host of other factors. If the institutionalized means of training is the driving force behind the needs assessment, it is likely that the needs assessment will find that more training of service providers is needed, even if other interventions may have a great effect on contraceptive use.

Institutionalized objectives are often determined by agencies that fund programs; no matter how good the needs-assessment effort may be in a technical sense, it may not, by the very nature of institutionalized objectives, be useful in improving the situation relative to selected verifiable ends.

Expert bias is the problem that those who are expected to carry out the needs assessment—the "experts"—may have predetermined notions about what the needs assessment should show. For example:

- Physicians assessing emergency medical care in a community may well determine that what is needed is expanded and improved medical services in emergency rooms.
- A representative of a law enforcement agency may conclude that the problem is the need for better control of highway accidents.
- The ambulance service may conclude that what is needed is a better distribution of emergency vehicles.
- A social scientists may conclude that the problem is the need to control domestic violence.

This is different from the problem of institutionalized means because in the case of institutionalized means a serious and detailed effort to examine the problem may exist, but only from the standpoint of a single or limited number of programmatic aspects. In the case of expert bias, the problem may never actually be examined at all, but simply be assumed to exist by an expert doing the assessment, who by virtue of expertise itself may not recognize the need to empirically verify the assumed problem.

Approaches to needs assessment

A number of strategies exist that can be used in the conduct of a needs assessment and in the determination of the relevance and adequacy of a program intervention. These include survey research, use of available data, Delphi and nominal group techniques, and expert judgments. The steps of the needs assessment process include the following:

1. Develop a general statement of what the program is expected to accomplish.
2. Determine the degree and nature of the problem that the program is expected to address and determine the level of accomplishment that may actually be realized.
3. Determine the strategies that should be employed by the program to address the identified problem.

Following is an illustration and discussion of each step.

1. Developing program expectations

The first step in the needs assessment is to develop a general statement about what the program or service activity is expected to accomplish. For example, in the area of maternal and child health services:

- Is the program expected to produce a set of activities to slow the rate of increase in the growth of the population?
- Is the program expected to reduce the number of unwanted pregnancies?
- Is the program expected to reduce the incidence of maternal and neonatal mortality and morbidity through child spacing?
- Is the program expected to increase the number of first-time acceptors of family planning methods?
- Is the program expected to increase the prevalence of family planning use?
- Is the program expected to increase the number of women who have favorable attitudes toward the use of family planning services?

In fact, the program organizers are likely to say that the program is expected to do all the things indicated in the preceding list, and more. Herein lies the first barrier for evaluation-based decision making, however.

Managers are unlikely to be willing to expend the resources necessary to define adequately, and then to measure routinely, each possible end previously indicated. A few of the ends may be measured and the rest are left to faith, and to the traditional—or perhaps worse, random-walk—decision mode. Agreement on the ends is only the first step in the needs assessment, however.

2. Determining the nature and degree of the problem

To realistically determine what is to be accomplished by the program requires a combination of techniques including a review of existing data, survey data of risk factors, community-based interviews, and an inventory of available healthcare resources within the community, specifically:

- *Review of existing state, local, and national health data.* Existing sources of data provide important yet often overlooked data sources to assess geographic, economic, and demographic characteristics of the community. These sources provide important insights to the principle causes of morbidity and mortality and utilization of health services within the community.

- *Telephone survey of behavioral risk factors.* While secondary data provides the base for determining need, assessing what people within the community think about their own health status and determining the health risk factors that may affect their health in the future is also important. This information can be obtained through a random telephone survey of a representative sample of the community. The survey should include a broad range of topics including levels of physical and mental health and levels of healthcare coverage.

- *Community focus group interviews.* These interviews are conducted to gain informatin on the perceptions of citizens' focus groups and to provide an opportunity to gain insight into health concerns of the community beyond that revealed in interview surveys. Focus groups must have a good representation of the community, including adolescents, business leaders, parents, senior citizens, homeless citizens, and other special population groups.

- *Healthcare resources inventory.* To determine the level of health resources available in the community, interviews need to be conducted with health professionals and community leaders. Information should include issues dealing with health insurance, types of providers available, and the overall availability of healthcare within the community.

3. Determining strategies

A third step in the needs assessment is to determine what programs or service activities should be employed to address the problems specified. One approach that has proven useful is the application of a rating technology using a computer program known as "Option Finder" (Flexner 1995; Halverson

1995). This approach involves all the relevant participants and stakeholders and provides an opportunity to vote interactively in the following sequence:

1. Review risk factors and their definitions and, taking one risk factor at a time, rate each factor on its perceived "seriousness" using a scale of 1 (little impact on community health) to 7 (major impact on community health).

2. Given the risk factor ranking relative to "seriousness," rate the risk factor list again on "willingness," or likelihood that the community can work together on addressing this particular risk, using a scale of 1 (little willingness to collaborate) to 7 (high willingness to collaborate).

3. Figure 8.4 displays a grid for comparing and identifying those factors that fell in the various quadrants giving a sense of the highest priorities to be addressed.

At this point, participants are encouraged to explore possible explanations for the data and why certain factors had been rated high and others low. The technology allowed facilitators to display the spread of votes and degree of variation in votes on each factor of special interest (as in high-impact risk factors that the group believed would not enlist high community effort, such as smoking).

Figure 8.4   Community Health Priority-Setting Grid

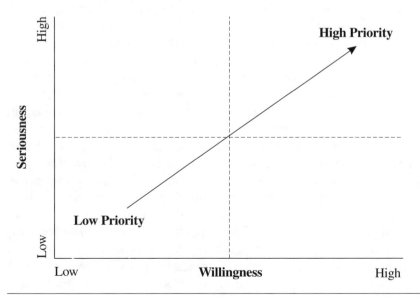

4. Focusing on risk factors in the High Priority quadrant, participants compare all risk factors two at a time (Paired Comparison), until a final priority list has been developed. For example, participants may arrive at a final list of priority risk factors that are of high impact and that they are willing to address: alcohol and drug abuse; parenting skills; access to healthcare; prenatal care; low-immunization levels; and seatbelt use.

5. Finally, a list of perceived health system gaps are identified and rated one by one, first by perceived "potential to improve community health in the county" (1 = little potential to 7 = high potential), then by perceived "feasibility to successfully implement necessary changes" (1 = not feasible to 7 = highly feasible). For example, health system gaps identified as being in the High Potential, High Feasibility quadrant may include services to prevent or deal with substance abuse, health system coordination, services to improve parenting skills, public information and education about health and health services, physician recruitment and distribution within the county, dentist recruitment and distribution within the county, and allied health worker recruitment. Given this listing, these gaps are compared two at a time to arrive at a priority listing.

Program Implementation

Given the priority of activity established by the needs assessment, the major issue of implementation is to ensure that the identified program activities are in place and on track. This is the issue of progress. While managers and evaluators often assume the extent of implementation, implementation varies by site, over time, and even among program recipients, as their characteristics interact with the attributes of the intervention (Scheirer 1989).

Assessment of progress is generally considered to be an issue of monitoring. For example, the program is expected to have progressed to a certain point by a certain time. The point to which the program is expected to have progressed will be associated with the assurance of anticipated funding; the delivery of program equipment; the construction of a facility; the hiring or training of personnel; and the provision of services to a client population. Figure 8.5 depicts the province of monitoring as an evaluation activity.

In general, what is monitored in the assessment of progress is the provision, deployment, and use of program inputs. Figure 8.5 shows a generalized view of program implementation from the standpoint of program inputs, process, outputs, and outcomes. Program monitoring as an evaluation activity is concerned particularly with program inputs and process. The questions raised in program monitoring will be particularly questions of whether such critical inputs as funding, equipment, facilities, and personnel have been

Figure 8.5 Schematic of Program Inputs, Process, Outputs, and Outcomes

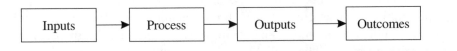

made available in the quantities and at the times specified by the program plan. Program monitoring will be concerned with whether the process of the program—which will include the way in which inputs are deployed and expended, and the timing of this use—conforms to the program plan. It also will be concerned with determining whether the persons expected to be served by the program have actually been served in the quantity and with the level of quality expected, and how the program can be improved.

In all of these monitoring activities, the evaluation-based approach to decision making has a clear role. The verifiable ends are, in this case, the inputs and deployment of inputs (program process) specified by the program plan, or evolving on a real-time basis in the minds of the program managers. Evaluation in this context is concerned with determining whether the actual deployment of resources fits the existing or evolving plan. If it does not, it is the responsibility of the program managers to make those decisions necessary to assure that the deployment and use of resources do fit the plan. Statisticians speak of type one error, the finding of a program result when none actually exists, and of type two error, the finding of no program result when a result does exist. Program evaluators also speak of a type three error, the assumption that a program was implemented when in fact it was not. Monitoring serves the purpose of allowing the manager to make the decisions necessary to assure that a program is implemented as expected and also serves the purpose of providing the basis for its continuous improvement. Monitoring fits into the evaluation-based mode of decision making, with the verifiable ends being the program plans for provision and deployment of inputs.

Results Assessment

The assessment of program results includes the three categories of evaluation—efficiency, effectiveness, and outcome. Efficiency and effectiveness are program characteristics that may be assessed in large part while the program is ongoing. Outcome is concerned with the long-term effects of a program and, in particular, program influence on such difficult-to-measure concepts as quality of life. In each category of evaluation, however, the evaluation-based approach to decision making should be very relevant to the managerial process.

Differences exist between the use of the evaluation process in the case of program results as compared to program implementation. Often with program implementation, evlauation information (i.e., results of program-monitoring efforts) will be available and may produce changes in a program, on a real-time and continuing basis. In the case of program results, evaluation information (i.e., assessments of efficiency, effectiveness, and impact) may come too late in the life of a program to inform decisions for significant changes in the program itself, but rather may be most valuable in decisions about how a similar program should be structured the next time.

Effectiveness

Effectiveness concerns the question of whether the expected program outputs are produced. From the standpoint of the evaluation-based decision-making model, a critical feature of this question is whether the objectives of the program are stated in such a way as to allow the evaluator to assess whether the objectives have been met—in short, to verify the achievement of program ends. If, for example, a family-planning program has been upgraded for the expressed purpose of increasing the length of time that women continue to use contraceptives, the verifiable program end is an increase in the length of time that women who begin family planning actually continue use. Legitimate questions can be raised as to how much of an increase in length of time is actually an increase; this is in part a technical question that can be resolved by recourse to statistics. After that question is resolved, getting data on continuation from records that are almost certain to be available in family-planning clinics should be relatively easy.

If the stated objective of the program is to increase the quality of care provided in the clinics, however, devising a verifiable measure of quality of service provided may be very difficult. The quality of training of providers and their knowledge and skills at training may be assessed, but these are essentially program inputs; what is to be assessed are outputs. Quality of service, as provided, may be assessed through the technique of observation or demonstration. This, however, is not only a costly activity, requiring a substantial amount of time in observation of the providers, but it also requires specifications of precisely what service provision actions are to be assessed, how they are to be assessed, and what measuring instruments are to be used. In the absence of such specifications, which is not a trivial matter, any decisions that result from the evaluation effort will have drifted back into either the traditional or the random-walk decision modes.

Although effectiveness concerns program outputs, this does not always mean that evaluation of effectiveness comes only at the end of the program.

Efforts to determine whether the program inputs are associated with greater continuity of contraceptive use may reasonably occur during the course of the program life, and the determination that no increase in continuity of use was occurring may lead directly to a decision to modify the program. The downside to this is that decisions to change a program in midcourse can have significant and unexpected results in terms of the determination that the program—as opposed to other factors, including the changes in the program—was actually the causal agent in the change in outputs. In this regard, assessment of effectiveness can also be seen to ocur on a real-time basis and to have an input on decisions made about program operation.

A number of ways exist in which effectiveness may be assessed, depending on the nature of the program itself and on the nature of the verifiable end under assessment. With varying degrees of internal validity, these include case studies, trend analyses, surveys, experiments, and simulation techniques.

Efficiency

The issue of efficiency is essentially one of whether the verifiable ends of the program are sufficient to justify the costs incurred. This may also be considered in the context of the question of whether the verifiable ends are realized through the program under assessment at a lower cost than they may be realized through another program. Both issues imply that the ends have in fact been reached, and that they can be verified. Assessment of the cost of increasing the length of time that family-planning acceptors continue to use family planning can move forward relatively easily if a way is found to determine the costs of the program. However, efforts to assess the cost of increases in quality in the same program depend on the ability to determine costs and on the other problematic issue of how to determine that quality has increased. In either case, however, to speak of the efficiency of a program that had failed to meet the verifiable ends specified would make little sense. Moreover, if program outputs cannot be stated as verifiable ends, assessment of efficiency is simply not possible.

On the strength of the possibly optimistic assumption that program ends can be stated in ways that allow them to be verified, the assessment of efficiency, like the assessment of effectiveness, has the potential to provide input to decisions made about the program at two times: while the program is under way, comparing actual costs to expected costs or to costs realized under some other scheme; and at the end of the program, with the same types of comparisons. Decisions taken as a result of the evaluation effort may influence the nature of the program as it is ongoing or may be used to determine how a future program to produce similar results should be structured. In either case, the assessment of efficiency is usually subsumed under the topics of cost-benefit or cost-effectiveness analysis.

Outcome

The evaluation of outcome stands in a somewhat different position relative to the evaluation decision model than do the other four aspects of evaluation. Outcome refers to the long-term results of the program—in particular, improvements in health and quality of life. The word outcome itself—while achieving almost spiritual meaning within the health services research and evaluation literature and frequently invoked by funding agencies, planners, and managers as the standard toward which all activity is to be judged—seems much too dramatic to describe even long-term results to be expected from most programs. The next section addresses some challenges associated with the use of outcomes as the gold standard in decision making.

Long-term effect and sustainability

Outcome must be thought of as the long-term effects of program activities. This definition itself makes an interest in an assessment problematic for the program manager. In general, managers are—and should be—concerned with decisions, and thus evaluations that bear on the decisions they will make about the continued progress of the program. They should do so to ensure that the results of the program are as expected, or—at the very least—to ensure that they can demonstrate where the program failed to meet its short-term objectives. The manager's job is not to ensure that two, five, or ten years after the program ends salubrious changes in health or education or quality of life will exist. In any case, program funders are not going to include the necessary resources to do such an assessment and thus ensure the sustainability of the program. On the basis of long-term outcomes, any assessment of outcomes seems clearly challenging, if not problematic.

Verifiable ends

The utility of the evaluation decision model depends on the specification of verifiable ends against which the results of the program can be assessed. A few items are in the nature of such long-term outcomes of a program as improved health, welfare, or quality of life. One is that to reach consensus on what the components of these things are is difficult (e.g., what goes into a measure of quality of life?). Another is that the components, even if agreed upon, are difficult or impossible to verify. For example, in the classic concept of health as expressed by WHO, the WHO constitution defines health as a "state of complete physical, mental and social well-being . . ." (WHO 1981). How many different aspects of complete physical, mental and social well-being would we have to specify to assure that we had all the important ones? When we had them, how would we measure them? The likely recourse would be to fall back on specific indicators like infant-mortality rates as a measure of well-being. Why not admit that the purpose of the program is to reduce infant-mortality rates, which is a verifiable end?

REFERENCES

Cochrane, A. 1972. *Effectiveness and Efficiency*. London: The Nuffield Provincial Hospitals Trust.

Deming, W. E. 1986. *Out of Crises*. Cambridge, MA: Massachusetts Institute of Technology.

Deming, E. 1993. *The New Economics for Industry, Education, Government*. Cambridge, MA: MIT Center for Advanced Engineering Study.

Deutsch, K. W. 1968. "Toward a Cybernetic Model of Man and Society." In *Modern Systems Research for the Behavioral Scientist*, edited by W. Buckley, 387–400. Chicago: Aldine Publishing Company.

Flexner, B. 1995. "Designing and Facilitating Option Finder-Supported Meetings." Mendota Heights, MN: Option Technologies, Inc.

Halverson, P. 1995. "Davidson County: Agenda or Health Project Final Report." University of North Carolina at Chapel Hill, School of Public Health.

Senge, P. M. 1990. *The Fifth Discipline: The Art and Practice of the Learning Organization*. New York: Doubleday.

Scheirer, M. A. 1989. "Implementation and Process Analysis in Worksite Health Promotion Search." In *Methodological Issues in Worksite Research*. Bethesda, MD: National Heart, Lung and Blood Institute.

Scott, W. R. 1998. *Organizations: Rational, Natural, and Open Systems, Fourth Edition*. Upper Saddle River, NJ: Prentice Hall.

Thompson, J. D. 1967. *Organizations in Action*. New York: McGraw-Hill.

Weiner, N. 1948. *Cybernetics or Control and Communication in the Animal and Machine*. New York: Wiley.

World Health Organization. 1981. "Health Programme Evaluation: Guiding Principles, Health for All, Series No. 6." Geneva.

Healthcare Fraud and Abuse

J. Stuart Showalter, J.D.

T he annual cost of healthcare in this country is more than $1 trillion, and the government estimates that as much as 10 percent of that amount may result from fraud (intentional deception) or abuse (unsound practices that result in increased costs).[1] Because the U.S. government is the largest single purchaser of healthcare, the elimination of fraud and abuse has been called the Department of Justice's number two law enforcement priority (second only to violent crime),[2] and ever more resources have been allocated to enforcement activities conducted by the Department of Justice (DOJ), United States attorneys, the Federal Bureau of Investigation, the Health and Human Services Department's Office of Inspector General (OIG), and other agencies. In addition, state attorneys general conduct their own investigations and prosecutions, often working closely with federal officials. Private citizens who have first-hand knowledge of fraud are even permitted to sue for the government and collect a percentage of the proceeds recovered, if any.

Verdicts and settlements in civil fraud cases can sometimes be hundreds of millions of dollars, and offenders who are prosecuted for criminal offenses can receive massive fines and lengthy jail terms. One example of the severity of the penalties is *United States v. Lorenzo*,[3] in which a dentist billed Medicare for "consultations" on nursing home residents. Although Medicare does not cover dental services or routine physicals, Dr. Lorenzo billed the government for his cancer-related examination of each patient's oral cavity, head, and neck, all of which is standard dental practice. The government proved that

Editor's Note: This chapter is from Chapter 9 of *Southwick's The Law of Healthcare Administration, Third Edition,* by J. Stuart Showalter, 1999, HAP

Dr. Lorenzo had submitted 3,683 false claims, resulting in overpayment of $130,719.20. The court assessed damages of nearly $19 million, almost 150 times the amount of the overpayment. A second example is *United States v. Krizek.*[4] Among other things, Dr. Krizek, a psychiatrist, charged the government for a full session (45 to 50 minutes) regardless of whether he spent 20 minutes or two hours with a patient. He argued that in practice the time evened out and the government was not harmed. In one instance, however, it was shown that he submitted 23 claims for full sessions in a single day. Dr. Krizek was fined $157,000 and assessed $11,000 in court costs.[5] Other examples include criminal convictions and civil fines of more than $100 million each levied against Caremark International, Corning (Damon) Laboratories, Roche Laboratories, National Medical Enterprises, and National Health Laboratories, and a settlement in excess of $30 million with the University of Pennsylvania. (The National Medical Enterprises case resulted in criminal and civil fines totaling $379 million.)

In such a volatile climate, it is little wonder that prevention of fraud and abuse became a serious topic for healthcare executives in the late 1990s and will continue to be so for the foreseeable future. A basic understanding of the major criminal and civil fraud statutes is therefore essential.

Some of the most common types of healthcare fraud and abuse follow.

- Filing claims for services that were not rendered or were not medically necessary.
- Misrepresenting the time, location, frequency, duration, or provider of services.
- "Upcoding" (i.e., assigning a higher current procedural terminology code or diagnosis-related group code than the procedure or diagnosis warrants).
- "Unbundling" (the practice of billing as separate items services, such as laboratory tests, that are actually performed as a battery).
- Violation of the "72-hour rule" (the rule stating that outpatient diagnostic procedures performed within three days of hospitalization are deemed to be part of the Medicare DRG payment and are not to be billed separately).
- Payment of "kickbacks" to induce referrals or the purchase of goods or services.
- Billing for services said to have been "incident to" a physician's services but that in fact were not provided under the physician's direct supervision.
- Self-referral (the practice of physicians referring patients for services to entities in which they have a financial interest).

The major statutes that these kinds of activities may violate include the civil and criminal False Claims Acts, the "anti-kickback" law, and the "Stark I" and "Stark II" self-referral laws. Depending on the facts of the case, mail and wire fraud statutes, the Racketeer Influenced and Corrupt Organizations Act (RICO), money-laundering statutes, and laws relating to theft, embezzlement, bribery, conspiracy, obstruction of justice, and similar matters may also be implicated. This chapter will focus on the major healthcare fraud statutes and will not address the kinds of laws noted in the previous sentence. Readers should be aware, however, that myriad legal standards (both state and federal) apply to healthcare organizations. The importance of competent legal counsel and a process to prevent criminal activity cannot be overemphasized.

FALSE CLAIMS ACTS

The major weapon in the federal government's arsenal in the war on fraud and abuse is the civil False Claims Act (FCA).[6] The law provides that a person is liable for penalties if he or she:

- "knowingly presents, or causes to be presented, to an officer or employee of the United States a false or fraudulent claim for payment or approval";
- "knowingly makes, uses, or causes to be made or used, a false record or statement to get a false or fraudulent claim paid or approved by the Government";
- "conspires to defraud the Government by getting a false or fraudulent claim allowed or paid"; or
- "knowingly makes, uses, or causes to be made or used, a false record or statement to conceal, avoid, or decrease an obligation to pay or transmit money or property to the government."[7]

Violations result in penalties ranging from $5,000 to $10,000 *per claim* plus three times the amount of damages sustained by the government, if any. The costs of bringing the action are charged to the defendant. If the claim was false, penalties and costs can be assessed even if the claim was not paid and the government suffered no damages.[8]

Interestingly, the FCA was enacted during the Civil War to stem the practice of certain suppliers overcharging the Union Army for goods and services. Because the issue of what constitutes a "claim" was apparently somewhat more straightforward then than it is now, the term is not defined in the statute. In healthcare, however, what amounts to a "claim" has been a matter of considerable dispute. For example, each CPT code on a HCFA 1500 form (the form used for Medicare Part B payments to physicians) could be considered a separate claim and, therefore, each false code could result in up to $10,000 in penalties. Twenty false CPT codes would, by this line of reasoning, allow a penalty of up to $200,000 to be assessed, plus damages and court costs.

This issue was addressed in the appeal of *Krizek*, in which the U.S. Court of Appeals for the D.C. Circuit held that each HCFA 1500 form was one "claim" irrespective of the number of false codes contained on it. The court felt that the form was merely one request for payment of the total sum it represented.[9] This result seems consistent with other cases defining a "claim" as "a demand for money or for some transfer of public property."[10]

The language of the statute, quoted above, requires the government to prove that the defendant acted "knowingly" in presenting the false claim or making a false record. For some time there was a question of whether this standard required proof of a specific intent to defraud the government. In 1986, however, Congress amended the FCA by stating that "no proof of specific intent to defraud is required" and that "knowingly" with respect to a claim means either (a) actual knowledge of its falsity, (b) deliberate ignorance of its truth or falsity, or (c) reckless disregard of its truth or falsity.[11] As stated in the committee report accompanying the 1986 amendments,

> The Committee is firm in its intentions that the act not punish honest mistakes or incorrect claims submitted through mere negligence. But the Committee does believe the civil False Claims Act should recognize that those doing business with the Government have an obligation to make a limited inquiry to ensure the claims they submit are accurate.[12]

Krizek illustrates the application of this standard. Although Dr. Krizek was not personally involved in the billing process, the court found that he had submitted the claims "knowingly."

> These were not "mistakes" nor merely negligent conduct. Under the statutory definition of "knowing" conduct, the court is compelled to conclude that the defendants acted with reckless disregard as to the truth or falsity of the submissions.[13]

This standard places healthcare providers (and their top management and governing board members) in the position of having an affirmative obligation to have a mechanism for verifying the accuracy of their organization's claims. A further incentive to do so, if one were needed, is the fact that the government may exclude from participation in the Medicare and Medicaid programs any individual who (a) has a direct or indirect ownership or control interest in a sanctioned entity and has acted in "deliberate ignorance" of the information or (b) is an officer or managing employee of a convicted or excluded entity, *irrespective of whether the individual participated in the offense*.[14] Any excluded person who retains ownership or control or continues as an officer or managing employee may be fined $10,000 *per day*.[15] The threat of "exclusion"—the Medicare and Medicaid programs' equivalent of the death penalty—and the potential for criminal convictions and massive fines have been major impetuses in the move to adopt "corporate compliance programs" in healthcare organizations. (Corporate compliance programs will be discussed later in this chapter.)

FCA cases are usually investigated by OIG and brought by a U.S. attorney. An unusual feature of the statute, however, allows private citizens to sue on their own behalf and for the government to recover damages and penalties. These *qui tam* lawsuits (the name comes from a Latin expression meaning "he who brings the action for the king and for himself") have become an important factor in FCA enforcement because, if successful, the "whistle blower" plaintiff (called a "relator" in legal parlance) can share in the amount of the award.

Any person with information about healthcare fraud can be a *qui tam* plaintiff, and "person" is defined to mean "any natural person, partnership, corporation, association, or other legal entity, including any State or political subdivision of a State."[16] The plaintiff must file the complaint (which is immediately sealed and thus not made public pending investigation) and file a copy with the U.S. attorney general and the appropriate U.S. attorney. The government then has 60 days (plus extensions for good cause) in which to determine whether to pursue the case. If the government decides to take over the case, the relator will receive between 15 and 25 percent of the amount recovered. If the government declines to pursue the matter, the relator may do so and, if successful, will receive between 25 and 30 percent of the recovery.

The potential *qui tam* plaintiff must meet certain conditions to file suit. The plaintiff must be the first to file, there must not already be any government proceeding relating to the same facts, and the suit must not be based on matters that have been publicly disclosed (unless the relator is the "original source" of those disclosures). If these jurisdictional barriers are met and the facts of the case warrant recovery, the *qui tam* plaintiff can proceed to assist the government or pursue the case individually, often to significant financial advantage. Furthermore, federal law provides a remedy for whistle blowers who are discharged, demoted, harassed, or otherwise discriminated against because of their having filed a *qui tam* case.[17] Given the financial incentives and the protection against employment-related retaliation, the *qui tam* lawsuit has become a popular and effective means of combating fraud and abuse.

Recent statistics show that the number of healthcare-related *qui tam* lawsuits increased from 14 in 1992 to more than 280 in 1997.[18] Additionally, "the threat of a FCA suit that may be brought by anybody (competitors, current and previous employees or patients) will be an effective deterrent against greed-motivated individuals who may be tempted to submit fraudulent claims."[19]

Occasionally, healthcare-related *qui tam* plaintiffs have argued that a claim involving a kickback or self-referral (described in more detail below) violates the FCA, even though the claim itself is not "false" on its face. The roots of such an argument can be traced to *United States ex rel. Marcus v. Hess*, a World War II-vintage case in which a government contractor's claims were held to be false because the contract under which they were submitted was entered into as a result of collusion.[20] Similarly, in *United States ex rel. Woodard v. Country View Care Center, Inc.*,[21] the defendants had submitted Medicare cost reports that included payments to "consultants" that were actually kickbacks. Not too surprisingly, because the defendant's reimbursement was based on the cost reports, the court held that the False Claims Act applied. *United States v. Kensington Hospital*,[22] filed after the advent of the prospective payment system, brought a new twist to the argument. The defendants asserted that because their Medicaid reimbursement was a set amount, the government could not have suffered any loss and the cost of the kickbacks did not make the claims false. Citing *Marcus* and other cases, the court disagreed, holding that the government was not required to show actual damages to prove an FCA violation.

In neither *Country View* nor *Kensington Hospital* did the plaintiffs specifically base their claim of FCA liability on the kickback or self-referral statute. Some subsequent cases, however, have done so and have survived initial scrutiny by the courts. For example, an Ohio federal court denied a motion to dismiss a *qui tam* suit involving alleged kickbacks to doctors who referred business to an imaging center. The government alleged that the claims were false even though there was no allegation that the procedures were unnecessary or that the claims misstated the facts regarding the services rendered.[23] And in *United States ex rel. Pogue v. American Healthcorp*,[24] a trial court refused to dismiss a FCA case based on violations of the kickback and Stark self-referral laws. The court agreed with the relator's contention "that participation in any federal program involves an implied certification that the participant will abide by and adhere to all statutes, rules, and regulations governing that program."[25] The court held in effect that Stark violations create prohibited financial relationships and that, therefore, the FCA applies.[26] In *United States ex rel. Thompson v. Columbia/HCA Healthcare Corp.*, however, an FCA case based on alleged violations of the kickback and Stark laws was dismissed by a federal district court because "[a]llegations that medical services were rendered in violation of Medicare anti-fraud statutes do not, by themselves, state a claim for relief under the FCA."[27]

In summary, the proposition that a False Claims Act case can be based solely on violation of the anti-kickback or self-referral laws seems to have gained some acceptance, but the ultimate resolution of the issue remains in doubt. Clearly, relators and the government will continue to make this argument until the point is conclusively established or rejected. In the meantime, it remains an ominous threat for healthcare organizations because the cost of litigating such cases is high and the potential exists for massive penalties. The resulting pressures to settle, rather than litigate, FCA cases may mean that the issue will remain unresolved for some time.[28]

In addition to the civil FCA, another provision of federal law makes false claims a criminal offense.[29] If convicted, an organization can be fined $500,000 or twice the amount of the false claim, whichever is greater. An individual can be fined the greater of $250,000 or twice the amount of the false claim and can be sentenced to up to five years in prison. The standards of proof are higher, of course, in criminal prosecutions than in civil cases. In a civil FCA action the standard is a "preponderance of the evidence." But in a criminal FCA case the government must prove *beyond a reasonable doubt* that the defendant knew the claim was false. Therefore, and because the penalties in civil actions are already quite severe, criminal false claims cases are brought less frequently than their civil counterparts.

THE ANTI-KICKBACK STATUTE

Concerned about the high cost of healthcare and the potential for overutilization of healthcare services, in 1972 Congress prohibited any person to solicit, receive, offer, or pay any form of remuneration in return for or to induce referrals for healthcare goods or services for which Medicare or Medicaid would make payment.[30] Effective January 1, 1997, the statute was amended to cover payment by *any* federal healthcare program.[31] Violations of the anti-kickback law are felonies punishable by criminal fines of $25,000 per violation or imprisonment for up to five years, or both. In addition, the OIG has the authority to exclude from the Medicare and Medicaid programs persons who have violated the act.[32] This action can be taken without criminal prosecution and using the more lenient "preponderance of the evidence" standard. Finally, a 1997 amendment provides for *civil* penalties of $50,000 per violation plus three times the amount of the remuneration involved in addition to the possible criminal sanctions noted above.[33]

The statute contains numerous exceptions to the prohibition of remuneration to induce referrals.[34] The prohibition does not apply to:

- properly disclosed discounts that are reflected in the cost reports;
- amounts paid by an employer to an employee to provide healthcare services;
- certain amounts paid by a vendor to agents of a group purchasing entity;
- waivers of coinsurance for Public Health Service beneficiaries; or
- certain remuneration through a risk-sharing arrangement (e.g., under capitation).

In addition, a 1987 amendment required the Department of Health and Human Services to promulgate regulations "specifying those payment practices that will not be subject to criminal prosecution [or] provide a basis for exclusion. . . ."[35] These regulations provide for certain "safe harbors"—categories of activities in which providers may engage without being subject to prosecution—but they are very technical and are interpreted quite narrowly. The safe harbors are as follows:

- investment in large, publicly traded entities and certain smaller entities, if numerous conditions are met;
- fair market value leases for rental of space or equipment;
- fair market value contracts for personal services;
- purchase of physician practices;
- payments to referral services for patients, so long as the payment is not related to the number of referrals made;
- properly disclosed warranties;
- properly disclosed discounts that are contemporaneous with the original sale;
- bona fide employment relationships;
- discounts available to members of a group purchasing organization;
- waivers of coinsurance and deductibles for indigent persons;
- marketing incentives offered by health plans to enrollees; and
- price reductions offered by providers to health plans.

As mentioned earlier, these regulations are quite technical, and an in-depth analysis of their provisions is beyond the scope of this chapter. It is sufficient to say that although the anti-kickback statute is one of the most important laws affecting healthcare today, it is also, unfortunately, one of the most complicated and ambiguous. Congress itself recognized this fact when it wrote in 1987: "[T]he breadth of the statutory language has created uncertainty among health care providers as to which commercial arrangements are legitimate, and which are proscribed."[36] Unfortunately, although the 1987 amendments that led to the safe harbors listed above were intended to provide guidance and clarity, the basic uncertainty persists.

The problem is illustrated by considering the meaning of the word "referral." Unfortunately, neither the statute nor its implementing regulations define the term, and we are left with considerable uncertainty regarding one of the statute's key terms. For example, is it a "referral" when one member of a multispecialty group practice sends a patient to another member of the same group? If the referring physician's compensation depends in part on the volume of services he or she orders from other group members, is he or she receiving, and is the group paying, remuneration for referrals? These questions have not been answered because no enforcement action has been taken to date regarding intra-group referrals, but a literal reading of the statute calls the practice into question. The creation of a group practice "safe harbor" under the Stark self-referral laws (discussed below) seems to suggest that regulators believe a referral has occurred under those circumstances. Because intra-group referrals will not be Stark violations, the government may refrain to take enforcement action under the anti-kickback law for the same behavior. Whether this proves to be the case remains to be seen, of course.

A similar situation is involved when a medical group owns a hospital. Under traditional indemnity insurance plans, the physicians will benefit financially if they admit patients to their own hospital, yet distribution of the hospital's profits to the physician-owners would appear to violate the literal language of the statute. A proposed regulatory safe harbor for such situations was abandoned in 1993. Thus, the issue remains unresolved.

Hanlester Network v. Shalala illustrates what amounts to remuneration as an inducement for referrals.[37] In *Hanlester,* physicians were limited partners in a network of three clinical laboratories, to which they referred their patients for laboratory work (see Figure 9.1). The laboratories contracted with Smith-Kline Bio-Science Laboratories (SKBL) to manage the facilities for a fee of $15,000 per month or 80 percent of the laboratories' collections, whichever was greater. (As it turned out, the 80 percent figure was generally higher than the fixed monthly fee.) Because performing the tests at SKBL's own laboratories was more economical, 85 to 90 percent of the Hanlester labs' testing was done at SKBL. Even though the cash payments under the arrangement flowed from the Hanlester labs to SKBL, the Ninth Circuit held, among other things, that the arrangement was a scheme by which SKBL in effect had offered a 20 percent discount (the prohibited remuneration) for the physicians' referrals to the SKBL labs. (Note that today the arrangement would also violate the self-referral laws, discussed below.)

Although neither the statute nor the regulations defines "remuneration," it is clear that the law reaches the provision of *anything* having a monetary value. The 20 percent "discount" in *Hanlester* is one example. Likewise, the provision of free goods or services has an economic benefit to the recipient and

Figure 9.1 Hanlester Network Structure

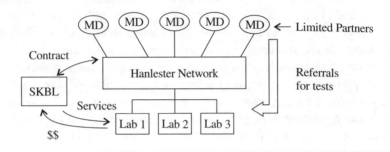

would be prohibited.[38] Furthermore, there is no exception for remuneration of a minimal nature. In one case, a physician was excluded from the Medicare program for having received a kickback in the amount of $30.[39]

Beyond prohibiting payment of remuneration to induce referrals, the anti-kickback law prohibits payment of remuneration to induce or in return for "purchasing, leasing, or ordering of, or arranging for or recommending the purchasing, leasing, or ordering of, any good, facility, service, or item for which payment is made in whole or in part by a federal health care program."[40] For example, it would clearly be illegal for a company that provides patient transportation to provide remuneration to the hospital employee who arranges for patient transportation to encourage that employee to choose that particular company. But query: Is it illegal for a hospital or clinic to provide free transportation to patients who are otherwise unable to come to the facility? In *United States v. Recovery Management Corp. III*, a psychiatric hospital pleaded guilty to an anti-kickback violation after it gave patients free air fares to and from the hospital as an inducement to choose the facility.[41] This case illustrates the fact that the anti-kickback statute applies even where no literal "referral" per se is involved (the referral in this case being the patient's choice of the facility), and it applies to the provision of anything of value that induces patients or providers to purchase or order services.

The practice of waiving coinsurance and deductible amounts is similarly prohibited as an inducement for referrals, except in limited circumstances. The 1996 Health Insurance Portability and Accountability Act (HIPAA; the Kassebaum-Kennedy Act) added civil money penalties that can apply to any person who "offers . . . or transfers remuneration . . . that such person knows or should know is likely to influence [the recipient] to order or receive [goods or services] from a particular provider, practitioner or supplier. . . ."[42] HIPAA defines "remuneration" to include:

the waiver of coinsurance and deductible amounts (or any part thereof), and transfers of items or services for free or for other than fair market value. The term remuneration *does not* include—

(A) the waiver of coinsurance and deductible amounts by a person if—

(i) the waiver is not offered as part of any advertisement or solicitation;

(ii) the person does not routinely waive coinsurance or deductible amounts; and

(iii) the person—

(I) waives the coinsurance and deductible amounts after determining in good faith that the individual is in financial need;

(II) fails to collect coinsurance or deductible amounts after making reasonable collection efforts; or

(III) provides for any permissible waiver as specified in section 1128B(b)(3) [of the Social Security Act] or in regulations issued by the Secretary;

(B) differentials in coinsurance and deductible amounts as part of a benefit plan design as long as the differentials have been disclosed in writing to all beneficiaries, third party payers, and providers . . . ; or

(C) incentives given to individuals to promote the delivery of preventive care as determined by the Secretary in regulations so promulgated.[43]

Thus the waiver of coinsurance and deductibles may be permissible in isolated instances meeting the criteria of HIPAA quoted above, but a practice of routinely waiving those amounts, and particularly of advertising that fact in the hope of stimulating business, would appear to violate the anti-kickback statute as an inducement for referrals.

The anti-kickback statute is one of the most important fraud and abuse statutes affecting healthcare today. Unfortunately, given the nearly infinite number of arrangements possible among healthcare-related organizations, it is also one of the most difficult to apply with any certainty. Because the penalties for violating the law can be extremely harsh, readers must be generally aware of its provisions and must be prepared to seek competent legal counsel whenever there is any question about the propriety of their conduct.

THE "STARK" SELF-REFERRAL LAWS

The Ethics in Patient Referrals Act (EPRA),[44] first enacted in 1989 and amended in 1993, was championed by Rep. Fortney "Pete" Stark of California. Its purpose, like that of the anti-kickback statute, is to discourage overuse of healthcare services and thus reduce the cost of the Medicare and Medicaid programs. As stated by HCFA:

Congress enacted this law because it was concerned that many physicians were gaining significant financial advantages from the practice of referring their

[Medicare and Medicaid] patients to providers of health care services with which they (or their immediate family members) had financial relationships. For example, if a physician owns a separate laboratory that performs laboratory tests for his or her patients and shares in the profits of that laboratory, the physician has an incentive to overuse laboratory services. Similarly, if a physician does not own any part of an entity but receives compensation from it for any reason, that compensation may be calculated in a manner that reflects the volume or value of referrals the physician makes to the entity.

The reports of 10 studies in the professional literature, taken as a whole, demonstrate conclusively that the utilization rates of medical items and services generally increase when the ordering physician has a financial interest in the entity providing the item or service. These self-referrals generate enormous costs to the Medicare and Medicaid programs and jeopardize the health status of program beneficiaries.[45]

The provisions of the EPRA—commonly referred to as "Stark I" and "Stark II" (or simply "Stark")—are extremely complicated, and their application must be analyzed on a case-by-case basis. The law can, however, be summarized as follows.

In general, Stark prohibits a physician (a medical doctor, doctor of osteopathy, dentist, podiatrist, optometrist, or chiropractor) from referring Medicare or Medicaid patients for certain "designated health services" to entities with which the physician or an immediate family member has a financial relationship. "Financial relationship" is defined as a compensation arrangement or an ownership or investment interest (such as through equity or debt). If such a relationship exists, the physician may not, unless an exception applies, refer patients to the entity for the following kinds of services:

- clinical laboratory services;
- radiology services (including MRIs, CAT scans, and ultrasound);
- radiation therapy services and supplies;
- physical and occupational therapy services;
- durable medical equipment and supplies;
- parenteral and enteral nutrients, equipment, and supplies;
- prosthetics, orthotics, and prosthetic devices and supplies;
- outpatient prescription drugs;
- home health services;
- outpatient prescription drugs; and
- inpatient and outpatient hospital services.

Violations of the Stark law can result in various sanctions, including denial of payment for the services, an obligation to refund any payments made, civil money penalties of up to $15,000 for *each* illegal referral, and possible exclusion from the Medicare and Medicaid programs. In addition, a physician or entity that enters into a cross-referral arrangement or other scheme to bypass Stark can be fined up to $100,000 for each such arrangement and can be excluded from the programs. Stark also imposes an obligation on each entity that provides designated health services to report the names and identification numbers of all physicians who have a compensation arrangement or an ownership or investment interest in the entity to the Secretary of Health and Human Services. Failure to do so can result in a civil money penalty of up to $10,000 for each day for which reporting was required. Unlike the anti-kickback law, which requires proof that the defendant acted "knowingly and willfully," making a prohibited referral is a per se violation of Stark and no proof of intent is required. The fact that a defendant acted in good faith or that he or she was unaware of the law is not a defense. The anti-kickback and Stark laws differ in one other respect: the former applies to *anyone*, whereas the latter applies *only* to physicians.

The basic provisions of Stark are extremely broad and complex, as HCFA recognizes:

> The law is . . . complex because it attempts to accommodate the many complicated financial relationships that exist in the health care community. The prohibitions are based on the general principle that if a physician has a financial relationship with an entity that furnishes items or services, he or she cannot refer patients to the entity. However, the law provides numerous exceptions to this general principle, and it is the exceptions that contain the most detailed and complicated aspects of the law. The exceptions are complicated because they attempt to achieve a balance that allows physicians and providers to maintain some of their financial relationships, but within bounds that are designed to prevent the abuse of the Medicare and Medicaid programs or their patients.[46]

As this quotation notes, Congress provided for certain exceptions to the self-referral ban because without them the law's sweeping language would have made many legitimate, laudable, and even necessary arrangements illegal. For example, the law excepts referrals for services provided by other physicians in the same group practice and most in-office ancillary services furnished "personally by the referring physician, personally by a physician who is a member of the same group practice . . . , or personally by individuals who are directly supervised by the physician or by another physician in the group practice. . . ."[47] Such in-office ancillary services must, however, be billed by the physician or the group practice,[48] and they must be provided in the group's building or in another building used by the group for the centralized provision of such services.[49]

Likewise, because the financial incentive for self-referral does not exist with prepaid health plans (HMOs, for example), the statute does not apply when a physician refers members of such plans for designated health services.[50] It also does not apply to referrals for services provided by a hospital in which the physician has an ownership or investment interest and at which the physician is authorized to perform services.[51] It is notable that physicians who are merely employed by a hospital rather than owners or investors cannot avail themselves of this exception; instead, a more detailed exception relating to employment relationships is provided later in the statute.[52]

In addition to the above exceptions, there are exceptions for certain kinds of financial relationships.[53] The financial relationships that will not trigger Stark can be summarized as follows:

- owning stocks or bonds in a large, publicly traded company or mutual fund;
- owning or investing in certain rural providers or hospitals in Puerto Rico;
- reasonable rent for office space or equipment;
- amounts paid under fair and bona fide employment relationships;
- reasonable payments for personal services provided to the entity or for other services unrelated to the provision of designated health services;
- compensation under a legitimate "physician incentive plan" (such as by withholds, capitation, or bonuses in managed care);
- reasonable payments to induce a physician to relocate to the hospital's service area;
- isolated transactions such as a one-time sale of property or a practice;
- an arrangement that began before December 19, 1989, in which services are provided by a physician group but are billed by the hospital; and
- reasonable payments by a physician for clinical laboratory services or for other items or services.

These exceptions to Stark are much more complicated than the simple list above implies. They have been the subject of much controversy and have generated many ambiguities. For example, it is unclear whether the "isolated transactions" exception would apply to the purchase of a physician's practice where payment for the practice is made in installments rather than in a lump sum. HCFA takes the position that the exception would not apply and that installment payments are prohibited. To avoid this interpretation, some have suggested making the payments not as installments but as an additional part of the physician's employment-related compensation. But the exception for employment relationships is limited to amounts paid for the provision of *services*. Thus, HCFA takes the position that the "employment relationships" exception is inapplicable as well. One can argue that *how* the physician is paid for the practice is irrelevant because in the employment relationship there is an inherent incentive to refer, and yet employment relationships are exempt from Stark. Nevertheless, HCFA persists in its interpretation, and because the question has not been litigated, it stands unresolved as an example of the law's ambiguity.

One can see another example of ambiguity in the case of plans for a patient's care by a home health agency (HHA). A physician employed by a hospital that owns a home health agency would presumably want to order home health services to be provided by the hospital's HHA. The question arises whether the physician's financial relationship with the hospital also constitutes a financial relationship with the HHA. HCFA opined privately in 1996 that it *does* and that, therefore, the physician cannot refer to the HHA. This opinion had not been the basis for enforcement action through the end of 1998, but proposed regulations issued in January 1998 seem to perpetuate this view. Specifically, in addressing the physician "ownership or investment interest" exception, the regulations indicate that the physicians may refer to hospitals in which they have an ownership or investment interest, but only for services provided *by the hospital*. They may not avail themselves of the "ownership or investment" exception with regard to services provided by the hospital-owned HHA. This interpretation, of course, raises a whole new set of ambiguities. What are "services provided by the hospital," for example? If the hospital uses a separate provider number to bill for some services (e.g., radiology), are those services to be considered provided by the hospital or by a separate entity?

As this example shows, each issuance of "guidance" and "clarifying" regulations—although helpful in some respects—adds new uncertainties, increases healthcare providers' uneasiness, and makes the practice of law in this area extremely difficult. Because of the ambiguities and complexities involved, the importance of expert legal counsel cannot be overemphasized.

CORPORATE COMPLIANCE PROGRAMS

As one can see from the above discussion, healthcare organizations must be sensitive to their potential for fraud and abuse or other criminal conduct. Violations of law can lead to convictions of the individuals involved and to monetary penalties levied against both the perpetrators and the organization, even if the crime occurred at the lowest levels and was contrary to express corporate policy. Not only are the perpetrators and the organization subject to prosecution, but officers and management can be convicted for the conduct of their subordinates under certain circumstances, even though they neither authorized the crime nor had knowledge of it. Under the "responsible official" doctrine, officers and managers may be held personally accountable if they deliberately or recklessly disregarded the possibility of the criminal conduct occurring. It is, therefore, clearly a mistake to believe "what I don't know can't hurt me."

One of the most effective tools to minimize an organization's and its board's and management's exposure is an effective corporate compliance program (CCP). This section describes the elements of a CCP and how one should be developed.

The CCP concept gained salience after the publication of the federal government's *Sentencing Guidelines for Organizations*,[54] which is used by federal judges during the sentencing phase of a trial when a corporation has been convicted of a violation of law. The *Guidelines* are intended to provide a measure of uniformity and predictability in federal criminal sentences. Although criminal violations can occur in many areas (such as antitrust, taxation, environmental, employment, and, in the case of healthcare providers, confidentiality of patient information), the most fertile ground for illegal activity in healthcare is, of course, fraud and abuse. As noted earlier, federal and state governments are cracking down on healthcare fraud because by some estimates up to 10 percent of the United States' annual healthcare spending may result from fraudulent activity. Enforcement activities have led to penalties in the hundreds of millions of dollars in individual cases, and fines of hundreds of thousands of dollars are common.

To protect against this frightening scenario, many providers have begun to implement corporate cmpliance programs—systematic efforts to prevent, detect, report, and correct criminal misconduct and provide ongoing review of policies, procedures, and operations. Properly structured, a corporate compliance program will address the healthcare organization's potential liability in all areas of law, not just fraud and abuse. If the CCP is effectively implemented and is supported and encouraged by its governing board and top management, the program becomes powerful evidence that the organization took steps to prevent criminal violations by its employees and agents. It also demonstrates good faith, a critical factor in determining what sentence will be assessed in the event of a conviction.

Without a CCP, a convicted organization will incur much stiffer penalties and will usually face a court-imposed compliance program more severe than the sentencing guidelines require. Under the *Guidelines*, however, an organization with an effective CCP will benefit from penalty reductions of up to 95 percent. The following example illustrates this point. Assume that two hospitals, each with 3,000 employees,[55] are convicted of defrauding Medicare through coding errors. Assume further that the frauds resulted in overpayment of $1,600,000 to each facility. Hospital A does not have a corporate compliance program, and, in fact, its management was found "willfully ignorant" of the existence of the fraudulent activity.[56] Hospital B, on the other hand, has an effective CCP, discovered the fraud, and reported it to the authorities immediately. According to the *Guidelines*, the potential penalties for the two hospitals will be computed as follows:

	Hospital A	*Hospital B*
Base fine (usually the amount of the overpayment)	$1,600,000	$1,600,000
Culpability score (determined from a table):		
Base score (identical for all defendants)	5	5
Willful ignorance factor (aggravating)	4	4
Effective CCP factor (mitigating)	0	−3
Self-reporting factor (mitigating)	0	−5
Total Culpability Score:	**9**	**< 0**
Culpability multiplier range (CMR) (from a table)	1.8 to 3.6	0.05 to 0.2
Minimum fine (low CMR × base fine)	$2,880,000	$80,000
Maximum fine (high CMR × base fine)	$5,760,000	$320,000

In addition to reducing the organization's criminal sentence in the event a violation occurs, an effective CCP may also provide early detection of conduct that could lead to civil enforcement efforts by the government, *qui tam* litigation, or other civil actions. The CCP's preventive activities allow management to take corrective action before suit is filed and to show due diligence if the matter goes to trial.

Notwithstanding the obvious benefits, CCPs do have certain drawbacks. One is their cost: depending on the size and complexity of the organization and the number of attorneys and consultants required, the direct expense involved in starting the program will be at least $250,000 and may easily exceed $1 million. When one factors in staff time, other fixed costs, and the cost of on-going implementation efforts, a CCP appears to be an expensive proposition indeed. Another disadvantage is that during the CCP development phase the organization may uncover past criminal activities. If so, the offenders will have to be dealt with and the conduct may have to be reported to the proper authorities. A final negative consideration is that, like all internal policies, the CCP will be viewed as the organization's self-established "standard of care." If the CCP is not followed, that fact could be seen as evidence of negligence or recklessness and could increase the sentence or verdict if a case goes to trial. Despite these considerations, the benefits of a CCP far outweigh the potential disadvantages.

The elements of an effective CCP are as follows. First, it must contain established compliance standards and procedures. This requires management to publish for its employees standards of conduct outlining legal requirements in all areas that affect the organization's business operations. Such areas include antitrust, document retention, employment and employee benefits, environmental compliance, Medicare/Medicaid fraud and abuse, occupational safety, patient protection, and taxation. Second, the CCP must be overseen by high-level personnel. Most organizations assign the function (either as a collateral duty or a full-time position) to an individual who reports to the chief executive officer and also has a relationship with the governing board. Third, the CCP must provide that no discretionary authority in the organization may be vested in persons who are known to be (or *should* be known to be) likely to engage in criminal conduct. In effect, this means that the organization must have a mechanism (such as a policy requiring criminal background checks) to prevent the hiring of persons who, for example, have previously been convicted of healthcare offenses or who have been excluded from Medicare and Medicaid.

The fourth element of an effective CCP is the communication of the standards of conduct and CCP procedures to employees and agents of the organization. This means that the organization must educate all employees and agents about the requirements of the CCP (its standards and related procedures) and must continually publicize the topic in employee newsletters and similar media. In effect, the CCP must have the commitment and understanding of everyone in the organization, including not only the board and senior management, but also lower-level employees. Without this level of support, the CCP may be viewed as a sham, which could lead to harsher penalties being assessed. Fifth, the CCP must establish reasonable methods to achieve compliance with the standards of conduct. These methods should include ongoing monitoring activities, periodic audits of various operational departments, and encouragement to employees to report suspicious activities (for example, through "hotlines" or anonymous written reports). Sixth, the CCP must provide for and the organization must carry out appropriate and consistent discipline (including possible termination of employment) for those who violate the standards of conduct or fail to report violations. And seventh, there must be appropriate and consistent responses to violations that are detected, including necessary corrective action to prevent recurrence.

CONCLUSION

Healthcare organizations, including their governing boards and senior management, must take seriously the possibility that criminal violations (including fraud and abuse) may occur in the course of their business. Although the cost of developing a corporate compliance program is significant, the consequences of not having a CCP can be dire if criminal conduct occurs, and significant benefits may accrue in the form of reduced exposure to *qui tam* suits and other civil actions. Each healthcare organization should begin immediately to adopt and implement effective corporate compliance programs covering their entire operation.

NOTES

Portions of this chapter appeared in Gunn, Goldfarb, and Showalter, *Creating a Corporate Compliance Program*, 79 HEALTH PROGRESS 60 (May–June 1998), and are reprinted here with permission.

1. General Accounting Office, *Report on Medicare Fraud and Abuse*, GAO/HR-95-8 (Feb. 1995).
2. U.S. Dept. of Justice, *Department of Justice Health Care Fraud Report, Fiscal Year 1994* (Mar. 2, 1995).
3. 768 F. Supp. 1127 (E.D. Pa. 1991).
4. 859 F. Supp. 5 (D. D.C. 1994).
5. 909 F. Supp. 32 (D. D.C. 1995) (memorandum opinion).
6. 31 U.S.C. §§ 3729-3731.
7. This last provision was added in 1986 to deal with "reverse false claims," situations in which a person attempts to avoid paying money owed to the government.
8. *See, e.g.,* Rex Trailer Co. v. United States, 350 U.S. 148 (1952) and Fleming v. United States, 336 F.2d 475 (10th Cir. 1964).
9. United States v. Krizek, 111 F.3d 394 (D.C. Cir. 1997).
10. *See, e.g.,* United States v. McNinch, 356 U.S. 595 (1958).
11. 31 U.S.C. § 3729(b).
12. S. Rep. No. 345, 99th Cong., 2d Sess. 7.
13. 859 F. Supp. at 13. *But see*, United States v. Nazon, No. 93-C5456m (N.D. Ill. Oct. 14, 1993).
14. Pub. L. No. 104-191, § 213, amending 42 U.S.C. § 1320a-7(b)(15).
15. 42 U.S.C. § 1320a-7a(a)(4).
16. 31 U.S.C. § 3733(l)(4).
17. 31 U.S.C. § 3730(h).
18. *See, Federal Enforcers Urge Healthcare Companies to Police Their Own Fraud*, Vol. 1, No. 12, HEALTH L. NEWS 4 (Dec. 1998). An organization known as Taxpayers Against Fraud reports that total *qui tam* recoveries of all kinds were approximately $1.5 billion from the time of the 1986 amendments through October 1996. Cases arising in the Department of Defense accounted for the largest number of *qui tam* cases filed, but the number of HHS-related cases has been increasing steadily. Of the cases pending in October 1996, "approximately 80% involve DOD or HHS, and they are equally divided between the two." Taxpayers Against Fraud, www.taf.org.
19. Paschke, *The Qui Tam Provision of the Federal False Claims Act: The Statute in Current Form, Its History and Its Unique Position to Influence the Health Care Industry*, 9 J.L. & HEALTH 163, 179 (1994–95).

20. 317 U.S. 537 (1943); *see also* United States v. Forster Wheeler Corp., 447 F.2d 100 (2d Cir. 1971) (invoices submitted on contract that was based on inflated cost estimates are false claims) *and* United States v. Veneziale, 268 F.2d 504 (3d Cir. 1959) (fraudulently induced contract may create liability when the contract later results in payment by the government).

21. 797 F.2d 888 (10th Cir. 1986).

22. 760 F. Supp. 1120 (E.D. Pa. 1991).

23. United States *ex rel.* Roy v. Anthony, 914 F. Supp. 1507 (S.D. Ohio 1994).

24. 914 F. Supp. 1507 (M.D. Tenn. 1996).

25. *Id.* at 1508-1509.

26. *Id.* at 1513.

27. 938 F. Supp. 405 (S.D. Tex. 1996). *See also* United States v. Oakwood Downriver Medical Center, 687 F. Supp. 302 (E.D. Mich. 1988) *and* United States v. Shaw, 725 F. Supp. 896 (S.D. Miss. 1989) (holding, in a case involving bribes to a Farmers Home Administration official, "[t]he bare fact that bribes were involved . . . does not necessarily lead to the further conclusion that false or fraudulent claims were made in connection with each of the loan applications or preapplications." *Id.* at 900.).

28. At least one consent judgment has been entered in a case of this type. In 1994, a company that ran home infusion centers agreed to pay $500,000 in settlement of an FCA case because it gave physicians incentives to refer patients to the centers. United States v. T[su'2'] Medical, Inc., Ga. No. 1:94-CV-2549 (N.D. Ga. Sept. 26, 1994).

29. 18 U.S.C. § 287.

30. 42 U.S.C. § 1320a-7b(b)(1)(A) and (2)(A).

31. Pub. L. No. 104-191, § 204, 110 Stat. 1999, codified at 42 U.S.C. § 1320a-7b(a).

32. 42 U.S.C. § 1320a-7(b)(7).

33. 42 U.S.C. § 1320a-7a(a)(7).

34. 42 U.S.C. § 1320a-7b(b)(3).

35. 42 U.S.C. § 1320a-7b.

36. S. Rep. No. 109, 100th Cong., 1st Sess. 27.

37. 51 F.3d 1390 (9th Cir. 1995).

38. Office of Inspector Gen., U.S. Dept. of Health & Human Servs., Advisory Op. No. 97-6 (Oct. 8, 1997).

39. Levin v. Inspector General, No. CR343 (HHS Dept. App. Bd. Nov. 10, 1994).

40. *See* 42 U.S.C. §§ 1320a-7b(b)(1)(B) and (2)(B).

41. Unreported decision cited in "Psychiatric Hospital Firm Pleads Guilty to Violating Anti-Kickback Statute," 4 BNA's HEALTH L. REP. 687

42. 42 U.S.C. § 1320a-7a(a)(5).

43. 42 U.S.C. § 1320a-7a(i)(6) (emphasis added).

44. Codified at 42 U.S.C. § 1395nn.

45. HCFA Trans. No. AB-95-3 (Jan. 1995), *reprinted in* BNA's HEALTH L. & BUS. SERIES No. 2400 at 2400:3401, 3402 (1997).

46. *Id.* at 2400:3403.

47. 42 U.S.C. § 1395nn(b)(2)(A)(i).

48. 42 U.S.C. § 1395nn(b)(2)(B).
49. 42 U.S.C. § 1395nn(b)(2)(A)(ii).
50. 42 U.S.C. § 1395nn(b)(3).
51. 42 U.S.C. § 1395nn(d)(3).
52. 42 U.S.C. § 1395nn(e)(2).
53. *See generally,* 42 U.S.C. § 1395nn(c)-(e) and the discussion below.
54. 56 Fed. Reg. 22,762, 22,786 (May 16, 1991).
55. The size of the organization is a factor in the *Guidelines'* sentencing formula.
56. Willful ignorance is an aggravating factor in the formula.

10

Influencing Public Policy Environments

Beaufort B. Longest, Jr., Ph.D., FACHE

ublic policies are important elements in the environments of all types of organizations, including those involved in healthcare (Buchholz 1989, 1993; Longest; 1988, 1994). One need look no further than the effect of federal Medicare and the combination of federal and state Medicaid policies to see the direct relationship of public policies to healthcare organizations. Beyond this rather obvious example of the effect of public financing policy, there are numerous other public policies that are important elements in the environments of healthcare organizations—policies that fund programs, regulate market-related decisions and behaviors, facilitate medical research and education, and so on.

Thus, strategymakers in healthcare organizations must be concerned both about effectively analyzing and about influencing their public policy environments. They must seek information about public policies and they must help shape public policies when the policies and their related issues are of strategic importance to their organizations. Typically, such strategymakers seek to ensure that their organizations develop information about relevant policy issues before impact is felt so that strategically sound preparations and adjustments can be made. They do this by using the environmental analysis process and supporting techniques described in the previous chapter.

In addition, they seek to influence the formulation, implementation, and modification of relevant public policies using the techniques described in

Editor's Note: This chapter is from Chapter 5 of *Seeking Strategic Advantage Through Health Policy Analysis* by Beaufort B. Longest, Jr., 1996, HAP this chapter. Strategymakers are fulfilling their obligations to manage the relationship between public policy and their organizations only when both their analysis and influence responsibilities are properly met.

The purpose of this chapter is to consider the processes through which strategymakers in healthcare organizations can legitimately and ethically influence the public policymaking process and through this the public policies that are relevant to their organizations.

This chapter also includes a discussion of specific methods to influence the policymaking process at the various points of possible intervention, and it concludes with consideration of the ethical issues inherent in intervening in the public policymaking process. Inclusion of these ethical considerations is important because, although there is nothing innately wrong with exerting influence on the public policymaking process, it must be noted that the process can be tainted by overzealous attempts to influence policies for self-serving purposes.

Before discussing where and how influence can be exerted, some background information on the issue of who is responsible for this activity in healthcare organizations and on the concept of influence in general is presented.

RESPONSIBILITY FOR INFLUENCING PUBLIC POLICY ENVIRONMENTS

The authority and responsibility for influencing the public policy environments of healthcare organizations are reserved predominantly for their strategymakers; that is, for their senior-level managers and members of their governing boards. Unlike the analysis of public policy environments as discussed in the previous chapter, influencing public policy environments is typically not assigned to separate departments or units at all, although there may be board committees with oversight responsibilities. Importantly, in most healthcare organizations this stands in contrast to the widespread organization design practice of establishing a department or unit to house the environmental analysis work, along with other strategymaking or strategic planning activities.

Some healthcare organizations do, however, run against the general trend of not assigning responsibility for influencing public policy environments to particular departments. Many of the larger, more complex healthcare organizations, such as academic medical centers or large integrated healthcare systems and networks, establish departments or units specifically charged to conduct work related to influencing the public policy environments of these organizations. These departments are typically called public affairs departments or government affairs or relations departments. Some very large organizations even divide government relations into separate departments, one for the federal government and another for the state government.

When departments that are devoted to influencing public policy environments exist as separate units in an organization's design, they are very likely to be staff units with their own director, who reports to the organization's president or another senior-level manager or strategymaker. Importantly, even when an organization has a staff department that is devoted to influencing its public policy environment, the role of the organization's strategymakers in this process is still vital. Such departments mainly serve to enhance the ability of the organization's strategymakers to succeed in *their* efforts to influence the public policy environment to the organization's advantage.

When actual healthcare organization designs include assigning the analysis and influence duties to different departments or units, it becomes very important that attention be devoted to coordinating both sets of work. The most important way to ensure effective coordination is for strategymakers to insist that the coordination occur. By taking ultimate responsibility, exerting authority over both departments and involving themselves in both sets of work, they can be certain that the expertise and insight held by the people involved in each set of work informs and supports those involved in the other work. For example, valuable information about what aspects of a public policy environment to scan and monitor might well come from people who are intimately involved in trying to influence an organization's public policy environment. Similarly, effective scanning, monitoring, forecasting, and assessing of public policy environments can help establish the most appropriate and promising targets for efforts to influence public policy environments to strategic advantage.

Looking Outside the Organization for Help

The challenges involved for strategymakers to analyze and correctly interpret the effect of relevant issues in their public policy environment and to influence this environment to the strategic advantage of their organization are quite substantial. In large measure, this is the case because so many others are simultaneously seeking to exert their own influence in pursuit of their own preferences in this environment. Strategymakers in healthcare organizations, even very large ones, cannot hope to meet these challenges successfully by relying exclusively on the use of their own internal resources.

Given the extensive and dynamic set of forces and actors at work in their organization's public policy environment, strategymakers must frequently turn for assistance to outside resources in fulfilling both their analysis and influence responsibilities. The primary source of such assistance is the interest groups to which strategymakers and their organizations belong. In this chapter, the focus is on the mechanisms and techniques available to strategymakers themselves to influence their organization's public policy environment.

No matter how a healthcare organization is designed internally to influence its public policy environment, or how its strategymakers use the help of outside interest groups, the bottom line of exerting influence in public policy environments is that eventually influence must actually be exerted. In the next section, the concept of influence is defined and examined.

THE CONCEPT OF INFLUENCE

Within the context of the political marketplace where public policymaking occurs, many participants seek to further their objectives. Their objectives can be self-interest objectives involving some economic or political advantage or public-interest objectives involving certain participants' perception of what is best for the nation or society. In both cases, the outcome depends greatly on the relative abilities of participants in the exchanges within the marketplace to influence or shape the actions, behaviors, and decisions of other participants. The relevant participants in the public policy environments of healthcare organizations are the "demanders" of public policies (i.e., the strategymakers in the healthcare organizations as well as people inside and outside their organizations who support their efforts) and the "suppliers" of public policies (i.e., those in the legislative, executive, and judicial branches of government with policymaking duties and roles as well as people inside and outside government who exert influence on their decisions).

The exertion of influence in these public policy environments is "simply the process by which people successfully persuade others to follow their advice, suggestion, or order" (Keys and Case 1990, 38). But to have influence one must first have power. Power, whether it occurs in economic or political markets, is necessary because in the context of market relationships and exchanges it is the potential to exert influence. More power means more potential to influence others. Therefore, to understand influence, one must first understand power. Those who wish to exert influence in the political marketplace must first acquire power. But how do they do so, and what are the various sources of power available to them?

Sources of Power in Political Markets

Strategymakers in a healthcare organization, just as those in other types of organizations, have three bases of power that permit them to influence their organization's public policy environment: positional power, the power to reward or coerce others, and the power that derives from the possession of expertise or information. Briefly:

- **Positional power** derives from a person's position in a social system or in an organization; this form of power is also called *formal power* or *authority*. It exists because societies find it advantageous to assign certain powers to individuals to enable them to perform their jobs or fulfill their roles effectively. Thus, elected officials, appointed executives, and judges, as well as strategymakers in healthcare organizations, association professionals, corporation executives, union leaders, individual voters, and many other participants in the political marketplace, possess certain legitimate power that accompanies their social or organizational positions.

- **Power to reward or coerce** others is based on a person's ability to reward compliance, or to punish noncompliance, with the preferred decisions, actions, and behaviors that are sought from others. This form of power stems in part from the positional power that a person holds. Superiors in organizations have this base of power over their subordinates and leaders in Congress have it over the members. Such power stems from the ability to supply or withhold from any person something of value to that person, whether money, vacations, promises of future employment for the person or their family members, and so on.

- **Expert power** derives from possessing expertise or information that is valued by others. Within the political marketplace, such expertise as that necessary for solving problems or performing crucial tasks can be extremely important.

Importantly, for the effective use and effect of power, these three bases in the political marketplace are interdependent, and they can and do complement each other. People whose positions in society or in organizations permit them to use reward power, and who do so wisely, can strengthen their positional power. Similarly, people in positions of power typically have more opportunities to reward or coerce others. Expertise, especially that based on exclusive access to information, is frequently a function of a person's position or access to people in certain positions. Such access can be facilitated through the power to reward or coerce.

Effective participants in the marketplace for policies are those who succeed at translating their power into influence and they tend to be aware of the sources of their power and to act accordingly. Effective participants seem to be those who "understand—at least intuitively—the costs, risks, and benefits of using each kind of power and are able to recognize which to draw on in different situations and with different people" (Morlock, Nathanson, and Alexander 1988, 268).

What enables certain people to use effectively the power to which they have access—that is, to translate power into influence in the political marketplace—is their interpersonal and political skills. It is not enough to have access to power; one must also know how to use it in order to influence others. Mintzberg, perhaps as much as anyone, has recognized this important fact. He attributes success in using power largely to a person's relative political skills, which he defines as

> the ability to use the bases of power effectively—to convince those to whom one has access, to use one's resources, information, and technical skills to their fullest in bargaining, to exercise formal power with a sensitivity to the feelings of others, to know where to concentrate one's energies, to sense what is possible, to organize the necessary alliances (Mintzberg 1983, 26).

The Appropriate Focus of Influence

Strategymakers in healthcare organizations should be guided in their efforts to influence policies by focusing on the same activities that they were advised in the previous chapter to use as the focus for their environmental scanning activities. That is, their influencing activities should be guided by the identification of policies that are of strategic importance to their organizations as well as by identification of problems, potential solutions, and political circumstances that might eventually lead to such policies. By focusing in this way, they will seek to influence relevant policymakers strategically in all three branches and in federal, state, and local levels of government. Furthermore, they will extend their efforts to influence to those who have influence with these policymakers. If they are to influence the policymaking process effectively, in addition to influencing policymakers directly, strategymakers must also concern themselves with shaping the conceptualizations of problems, the development of potential solutions to the problems, as well as with the political circumstances that help drive the policymaking process. The suppliers of public policies, and those who can influence them, form the appropriate focus for strategymakers who seek to influence the public policies that will affect their organizations.

In short, strategymakers should exert their influence throughout the entire public policy environment of their organization. A good map to this complex terrain can be very useful.

A MAP TO PLACES WHERE THE PUBLIC POLICYMAKING PROCESS CAN BE INFLUENCED

The model of the policymaking process shown in Figure 10.1 can be used to identify the places in the process where strategymakers, either working independently, or, as is more often the case, working in concert with others with similar interests through associations or other collaboratives, can exert influence.

Figure 10.1 A Model of the Public Policymaking Process in the United States

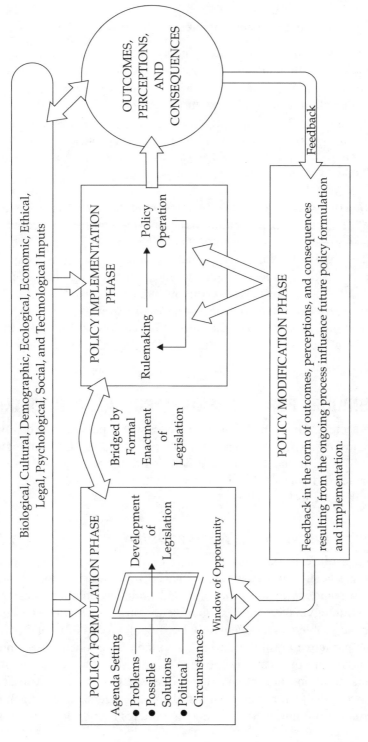

Source: Health Policymaking in the United States (p. 160), 1994 by B. B. Longest, Jr. Adapted by permission of AUPHA/Health Administration Press.

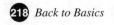

Figure 10.1 includes three interconnected phases:

- policy formulation, which incorporates activities associated with agenda setting and subsequently with the development of legislation;
- policy implementation, which incorporates activities associated with rulemaking and policy operation; and
- policy modification, which exists because perfection cannot be achieved in the other phases and because policies are established and exist in a dynamic world where events and circumstances routinely render existing policies inadequate.

Thinking of Figure 10.1 as a map enables strategymakers to see that the places where efforts to influence public policymaking can be focused are agenda setting, legislation development, rulemaking, and policy operation.

The circular flow of the relationships among the various components of the policymaking process reflects the fact that policymaking is an ongoing process in which almost all decisions are subject to subsequent modification. This feature greatly increases opportunities for strategymakers in healthcare organizations, as well as for others, to influence policies. In effect, those who would influence public policies usually have more than one opportunity to do so.

TECHNIQUES FOR INFLUENCING PUBLIC POLICYMAKING

In this section, following the map of places where policies can be influenced shown in Figure 10.1, a variety of techniques through which strategymakers can exert their influence are identified and described. As will be seen, the techniques differ according to the place in the overall policymaking process where they are used.

Exerting Influence on Agenda Setting

A logical place to begin is on the left side of the policymaking model, where the health policy agenda is shaped by the interaction of problems, possible solutions to the problems, and political circumstances (Kingdon 1995). Strategymakers can exert influence on policymaking by helping to define the problems that eventually become the focus of public policymaking, by participating in the design of possible solutions to these problems, and by helping to create the political circumstances necessary to convert potential solutions into actual policies. In short, policies can be influenced by influencing the factors that establish the policy agenda itself. Each of these important opportunities for influencing policies is considered in turn.

Problems

The scope of problems that can be addressed through the public policymaking process is massive. Even the fraction of all these problems that are of strategic importance to strategymakers in healthcare organizations is large and diverse. After all, health is determined in human populations by several factors acting in combination: the physical, sociocultural, and economic environments in which people live; their lifestyles, behaviors, and genetics; as well as by the type, quality, and timing of healthcare services that they receive (Evans and Stoddart 1994). Problems, real or perceived, in all these areas are of interest to strategymakers. But how do they influence agenda setting around the array of problems in which they have strategic interest? The answer requires a consideration of how the problems that eventually stimulate policymaking come to occupy places on the agenda.

Some problems that drive policymaking emerge because a condition or situation reaches a critical mass or a highly visible or unacceptably troublesome level. Examples include the prevalence of HIV in the population and the growing number of those without health insurance. Another example is the increasing cost to the federal government of the Medicare program and to the states for operating their Medicaid programs. Other problems emerge by virtue of specific events that force attention to them, such as medical waste products washing up on beaches or the discovery of a new drug for treating a relatively rare disorder that is so expensive few people can purchase it on their own. Still other problems are spotlighted by their widespread applicability to many people (e.g., the high cost of prescription medications) or by their sharply focused effect on a small but powerful group (e.g., the high cost of medical education).

Strategymakers in healthcare organizations, because of their positions and of the environmental scanning activities they engage in can be among the first to observe certain types of problems, sometimes in their early stages. This gives them an important means through which to help shape the policy agenda. Strategymakers are often well-positioned, especially when they act in concert, to document problems—to gather, catalog, and correlate facts that depict the actual state of a problem and to share this information with policymakers. Problem definition and documentation can exert a powerful influence on the agenda setting that precedes all public policymaking.

An example of problem definition by strategymakers in healthcare organizations that eventually led to a specific policy to address the problem can be seen in the background of Maine's Hospital Cooperation Act of 1992 (Cerne 1993; Kania 1993). Prior to establishment of this legislation, if hospitals in Maine sought to form coalitions to purchase and share expensive technologies or to cooperate in other cost-reducing efforts, they risked violating antitrust laws. As the costs of new technologies grew and as the pressures to contain healthcare costs increased, some of Maine's hospital strategymakers sought legislation that would offer them at least limited protection from the antitrust restrictions so that they could establish cooperative agreements to share expensive technologies or scarce professional personnel to contain healthcare costs.

Through the coordinating efforts of the Maine Hospital Association, the strategymakers' account of the problems they faced in containing costs and of the limitations imposed on cooperative and collaborative solutions by the threat of antitrust sanctions was sufficiently documented. The documentation allowed them to prove the problem and as a result it became part of the public policy agenda in Maine. Eventually, the legislature enacted P.L. 814, the Hospital Cooperation Act of 1992, in response (Michaud 1992).

This policy permitted, under specified circumstances, cooperative agreements among or between hospitals in Maine. In the language of the legislation, "cooperative agreement means an agreement among two or more hospitals for the sharing, allocation or referral of patients, personnel, instructional programs, support services and facilities or medical, diagnostic or laboratory facilities or procedures or other services traditionally offered by hospitals." This policy was enacted through a string of policymaking activities that began with the strategymakers in Maine hospitals documenting to the state legislature that a problem existed that could be at least partially addressed through a policy change.

Possible Solutions

The mere existence of problems, however, no matter how serious or widely acknowledged they are, or how well documented, is not sufficient to trigger the active development of policies to address them. For this to happen, there must also exist possible (or what at least appears to be) solutions to the problems. Enactment of Maine's Hospital Cooperation Act was facilitated not only by the documentation of a problem, but also by the availability of a feasible solution to the problem.

Possible solutions to problems are generated through the development of ideas for solving problems, refinement of the ideas, and, ultimately, selection from among the options. Here again, healthcare strategymakers can be influential in setting the policy agenda as was done in Maine.

Strategymakers in healthcare organizations are, in fact, frequently well positioned to play important analytical and prescriptive roles in determining viable solutions to many problems. Sometimes their organizations can even serve as laboratories for demonstrating the utility of a potential policy solution to a problem. Examples of this abound. The experience of Maine hospitals with their Hospital Cooperation Act has been instructive for healthcare organizations and legislatures in other states regarding this approach as a potential solution to their own similar problems. A rather comprehensive list of healthcare organization-based demonstrations with policy relevance can be found in Shortell and Reinhardt (1992), including:

- a demonstration through which an insurer will reimburse participating hospitals through a payment system that links patient outcomes with provider reimbursements;
- a demonstration of the extent to which an intensified program of post-hospital care for high-risk patients can improve their prospects for full, uneventful recoveries and reduce total costs per episode of illness; and
- a feasibility study of the creation of a geriatric day hospital as a cost- and outcome-effective alternative to inpatient, nursing home, and home care within the broader, interdisciplinary geriatrics program of an academic medical center.

Although the existence of problems and possible solutions to them are two prerequisites for policymaking, they do not ensure the development of policy. Public policies are made within a political context. Thus, strategy-makers can also influence the policy agenda through their involvement in the political circumstances that help shape the agenda.

Political Circumstances

A variety of political circumstances help create windows of opportunity through which policy issues move to the stage at which legislation may be developed to address them (see Figure 10.1). These political circumstances include such factors as:

- the public attitudes, concerns, and opinions surrounding issues;
- the policy preferences of various individuals and interest groups, in-cluding strategymakers in healthcare organizations, and their relative ability to influence political decisions;
- the positions of key political leaders on issues; and
- the scope and complexity of competing issues on the policy agenda at any particular point.

Strategymakers have available to them two especially powerful methods of influencing the political circumstances that affect a particular policy issue. First, they can present and push their views, often through interest groups, and often in the form of lobbying. Second, they can seek to exert their influence by filing or joining others in filing lawsuits in which they challenge existing policies, seek to stimulate new policies, or try to alter certain aspects of the implementation of policies.

Advocating viewpoints and lobbying to influence the policy agenda

In efforts to advocate their views and to lobby for their preferences, strategymakers in healthcare organizations are supported by one of the most significant features of the political economy of the United States: the existence of the concentrated interests of those who earn their livelihoods in this domain or who are positioned to gain specific advantageous benefits for the organizations they govern and manage.

One direct result of the existence of concentrated interests is the formation of organized interest groups (Miller 1985; Ornstein and Elder 1978). An interest group "is an organization of people with similar policy goals who enter the political process to try to achieve those aims" (Lineberry, Edwards, and Wattenberg 1995, 216). Interest groups can seek to influence the formulation, implementation, and modification of policies for the purpose of providing the group's members some advantage, although in this section the focus is on their role in helping to shape the policy agenda as part of the formulation phase of the policymaking process depicted in Figure 10.1.

Because all interest groups seek policies that favor their members, their agendas and behaviors are rather predictable. Feldstein (1988) argues, for example, that healthcare provider interest groups seek to accomplish through legislation such purposes as increasing the demand for members' services, limiting competitors, permitting members to charge the highest possible prices for their services, and lowering their members' operating costs as much as possible. In contrast, an interest group representing a group of consumers of healthcare services (e.g., the American Association of Retired Persons, or AARP) would seek through public policies to minimize the costs of services to members, ease their access to services, and increase the availability of services their members want.

Interest groups play powerful roles in setting the nation's health policy agenda, as they do subsequently in the development of legislation and in the implementation and modification of policies. These groups can play their roles proactively by seeking to stimulate new policies that serve the interests of their members, or they can play their roles reactively by seeking to block policy changes they do not believe serve their members' best interests. Interest groups are an inherent part of the public policymaking process in the United States. Recent decades have brought an expansion of astonishing proportions in their involvement in the policymaking process (Scholzman and Tierney 1986); these groups seem especially ubiquitous in the health sector.

All strategymakers in healthcare organizations have ready access to membership in interest groups and to the collective influence such memberships afford. Those in hospitals, for example, can join the AHA and their state hospital associations. If they prefer a collective voice more specifically focused on their policy interests, managers in teaching hospitals can link their organizations to the Council of Teaching Hospitals (COTH), those in children's hospitals can join the National Association of Children's Hospitals and Related Institutions, and those in investor-owned hospitals can align themselves with the Federation of American Health Systems (FAHS). These and many other interest groups provide their members a way to link their policy preferences into more powerful, collective voices that greatly increase the likelihood of significant impact on the policy agenda.

Examples of several ways that strategymakers, working through interest groups, have sought to influence the policy agenda are reflected in actions taken by the AHA and other interest groups in the face of congressional consideration in 1995 of possible substantial reductions in federal spending on the Medicare program. These deliberations occurred in the context of an overall effort to balance the federal budget over a seven-year span. One example is the congressional testimony given by Richard Davidson, president of the AHA, on the issue of the long-term implications of severe cuts in federal support for the Medicare program. Testifying before the Senate Finance Committee on May 17, 1995, and reported in the May 22, 1995, issue of *AHA News*, Mr. Davidson said that "On Medicare's 30th anniversary, lawmakers should think about the next 30 years, not the immediate future." His testimony included other points in support of the preferences of the AHA's membership regarding the policy agenda for the Medicare program: He said, "Spending reductions in GOP budget plans under congressional consideration would only breathe a few years of life into Medicare's ailing hospital trust fund." In this testimony, he also renewed the AHA's call for the creation of a permanent, independent citizen's commission that would try to match Congress's spending targets with the kind of benefits that such allocations would buy.

Also on May 17, 1995, the AHA and the FAHS, joined by 20 other healthcare provider interest groups, sent a letter to all members of the House of Representatives stating that, "We know that savings in the [Medicare] system can be achieved, and we are willing to accept some reductions through restructuring. The proposals put forward by the House Budget Committee, however, [which were designed to slow the growth in federal spending on the Medicare program by $283 billion over seven years] go too far, too fast." Finally, on that day, the AHA and the federation ran a series of ads in newspapers widely read by federal policymakers asking the policymakers to work with these interest groups "to reform, restructure and save money in Medicare—not gut it."

These and other related activities represented attempts by the involved interest groups to help redefine Medicare cost escalation as a long-term problem that would interfere with people getting the services they need rather than a short-term budgetary problem and to offer an alternative solution (the proposed citizen's commission) to addressing the problem. In short, they sought to influence the health policy agenda as it pertains to the Medicare program and, through this, to help shape Medicare policy. This is a vivid example of the role that interest groups play shaping the health policy agenda.

Using the courts to influence the policy agenda

The use of both state and federal courts, as a means to influence public policymaking in the health domain, is increasing. In recent years, the courts have heavily influenced the health policy agenda in four areas: the coverage decisions made by insurers in both the private and public sectors, the Medicaid program's payment rates to hospitals and nursing homes, the antitrust issues involved in hospital mergers, and issues related to the charitable mission and tax-exempt status of nonprofit hospitals (Anderson 1992; Potter and Longest 1994).

A court provides one very important structural advantage to those who seek to influence the health policy agenda: a narrow focus on the issues involved in a specific case. Strategymakers who initiate court cases have the opportunity to control, at least to a significant degree, the issues to be addressed and to have their sides of the issues receive detailed attention. This stands in stark contrast to the wide-open, if not chaotic, political arena in which most efforts to influence the policy agenda must take place.

An example of how strategymakers in healthcare organizations can use a court to influence the public policy agenda can be seen in the ruling by the U.S. Supreme Court in April 1995 that the federal Employee Retirement Income Security Act (ERISA) does not impede states from setting hospital rates. The case that resulted in this ruling arose out of New York's practice of adding a surcharge to certain hospital bills to raise money to help fund healthcare for some of the state's low-income citizens. The state's practice was challenged by the strategymakers in a group of commercial insurers, HMOs, and by New York City (Green 1995a). A number of healthcare interest groups filed a joint *amicus curiae* ("friend of the court") brief in the case in which they asserted that Congress, in enacting ERISA, never intended for it to be used to challenge state health reform plans and initiatives. The Supreme Court's ruling is seen generally as supportive of state efforts to broaden healthcare services to their poorer residents through various reforms and initiatives. In this sense, it helps broaden the potential solutions available to address the problem of providing healthcare to the nation's uninsured citizens. That is, the court's ruling in this case has helped shape the public policy agenda regarding this issue.

Strategymakers are far more likely to influence public policies, and the effects of the policies on their organizations, through state courts and lower federal courts than through their relatively rare opportunities to do so before the U.S. Supreme Court. Recent examples of this technique can be seen in courts in Pennsylvania in cases involving the tax-exempt status of healthcare organizations. In one 1995 case, the Indiana County (PA) Court of Common Pleas rebuffed the strategymakers of Indiana Hospital in their appeal to have the hospital's tax-exempt status restored after the exemption had been revoked by the county in 1993. In making its ruling, the court held that the hospital failed to meet one of the state's tests adequately through which an organization qualifies for tax exemption. Among other rules, the state requires a tax-exempt organization "to donate or render gratuitously a substantial portion of its services."

In so ruling, the Indiana County Court took note of the fact that Indiana Hospital's uncompensated charity care in fiscal year 1994 had been approximately two percent of its total expected compensation and contrasted this with an earlier case resulting from the revocation of the tax-exempt status of a nursing home in the state. The state Supreme Court decision in the St. Margaret Seneca Place nursing home case had been that the nursing home did meet the state's test because it demonstrated that it bore more than one-third of the cost of care for half its patients. The variation in these and several other Pennsylvania cases in the courts' interpretation of the meaning of the state's partial test for tax-exempt status (i.e., the requirement that a tax-exempt organization is "to donate or render gratuitously a substantial portion of its services") has led a coalition of tax-exempt organizations in the state to seek clarifying legislation on this and other points regarding the determination of tax-exempt status. As a result of their efforts, Senate Bill 355, the Institutions of Purely Public Charity Act, has been introduced in the Pennsylvania legislature.

Exerting Influence in the Development of Legislation

Once health policy issues achieve prominence on the policy agenda, they can proceed to the next stage of the policy formulation phase—development of legislation (see Figure 10.1). At this stage, specific legislative proposals go through a process involving a carefully prescribed set of steps that can, but do not always, lead to policies in the form of new legislation, or as is more often the case, amendments to previously enacted legislation. In fact, only a small fraction of policy issues result in the development of specific legislation that is intended to address the issues. And even then, only some of the attempts to enact legislation are successful. While the path for legislation is indeed long and arduous, it is replete with opportunities for strategymakers to influence legislation development.

Both as individuals and through the interest groups to which they belong, strategymakers participate directly in actually drafting legislative proposals and frequently participate in the hearings associated with the development of legislation. An example of this latter technique for influencing the development of legislation can be found in the consideration by the Pennsylvania legislature in 1995 of so-called "any willing provider" legislation.

As part of the legislation development process, the Pennsylvania House of Representatives Insurance Committee held a series of hearings in 1995 on the potential legislation, House Bill 630. This bill would have created a circumstance in which managed care networks and health plans would have found it much more difficult to exclude providers from their networks, thus reducing their ability to contract selectively for the utilization of the services of providers whom they judged to be acceptably efficient in their professional practice and who met their quality standards. Healthcare strategymakers' concerns about such legislation were intense at the time of these hearings, both in Pennsylvania and across the nation. In fact, grouping their concerns about any willing provider laws with their concerns about mandatory point of service laws into a broader set of concerns they refer to as "selective contracting restrictions," the strategymakers in the nation's managed care plans identified such restrictions as the top item on their public policy agenda for 1995 (Ernst & Young 1995).

At the first of four hearings in the series, which was sponsored by the Pennsylvania House of Representatives Insurance Committee, a strategymaker from one of Pennsylvania's larger healthcare systems, representing the Hospital Association of Pennsylvania, testified that the proposed legislation was anti-competitive in that it would "destroy the gatekeeper concept that is central to managed care, severely limiting a managed care organization's ability to control health care costs and the quality of their networks" (Hospital Association of Pennsylvania 1995, 2).

Strategymakers or their spokespersons from several other organizations and healthcare interest groups also testified at this hearing in an effort to influence the development of this legislation, including Blue Cross of Northeastern Pennsylvania, the Insurance Federation of Pennsylvania, Pennsylvania

Nurses Association, Geisinger Health Plan, and HealthAmerica (an HMO). The views on this legislation of the Patient Advocacy Coalition, several individual physicians, and a pharmacist were also presented at this hearing.

Influencing Rulemaking

Enacted legislation rarely contains enough explicit language to guide its implementation completely. Rather, laws are often vague on implementation details, leaving the implementing agencies and organizations to establish the rules and regulations needed to put the legislation into operation. The promulgation of rules, as a formal part of the implementation phase, is guided by certain rules. Key among these at the federal level, with parallels in most of the states, is the requirement that the organization responsible for implementing a law (e.g., the HCFA) publish an NPRM in the *Federal Register*. A NPRM is, in effect, a draft of a rule or set of rules under development. Publication of this notice is an open invitation to those with an interest in the rules and regulations applicable to implementing a particular policy to react to proposed or draft rules before they become final.

The procedure of commenting on draft rules is one of the most active points of involvement for the strategymakers for healthcare organizations and others who have a stake in a particular policy in the entire policymaking process. This point of involvement can produce significant results. Changes in proposed rules often result from what Thompson (1991, 149) calls the "strategic interaction" that occurs between implementing organizations and those affected by their rules during rulemaking. For example, among the numerous rules proposed in implementing the 1974 National Health Planning and Resources Development Act (P.L. 93-641) were some that sought to reduce obstetrical capacity in the nation's hospitals. One proposed rule, in 1977, called for hospitals to perform at least 500 deliveries annually or close their obstetrical units. Notice of this proposed rule elicited immediate and vigorous objections, especially from the strategymakers from hospitals in rural areas where obstetrical care was needed but where meeting the rule's threshold of 500 deliveries annually could be difficult or impossible. As a result, the final rules were far less restrictive, in fact making no reference at all to a specific number of deliveries that hospitals in rural areas should perform (Zwick 1978).

A more recent example of the ability of strategymakers from health-care organizations to influence public policymaking through influence on rulemaking can be seen in an apparent change in the way the FTC plans to interpret certain rules in antitrust cases involving hospitals. Historically, the FTC focused on product and geographic markets and on competitive effects in their antitrust enforcement efforts aimed at hospital mergers. It has not viewed efficiency as a major factor in its analyses of possible hospital mergers. Now, however, following a long period during which healthcare strategymakers, working through their interest groups and through arguments presented in antitrust cases involving hospital mergers, have argued that improved efficiencies gained through mergers are an extremely important means of helping to contain healthcare costs, it appears that these views have affected the FTC. A reported account of a public speech given by FTC Commissioner Christine Varney in Chicago on May 2, 1995, states that she discussed plans whereby

> the agency is abandoning its "linear" method to hospital-merger antitrust enforcement for a more "holistic" approach that accommodates the field's peculiarities.
>
> Varney said this uniqueness, paired with the special nature of hospital-merger analysis, "virtually mandates that antitrust enforcers carefully examine asserted efficiencies before determining whether to challenge a particular hospital merger."
>
> From now on, Varney said, improved hospital efficiency resulting from mergers will be presumed to benefit consumers when mergers do not threaten competition (Green 1995b).

In addition to exerting their influence directly by commenting on the rules that will guide the implementation of policies, strategymakers can also use two other means to influence policymaking at this stage. When the development of rules and regulations is anticipated to be unusually difficult or contentious, or when rules and regulations are anticipated to be subject to continuous revision, special task forces may be established to help with their development. For example, after passage of the Health Maintenance Organization Act (P.L. 9–227) in 1973, the Department of Health, Education, and Welfare (DHEW) (now DHHS) organized a series of task forces, including on them some people who were or would become strategymakers in this industry, to help develop the proposed rules for implementing the law. This approach, which involved strategymakers in the development of rules, produced rules that were much more acceptable to those who would be affected by them than might otherwise have been the case.

Another approach to support rulemaking is the creation of advisory commissions to assist with the ongoing rulemaking effort directly. This, too, provides a means through which strategymakers can exert their influence. For example, following enactment of the 1983 Amendments to the Social Security Act (P.L. 98-21), which established the PPS for reimbursing hospitals for the care of Medicare beneficiaries, Congress established ProPAC to provide nonbinding advice to the HCFA in implementing the reimbursement system. Later, a second commission, the PPRC, was established to advise Congress and HCFA regarding payment for physicians' services under the Medicare program. These commissions have been useful in helping HCFA to make required annual decisions regarding reimbursement rates, fees, and other variables in the operation of the Medicare program.

Although the opportunities for direct service on such commissions are limited to very few people, others can influence their thinking. Strategy-makers can seek to influence the thinking of commission members, and thus the advice commission members ultimately provide to Congress and to HCFA, by sharing their ideas, experiences, and data as inputs to commission deliberations.

Influencing Policymaking at the Stage of Policy Operation

The policy operation stage of implementing policies involves the actual running of programs and activities embedded in or stimulated by enacted legislation. Operation is the responsibility, primarily, of the appointees and civil servants who staff the government, and who influence policies by their operational decisions and actions made in implementing them. Thus, strategy-makers can influence policies by influencing those who manage the operation of policies. This form of influence arises from the working relationships that can be developed between those responsible for implementing public policies and those whom their decisions and activities directly effect, such as the strategymakers in healthcare organizations.

The opportunities to build these relationships are supported by a prominent feature of the careers of bureaucrats—longevity (Kingdon 1995). Elected policymakers come and go, but the bureaucracy endures. Strategymakers, and other participants in their healthcare organizations, can and do build long-standing working relationships with some of the people responsible for implementing the public policies that are of strategic importance to these organizations.

The most solid base for these working relationships is the exchange of useful information and expertise. A strategymaker, speaking from an authoritative position based on actual operational experience with the implementation of a policy, can influence the policy's further implementation with relevant information. If the information supports change, especially if it buttressed with similar information from others who are experiencing the effect of a particular policy, reasonable implementors may well be influenced to make needed changes. This is especially likely if there is a well-established working relationship based on mutual respect for the roles of and the challenges facing each party.

Sometimes the relationships between strategymakers in healthcare organizations, usually operating through their interest groups, and those responsible for implementing policies important to them are expanded to include members of the legislative committees or subcommittees with jurisdiction over the policies. This triad of mutual interests forms what has been termed an *iron triangle*, so called because the interests of the three parts of the triangle "dovetail nicely and because they are alleged to be impenetrable from the outside and uncontrollable by president, political appointees, or legislators not on the committees in question" (Kingdon 1995, 33).

The enormity of the bureaucracy with which they might need to interact is an obvious and very limiting problem for strategymakers wishing to influence the policymaking process though influencing either the rulemaking or policy operation stages of policy implementation. Consider how many components of the federal government are involved in rulemaking and policy operation that is directly relevant to healthcare organizations. Add to this the units of state and local government that are relevant and the challenge of keeping track of where working relationships might be useful as a means of influencing policymaking—to say nothing of actually developing and maintaining the relationships—and the magnitude of the process becomes clear. Obviously, selectivity in which of these relationships might be of most strategic importance, as well as reliance upon the interest groups to which they belong to do much of the relationship building, helps strategymakers face such a daunting challenge.

Exerting Influence Through Policy Modification

Policy modification occurs when the outcomes, perceptions, and consequences of existing policies feed back into the agenda-setting and legislation development stages of the formulation phase and into the rulemaking and policy operation stages of the implementation phase and stimulate changes in legislation, rules, or operations (see the feedback loop running along the bottom of Figure 10.1). Although some health policies are developed *de novo*, the vast majority of them result from the modification of existing policies in rather modest, incremental steps.

Following the feedback loop shown in Figure 10.1, it can be seen that because agenda setting involves the confluence of problems, possible solutions, and political circumstances, policy modification can occur at this stage in a number of ways. As problems become more sharply defined and better understood through the actual experiences of those who are affected by the policies, modifications can be triggered. Strategymakers and others involved in healthcare organizations are the best sources of feedback on the consequences of policies for their organizations and, in some cases, the populations they serve. Similarly, possible new solutions to problems can be conceived and assessed through the operational experiences of strategymakers with particular policies, and, especially, when the results of demonstrations and evaluations provide concrete evidence of the performance of particular solutions that are under consideration. Finally, the interactions among the branches of government and strategymakers and their interest groups who are involved with and affected by ongoing policies become important components of the political circumstances surrounding the amendment of these policies.

The outcomes, perceptions, and consequences that flow from the ongoing policymaking process also help modify policies by directly influencing the development of legislation. Actual experience with the effect of the implementation of policies that affect their organizations help strategymakers to identify routinely needed modifications to such policies. The history of the Medicare program is a good example of this phenomenon. Over the program's life, services have been added and deleted; premiums and copayment provisions have been changed; reimbursement mechanisms have been changed; features to ensure quality and medical necessity of services have been added, changed, and deleted; and so on. The inputs of strategymakers from healthcare organizations, based upon their experiences with Medicare policy, played a role in each of these amendments to the original legislation, although other influences also helped guide these changes.

Strategymakers also have extensive opportunities to influence the modification of policies in their implementation phases, in both the rulemaking and policy operation stages. The modification of rules, as well as changes in the operations undertaken to implement policies, often reflect the actual reported or documented experiences of those affected by the rules and operations. Strategymakers can provide this feedback directly to those with rulemaking or operational responsibilities. They can also take their views on the rules and operational practices that affect their organizations to the courts or the legislative branch. Both can also be pathways to modifications.

The implementation of the Occupational Safety and Health Act (P.L. 91-596) in 1970 illustrates well how readily the strategymakers in healthcare organizations, as well as in many other types of organizations, can use the courts to influence rules and operational practices (Robinson and Paxman 1991). This legislation set in motion a massive federal program of standard setting and enforcement that sought to improve safety and health conditions in the nation's workplaces. As Thompson (1981) has noted, managers and labor leaders "have repeatedly appealed decisions by the Occupational Safety and Health Administration (OSHA) to the courts. The development of this program in some respects reads like a legal history."

Similarly, the rules promulgated to implement the Medicare and Medicaid legislation, as well as the operational decisions and actions of HCFA as the implementing organization, have frequently been challenged in the courts. Public policies of relevance to the strategymakers in healthcare organizations in such diverse areas as human resources, clinical laboratories, and mergers and acquisitions have also been challenged in court.

As demonstrated by the examples given above, there are abundant opportunities for strategymakers to influence public policymaking. Their influence can be exerted in both the agenda-setting and legislation development stages of the formulation phase and in both the rulemaking and policy operation stages of the implementation phase of the policymaking process. Furthermore, there are continuing opportunities for influencing policies as the outcomes, perceptions, and consequences that result from them trigger policy modification. In effect, those who would influence policies have an opportunity to do so in the initial iteration of the process in regard to any particular policy, but they also get additional opportunities to exert their influence through the subsequent modification of existing policies. The multiple opportunities for strategymakers to influence public policymaking are summarized in Figure 10.2.

In addition to having a number of places in the policymaking process to exert influence, strategymakers have three sources of power available to them in their influence activities: positional, capacity to reward or coerce, and expertise. Figure 10.3 combines the places where influence can be exerted within the policymaking process with the sources of power that can be used in exerting influence to illustrate in summary fashion the great variety of opportunities available to strategymakers to influence their organization's public policy environment.

The numerous opportunities that strategymakers in healthcare organizations have to influence policy and the variety of influence mechanisms described in this chapter, however, say little about the actual manner in which such influence can or should be exerted. The code of ethics of the American College of Healthcare Executives (ACHE) provides some guidance for strategymakers in their efforts to influence public policymaking by stating that they should "participate in public dialogue on healthcare policy issues and advocate solutions that will improve health status and promote quality healthcare" (American College of Healthcare Executives 1994: Section IV, C). But more needs to be said about the ethics of influencing public policy. There is an abiding danger that these activities can involve unethical behavior.

Figure 10.2 Opportunities for Strategymakers to Influence Policymaking

I. Influencing Policy Formulation
    A. Agenda Setting
        1. Defining and documenting problems
        2. Developing and evaluating solutions
        3. Shaping political circumstances through lobbying and the courts
    B. Legislation Development
        1. Participating in drafting legislation
        2. Testifying at legislative hearings
II. Influencing Policy Implementation
    A. Rulemaking
        1. Providing formal comments on draft rules
        2. Serving on and providing input to rulemaking advisory bodies
    B. Policy Operation
        1. Interactions with policy operators
III. Influencing Policy Modification
    A. Documenting the case for modification through operational experience and formal evaluations

Figure 10.3 The Opportunities to Exert Influence in Public Policy Environments

	Problem Definition	Identifying Solutions	Political Circumstances	Legislation Development	Rulemaking	Policy Operation
Power Based on Position						
Power to Reward/Coerce						
Power Based on Expertise						

ETHICAL CONSIDERATIONS IN INFLUENCING POLICY

Ethics play an important part in public policymaking, albeit only a part. Ethical principles can provide the moral background for a health policy, but in addition, "the policy itself must be informed by empirical data and by special information available in the fields of medicine, biology, law, psychology, and so on" (Beauchamp and Childress 1989: 14).

Ethical behavior, for any and all participants in policymaking (including strategymakers who seek to influence policy), can be guided in important ways by four philosophical principles: respect for the autonomy of others, justice, beneficence, and nonmaleficence. Each of these is considered below, beginning with the concept of respect for autonomy. This concept is based on the notion that individuals have the right to their own beliefs and values and to the decisions and choices that further these beliefs and values. Regarding healthcare, where respect for the autonomy of other people is of extreme importance, this principle pertains to the rights of individuals to independent self-determination regarding how they live their lives and to their rights regarding the integrity of their bodies and minds.

Respect for autonomy is important in such contemporary health policy considerations as those involving privacy and individual choice, including behavioral or lifestyle choices. Policies that do not reflect a respect for the autonomy of others are paternalistic. One vivid example of the kind of policies that result from adherence to the principle of autonomy in health policymaking is the 1990 Patient Self-Determination Act. This policy was designed to facilitate the efforts of people to exercise their right to make decisions concerning their medical care, including the right to accept or refuse treatment, and the right to formulate advance directives regarding their care. Strategymakers, and others, who supported this policy were acting in a manner consistent with respect for the autonomy of others.

The principle of respect for autonomy includes several other elements that are especially important in guiding ethical behavior in those who in-fluence policymaking. One of these is honesty: telling the truth. Respect for people as autonomous beings implies honesty in relationships with them. The element of confidentiality is closely related to honesty in such relationships. Confidences broken in the policymaking process can impair the process. A third element of the autonomy principle with relevance to the policymaking process is fidelity. This means doing one's duty and keeping one's word, which is often equated with promise keeping. When strategymakers who seek to influence policy tell the truth, honor confidences, and keep promises, their behavior is more ethically sound than if these things are not done.

Justice is a second ethical principle of significant importance to those who influence policymaking. The practical implications for public policymaking of the principle of justice are felt mostly in terms of distributive justice; that is, in terms of fairness in the distribution of healthcare benefits and burdens in society. Attention to the ethical principle of justice, of course, raises the question of what is fair. Allocative policies that adhere closely to the principle of justice allocate burdens and benefits according to the provisions of a morally defensible system rather than through arbitrary or capricious decisions. Regulatory policies guided by the principle of justice fairly and equitably affect those to whom the regulations are targeted.

Two other ethical principles have direct relevance to policymaking and to efforts by strategymakers to influence this process: beneficence and nonmaleficence. Beneficence in policymaking means acting with charity and kindness. This principle is incorporated into acts through which benefits are provided, and thus beneficence characterizes most allocative policies. But beneficence also includes the more complex concept of balancing benefits and harms, for using the relative costs and benefits of alternative decisions and actions as one basis upon which to choose from among alternatives. The growing emphasis on cost-effectiveness in healthcare and the development of policies to achieve this goal will increasingly call into play the principle of beneficence in developing ethically sound policies. Strategymakers will be in danger of violating this principle of ethical behavior when they seek policies that exclusively serve the interests of their organizations rather than maximizing the net benefits to society as a whole.

Nonmaleficence, a principle with deep roots in medical ethics, is exemplified in the dictum *primum non nocere*—first, do no harm. When strategymakers who influence policy are guided by this principle, they seek to minimize harm to society as a whole. The principles of beneficence and nonmaleficence are clearly reflected in health policies that ensure the quality of healthcare services and products. Such policies as those establishing Professional Review Organizations (PROs) to review the quality of care provided to Medicare patients and the policies that the FDA uses to ensure the safety of pharmaceuticals are examples. Policies that support the conduct and use of outcome studies of clinical care are also examples.

Although adherence to the principles of respect for the autonomy of other people, justice, beneficence, and nonmaleficence does not ensure that policies supported by strategymakers necessarily are in the best strategic interests of their organizations, such adherence does place the strategymakers on relatively high ethical ground.

SUMMARY

The public policies that are relevant to healthcare organizations are made through a highly complex, interactive, and cyclical process that incorporates formulation, implementation, and modification phases of activities. The process is played out in the context of a political marketplace with diverse participants. Participants include elected and appointed members of all three branches of government as well as civil servants who staff the government on the one hand, and strategymakers and others whose organizations are affected by policies or who are personally affected by policies, and the interest groups to which they belong, on the other hand. The policymaking process includes a number of opportunities for the latter group of participants to influence the policies made by the former group.

In this chapter, the model of the public policymaking process has been used to provide a map to the places in the process where strategymakers can exert their influence (see Figure 10.1). In the agenda-setting stage of policy formulation, strategymakers can help define the problems that policies might address, they can participate in designing possible solutions to them, and they can help create the political circumstances necessary to advance the potential solutions to actual policies. Their central roles in the health sector equip the strategymakers of healthcare organizations to be well informed about certain kinds of healthcare problems that should be addressed through public policies. The resources at their command and their abilities to permit their organizations to serve as demonstration sites for assessing possible solutions facilitate their roles in identifying feasible solutions to problems. And their abilities, as individuals and through interest groups, to lobby for their preferences and to use the courts as allies in seeking to have their policy preferences enacted provide effective mechanisms through which these strategymakers can participate in shaping the political circumstances surrounding a policy issue.

Strategymakers can also exert influence on policymaking in the legislation development stage of the process. Here, again acting both as individuals and through their interest groups, they can participate in the actual drafting of legislative proposals and they can provide testimony in the hearings in which legislation is developed.

Rulemaking, procedurally, is designed to include input from those who will be affected by the rules, such as strategymakers in the health sector. This input can be made through formal comment on proposed rules. Influence can also be exerted through inputs to task forces and commissions established by rulemaking agencies as a means to obtain advice on their work. In the policy operation stage, strategymakers can influence policies by influencing those with policy operation responsibilities. This is done best through establishing and maintaining effective working relationships with members of the implementing bureaucracy.

This chapter notes that strategymakers can exert their influence in the initial iterations of the process through which policies are made. But, importantly, because policymaking is a cyclical process in which the results of policies continuously feed back into the process where they trigger modifications, there are subsequent opportunities to influence policies—again in the agenda-setting, legislation development, rulemaking, and policy operation stages of the process. In effect, strategymakers have multiple opportunities to influence policymaking and resultant policies.

Given the importance of public policies to the strategic success of healthcare organizations, their strategymakers should avail themselves of the many opportunities to influence relevant policies that are described in this chapter. However, their efforts should be guided by ethical considerations. Four principles that can be useful in guiding strategymakers to more ethical policy-influencing behaviors and activities are respect for the autonomy of other people, justice, beneficence, and nonmaleficence.

REFERENCES

American College of Healthcare Executives. *Code of Ethics*. Chicago: American College of Healthcare Executives. As Amended on August 9, 1994.

Anderson, G. F. 1992. "The Courts and Health Policy: Strengths and Limitations." *Health Affairs* 11 (Fall): 95–110.

Beauchamp, T. L., and J. F. Childress. 1989. *Principles of Biomedical Ethics*, 3rd ed. New York: Oxford University Press.

Buchholz, R. 1989. *Environments and Public Policy*. Englewood Cliffs, NJ: Prentice Hall.

———. 1993. *Management Response to Public Issues*, 3rd ed. Englewood Cliffs, NJ: Prentice Hall.

Cerne, F. 1993. "Hospital Cooperation Act Opens Door to Increased Collaboration." *Hospitals* 67 (5): 27.

Ernst & Young LLP. 1995. "Anti-Selective Contracting Laws." *CapitolWATCH* 95(5): 2.

Evans, R. G., and G. L. Stoddart. 1994. "Producing Health, Consuming Health Care," 27–64. In *Why Are Some People Healthy and Others Not? The Determinants of Health of Populations*, edited by R. G. Evans, M. L. Barer, and T. R. Marmor. New York: Aldine De Gruyter.

Feldstein, P. J. 1988. *The Politics of Health Legislation: An Economic Perspective*. Ann Arbor, MI: Health Administration Press.

Green, J. 1995a. "High-Court Ruling Protects Hospital-bill Surcharges." *AHA News* 31 (18): 1.

———. 1995b. "FTC Ruling Clears Way for Hospital Mergers." *AHA News* 31 (19): 1.

Hospital Association of Pennsylvania. 1995. "HAP Testifies Any Willing Provider Legislation Can Do More Harm Than Good." *Pennsylvania Hospitals Nineties* 6 (10): 1.

Kania, A. J. 1993. "Legislation Gives Maine Hospitals OK for Collaboration." *Health Care Strategic Management* 11 (5): 12–13.

Keys, B., and T. Case. 1990. "How to Become an Influential Manager." *The Executive* 4 (November): 38–51.

Kingdon, J. W. 1995. *Agendas, Alternatives, and Public Policies*, 2nd ed. Boston: Little, Brown & Company.

Lineberry, R. T., G. C. Edwards, III, and M. P. Wattenberg. 1995. *Government in America: People, Politics, and Policy*, Brief Version, 2nd ed. New York: HarperCollins College Publishers.

Longest, B. B., Jr. 1988. "American Health Policy in the Year 2000." *Hospital & Health Services Administration* 33 (4): 419–34.

———. 1994. *Health Policymaking in the United States*. Ann Arbor, MI: Health Administration Press.

Michaud, S. R. "Breaking New Ground: Antitrust Policy and Health Care Provider Coalitions." A public lecture in the Lecture Series in Health Management and Policy sponsored by the Health Policy Institute at the University of Pittsburgh, October 20, 1992.

Miller, S. 1985. *Special Interest Groups in American Politics*. New Brunswick, NJ: Transaction Books.

Mintzberg, H. 1983. *Power In and Around Organizations*. Englewood Cliffs, NJ: Prentice Hall.

Morlock, L. L., C. A. Nathanson, and J. A. Alexander. 1988. "Authority, Power, and Influence." 265–300. In *Health Care Management: A Text in Organization Theory and Behavior*, 2nd ed., edited by S. M. Shortell and A. D. Kaluzny. New York: John Wiley & Sons.

Ornstein, N., and S. Elder. 1978. *Interest Groups, Lobbying and Policymaking*. Washington, DC: Congressional Quarterly Press.

Potter, M. A., and B. B. Longest, Jr. 1994. "The Divergence of Federal and State Policies on the Charitable Tax Exemption of Nonprofit Hospitals." *Journal of Health Politics, Policy and Law* 19 (Summer): 393–419.

Robinson, J. C., and D. G. Paxman. 1991. "Technological, Economic, and Political Feasibility in OSHA's Air Contaminants Standards." *Journal of Health Politics, Policy and Law* 16 (Spring): 1–18.

Scholzman, K. L., and J. T. Tierney. 1986. *Organized Interests and American Democracy*. New York: Harper & Row.

Shortell, S. M., and U. E. Reinhardt, eds. 1992. *Improving Health Policy and Management: Nine Critical Research Issues for the 1990s*. Ann Arbor, MI: AHSR/Health Administration Press.

Thompson, F. J. 1981. *Health Policy and the Bureaucracy: Politics and Implementation*. Cambridge, MA: Massachusetts Institute of Technology Press.

———. 1991. "The Enduring Challenge of Health Policy Implementation." 148–69. In *Health Politics and Policy*, 2nd ed., edited by T. J. Litman and L. S. Robins. Albany, NY: Delmar Publishers Inc.

Zwick, D. I. 1978. "Initial Development of Guidelines for Health Planning." *Public Health Reports* 93 (5): 407–20.

11

Universal Truths of Practical Governance

J. Larry Tyler, FACHE, and Errol Biggs, Ph.D., FACHE

Regardless of the size, location, or ownership of your organization or the structure and articulated responsibilities of your board, "universal truths" of effective healthcare governance exist. These universal truths were borne out both in our research and our conversations with CEOs and board chairs across the country. We have categorized these truths, or tenets, as follows: Universal Truths for CEOs, Universal Truths for Board Chairs, and Universal Truths for Boards. As you read further, why we made these distinctions will become clearer.

UNIVERSAL TRUTHS FOR CEOS

Universal Truth 1: You can never communicate too often or too much.

Any CEO who has enjoyed a positive relationship with his or her board and, more specifically, with the board chair does a substantial amount of talking to these individuals outside of the boardroom.

We talked with one CEO who meets with his board chair and vice chair one-on-one at least every two weeks and often weekly to review the agenda for the next board meeting, discuss any pending regulatory concerns, and so forth. He also tries to meet individually with each board member at least once a month.

Editor's Note: This chapter combines the chapters "Universal Truths," and "The CEO's Role," from the book *Practical Governance*, by J. Larry Tyler and Errol Biggs, 2001, HAP.

We are not suggesting, however, that CEOs need to adhere to such a rigorous schedule of one-on-one meetings. In fact, unless your board is relatively small—under ten members—such frequent one-on-one meetings are probably not realistic. Rather, when CEOs communicate with their boards between board meetings they put themselves at a tremendous advantage. Informal conversations, in particular, provide CEOs an opportunity to lay out complex or controversial issues without the time constraints of a board meeting. This means that CEOs are able to discuss thoroughly the topic at hand and to give the individual board member a chance to reflect on the conversation before the next meeting. In this way, the CEO paves the way for a more informed discussion and, more importantly, for more judicious decision making when the issue is considered by the full board.

Universal Truth 2: Your board does not want to be blindsided.

If you remember nothing else, remember this: Boards do not like surprises. This truth tenet isn't rocket science, especially in the business world. Similarly, surprises breed contempt. Just think of how you have reacted when a member of your management team dropped a bomb on you. Chances are you were less than pleased.

Surprises that will not be appreciated by the board include:

- Anything, absolutely anything, that has to do with financials;
- Human resources issues that threaten to put the organization in peril—for example, allegations of sexual harassment or a looming labor dispute;
- Medical staff dissatisfaction with management—to the extent that they plan to act on it;
- Issues that, if they hit the media, are likely to stir up negative publicity and a community backlash.

Universal Truth 3: You serve at the pleasure of your board.

We are confident that any CEO who has lost sight of this truth one-too-many times is no longer CEO of his or her organization, as one CEO puts it: [as CEO] "I'm the hired help." In some instances, your board chair may not be at the top of his or her game or your entire board may not see the big picture. Well, then, your job is to help them, not to step in to "save the day." In the vast majority of cases, these board members are *volunteering* their time and energy to serve your organization. You, on the other hand, are *paid* to guide the board in making informed decisions and to oversee the successful implementation of its directives. You may have a wonderful rapport with each board member, but if you forget the pecking order, your relationship could quickly sour and your days as CEO may be numbered. A related piece of advice: Pick your battles carefully. Occasions will arise when you feel compelled to speak up and take a stand. Just be sure that when you choose to go out on the limb, you do so for an issue or cause that is worth taking a stand on regardless of the consequences of your action.

Universal Truth 4: You must see the future and help your board see it, too.

In most organizations, the vast majority of board members come from the community. Before they served on the board, their understanding of healthcare was likely limited to their everyday experiences. For example, although they and their families may have been covered by a managed care plan, their understanding of the implications of these plans for hospitals and physicians was minimal.

Just as CEOs in the 1980s had to anticipate the effect of managed care on their organizations and to focus their boards on taking appropriate action, so too must the CEO of today look forward—beyond the limited view of his or her board—to ensure that today's governance team prepares the organization for tomorrow's challenges. In other words, you need a vision and the ability to communicate it effectively to your board. Predicting the future of healthcare is far from an exact science, which leads us to the next universal truth.

Universal Truth 5: You are paid to take risks, albeit calculated risks.

Any board that thinks and says that your job is to tell it what it wants to hear is a board that will soon be governing a sinking ship. At first blush, we may seem to be directly contradicting Universal Truth 3—serving at the pleasure of your board—but that is not the case. Although you should not grandstand or attempt to coerce your board in any way, the board expects you to speak up and suggest courses of action that may, on occasion, stir things up.

For example, like many other organizations a decade ago, you may have scrambled to participate in a large number of managed care contracts to protect your hospital's market share. Now, you realize that although managed care is likely here to stay, your organization must be much more selective about which plans it participates in, which is a strategic crap shoot (if such a thing exists). Certainly, if you were the CEO when your organization first entered into managed care contracts at a frenetic pace, you run the risk that the board will question why you have changed your position. You could possibly "save face" by not bringing the issue to their attention. As CEO, though, saving face should never be on your list of options.

Whether or not you have a contract that offers you financial protection for risk taking, taking risks—personally and on behalf of your organization—is an inherent responsibility of your job description. Phillip Goodwin, president and CEO of CamCare, Inc., a five-hospital integrated delivery network in Charleston, West Virginia, brings the point home. At his urging, the board authorized the development of an HMO about six years ago. Although the HMO has succeeded in terms of care management and per-patient cost reductions, it has continued to be a financial drain on the system. "The HMO has been bleeding the system dry," Goodwin explained. "I had to put the issue square on the table. I had to make it clear to the board that we are not going to be able to sustain the capital financing of this plan in our market. Even though I had initially pushed to acquire the HMO, I had a responsibility to now tell them we were going to have to seek an alternative."

Goodwin says that the board's reaction to his assessment was mixed. Some board members disagreed; some agreed philosophically, but did not want to give up on the HMO; and some concurred entirely. "We never had open conflict, but there were definitely some pretty tense discussions. It had the potential for being one of those situations where the CEO comes back from vacation and finds out that the Executive Committee wants to meet with you—right away—and it isn't good news."

UNIVERSAL TRUTHS FOR BOARD CHAIRS

Universal Truth 1: Your CEO looks to you to lead.

During our interviews, we heard more good things than bad about our CEOs' board chairs. In some cases, our interviewees probably felt compelled to say the politically correct thing, but we got the impression that, in most cases, the high marks they gave their board chairs were sincere. That said, we also heard from those who said their board chairs are "very nice people." We quickly figured out that "very nice" was code for "not terribly effective in their role." We also heard, "well, he [or she] certainly has a strong personality," which we decoded to mean, "the board chair's leadership style is akin to a dictator's." One CEO even compared his former board chair's style to "Tito in Yugoslavia." Simply if you are a board chair, or about to become one, you need to know that the CEO wants you to lead, not acquiesce and not force feed. This is a delicate balance to strike but a necessary one.

Universal Truth 2: You must do your part to cultivate an effective working relationship with the CEO.

The CEO technically works for you and the board as a whole. But the employment relationship does not mean that the CEO is solely responsible for making your relationship with each other a good one. Your responsibility extends beyond the boardroom. You must support the CEO in both formal and informal settings and, on those occasions when you're at odds with the CEO, you should first discuss it face-to-face and in private. Further, your CEO will likely turn to you for counsel or support throughout the course of your service. You need to be accessible and responsive. The bottom line is that if you don't do your part to cement the relationship, the repercussions will not simply affect the CEO but will carry over into the boardroom and affect the entire board's effectiveness.

Universal Truth 3: You must be a mentor.

Anyone who has served on a board for any length of time knows that board chairs vary greatly in style and effectiveness. In many cases, the board chair's attributes are learned attributes. In other words, the new chair was once a regular board member who likely observed the leadership style of the chairs who came before. That's right, people are watching. You are in the spotlight and have the ability to influence the leadership style of future board chairs of your organization. If you are well prepared, others notice. If you are even-handed, others notice. If you are a visionary, others notice. Be all three, and the CEO and next board chair will thank you.

Universal Truth 4: Your legacy is as much what you don't do as what you do.

During our CEO interviews, we heard multiple references to the "last board chair." In many cases, those recollections were not overwhelmingly positive. We heard about board chairs who were "nice guys" and "very well liked," but in the next breath, they were described as not terribly effective or, worse yet, not able to prepare the board or the organization very well for the future. Our CEO interviewees made clear that if they had to choose between a board chair who was affable or one who made sure the tough questions were asked and addressed, they would all choose the latter. In the final analysis, your legacy is what the board accomplishes during your tenure—or what it does not.

Universal Truth 5: You are the board's conscience.

Today, the board may face as many gray issues as it does black-and-white issues. As board chair, you have the responsibility to call it as you see it. If your board has entered, or is about to enter, a gray area with potential ethical or legal implications, you need to flag the issue and make sure the board remains on solid ground. Implicit in this role is the fact that your behavior must be beyond reproach—always. You must guard against self-dealing at

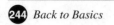

all costs and make sure that you never put yourself in a position where your motives are questioned. Once again, you are a mentor and others will follow your lead—good or bad.

UNIVERSAL TRUTHS FOR BOARDS

Universal Truth 1: You may be a volunteer, but your organization is counting on your commitment to the job.

In other words, don't sign on unless you are willing to put in the time between board meetings to do what is necessary to be an effective board member. Our CEO interviewees acknowledged that as board members in today's complex healthcare environment, you face the unprecedented demands on your time and energy. Most of you meet as a board at least once every other month and serve on board committees that meet at least as often. But your CEOs tell us that just showing up for these meetings is not enough. If you don't read your board packet in advance and if you don't pull your weight on committees, you are not only ineffective on the board, you may, in fact, be an impediment to the entire board's effectiveness.

Universal Truth 2: Your role is policy setting, not management of the organization.

This universal truth should not come as a surprise even to newcomers to the board. Yet, even though board members say they understand that they should not get involved in hospital operations, most board members at one time or another seem to wander in this direction. This propensity to get involved in issues out of one's domain is actually easy to understand. As a board member, particularly one who comes from the community, you may be immersed in operational issues in the course of everyday life. You may even be somewhat of an expert on human resources issues, finance, or marketing. You have attained a comfort level with operations. But you are new to the world of healthcare and perhaps somewhat uneasy establishing policy in an arena that is not totally familiar to you, and that may be downright confusing.

As a result, you gravitate to topics and issues with which you are comfortable. Suddenly, you are involving yourself in hiring and firing decisions, in developing the organization's branding strategy, and in other issues where the CEO doesn't really want or need your input. As one CEO puts it: "Some board members are like screwdrivers; everything they see looks like a screw."

Remember that your boad, or a previous one, has hired the CEO to manage hospital operations. If you don't believe he or she is up to the challenge, then the solution is to address that problem, not to take over the reins.

Universal Truth 3: Your personal agendas serve no one's interests, not even your own.

If you have served on a board for any length of time you no doubt have witnessed the board member who has his or her own agenda. Sometimes the personal agenda is so glaringly apparent that the board chair, CEO, or you or another board member has intervened. In many cases, however, the board member's personal agenda is not necessarily a blatant conflict of interest, but is inappropriate just the same. As a board member, you need to realize that when you put your agenda on the table, chances are everyone else in the room will realize that you are championing your personal cause whether or not they call you on it. In other words, when you pursue a personal agenda, not only are you unlikely to emerge victorious, but, worse yet, you are likely to lose credibility with your board colleagues.

Universal Truth 4: You owe it to your organization to admit when you were wrong and to take corrective action.

Any board that says it's batting 1,000 is probably not doing much to lead its organization into the future. Just as the CEO must take calculated risks, so must the board. And unless you are clairvoyant, you will make some miscalculations along the way. The important thing to do is to practice due diligence before you take the risks, to monitor the effectiveness of your actions, and to pull the plug when your best intentions are having damaging consequences. If you have any doubt that this is the right course of action, just reflect on how you feel when our government policymakers "let the wheels fall off the bus" before admitting they were wrong and taking corrective action. Beside creating ill will, this approach to healthcare governance is, at its extreme, a tremendous breach of the board's fiduciary responsibility. It's ill-advised, imprudent, and just bad governance.

Universal Truth 5: You must not lose sight of the community; boards that do fail their organizations.

This universal truth does not apply only to not-for-profit healthcare organizations; it applies equally to those in the investor-owned sector. Although some boards are almost always focused on the community, others still become so immersed in the intricacies of governing a complex healthcare organization that they lose sight of the implications of their decisions on the communities their organizations serve. The danger of such myopic vision is obvious: If

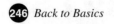

your organization loses the trust of the community, your organization sooner or later will pay the price. Whether you start losing patients, your stock price declines, your endowments diminish, or your medical staff limits admissions to your hospital, the consequences won't be pleasant.

These are only a handful of the universal truths of practical governance. We could have highlighted many more, perhaps enough for an entire book. These universal truths may appear to be largely negative or accusatory in nature, and perhaps there is some truth to that.

The good news is that plenty of boards are models for practical governance. The CEO, board chair, and the board as a whole understand their respective roles and execute them well. We share their stories in the pages that follow.

THE CEO'S ROLE

Earlier in this chapter, we identified five universal truths pertaining to a CEOs role in practical governance. In the following section, we explore each truth in greater detail.

The Great Communicator

Being an effective communicator may be more art than science, but in the case of communicating formally with the board, the CEO should have some standardized mechanisms in place to ensure the timely flow of "need-to-know" information. To this end, let's focus first on arguably the most essential CEO–board tool of communication: The board meeting agenda packet.

Board agenda packet

If your process for developing and disseminating materials for your board meetings is not like a well-oiled machine, you're ready for a tune up. Perhaps the best way to assess the caliber of your board meeting packet is to ask yourself: If I were a board member, would these materials meet my needs?

Criteria you would want to use to determine if the agenda packet makes the grade include:

- Did I receive the materials sufficiently before the meeting to allow for my thorough review? (Ideally, the board should receive the packet at least a week before the meeting.)
- Does the agenda clearly point to the items that require board action?
- If issues that the board has not addressed are on the agenda, are materials that provide sufficient and balanced background on the issue(s) enclosed?
- Are the financials timely, accurate, and understandable?

- Do the board packets contain reports started months, or even years ago, and are no longer relevant?
- Are all of the enclosed memos and reports clearly written and to the point? (We have known CEOs who boasted about the number of tabs and weight of their board packets.)

You have a responsibility to produce board materials that, at a minimum, meet the above criteria. To the extent that you can make other enhancements, so much the better. For example, a number of CEOs now include a quarterly or annual report of key financial and quality indicators of organizational performance in their board packets. (Given that the Joint Commission on Accreditation of Healthcare Organizations requires boards to be involved in improving performance, we believe such "quality" reports should be required for inclusion in packets.)

We want to emphasize that board meetings should be held no more than six times annually. If you think that your full board needs to meet more frequently, we recommend that you revisit your process for getting board work done. Chances are that you have not effectively delegated work to committees and subcommittees, or that you are asking the board to consider issues that can appropriately be handled elsewhere.

Day-to-Day Communications

As CEO, your informal communications are just as important as your formal communications. Your ability to stay "connected" to the staff, including the medical staff, is critical in your effectiveness as a conduit between the organization and the board. You want to be accessible and approachable to catch wind of issues before they become larger than life. You want to run interference so that issues that should never come to the board's attention are addressed expeditiously by you or your staff. You want to present yourself as—and truly be—your staff's biggest advocate. But you must do so in a way that does not diminish your responsibilities to the organization as a whole.

Most CEOs say that they understand the importance of their informal communications with staff. They perceive themselves as accessible and responsive people. Unfortunately, many CEOs need a reality check. The truth is that many CEOs are weighed down by a multitude of demands and pressures, and tend to be accessible and responsive only when they have time. As a result, informal communication quickly moves down on their list of priorities; that is, until they are blindsided by an issue that makes its way to the board without their knowledge.

One CEO we spoke with recalled when this scenario happened to him. Suddenly, the executive committee of his board held a meeting with his medical staff leadership without him. The medical staff leaders had called the meeting to appeal to the board to fire the CEO because they had lost faith in him. The board in this case probably should not have agreed to the meeting, particularly without inviting the CEO to attend. Luckily for the CEO, despite the apparent breach of protocol by the board, the executive committee stood behind him. After this harrowing experience, you can bet that the CEO has moved informal communication up on his list of priorities.

So how do you know whether your informal communications are effective, sufficient, or somehow lacking? Typically, your management team knows, although it isn't necessarily comfortable with sharing its observations with you, particularly when it thinks you could be doing better. If you truly want to know how you are doing and are prepared to make improvements as indicated, you may want to consider a 360° assessment; this is a process whereby you, your board, and your management team all assess your leadership effectiveness and communications style. You may find that your perceptions are not shared.

Informal communications with board members

CEOs who enjoy positive relationships with their boards are CEOs who take the time to talk with board members outside of meetings. Certainly, having weekly, or perhaps even monthly, one-on-one meetings with your board is unrealistic, unless the board is relatively small. But even one-on-one meetings once a year with each board member can be extremely beneficial. Conversely, if the only time that board members get a chance to talk with you is in the boardroom, you are making a mistake.

The vast majority of your board members are giving their time and energy to your organization because they believe in it and want to make a positive difference on behalf of the community it serves. Similarly, they need to know that you care as much as they do. If they only see you in the boardroom, your commitment will be much tougher to sell.

If you are a new CEO, sit down with as many board members as possible before your first board meeting. Sure, this meeting will eat up a lot of time— time you would rather devote to getting up to speed on a multitude of things— but it will be time well spent because you get a first-hand understanding of the personalities and priorities of individual board members. You also want to begin to get a sense of which board members are leaders and which are followers.

Veteran CEOs will advise you to make time—not just initially, but routinely—for your board chairs. In other words, carve out time to review the upcoming board agenda with your chairs before each meeting; schedule a standing lunch or at least a standing phone call at least once a month, or more frequently if your board meets more often than every other month; and be accessible every minute, day in and day out. Although, as we mentioned earlier, you serve at the pleasure of your board, the board chairs we interviewed all said that they consider support for the CEO a big part of their job. The only way they can serve you effectively is by talking with you, learning from you the operational implications of past or potential policy decisions, and believing that you truly value their counsel.

THE NO-SURPRISE SCHOOL OF LEADERSHIP

In today's healthcare organizations, deciding on which issues to bring to the board's attention and when the appropriate time to do so is not always easy. First-time CEOs find this determination to be particularly challenging and often err on the side of asking for board involvement in decisions that are much too operational in nature. (A few decision-making meetings with the board about paint colors for the nursery or menu planning for a hospital fundraiser quickly cure this tendency.)

The other extreme case is when the CEO operates under the dangerous misconception that he or she knows best in virtually all situations and involves the board only in the purest policy issues. Certainly, the board's job is to set policy, not to become involved in operations. But some issues are in that gray zone—they may first appear as operational issues but, upon closer inspection, in fact have policy implications. Take, for example, a labor dispute. Labor disputes typically begin because a group of employees are unhappy with compensation, benefits, or other aspects of their job. At first, dissatisfaction may be voiced informally and make its way to the CEO anecdotally. In some of these cases, concerns can be addressed by management without the board's knowledge or input. But if the grievances are numerous and the dissatisfaction is widespread, chances are that a quick fix won't work. As CEO, you can bide your time and see if things quiet down; after all, if all is well, you "saved" the board from having to spend time on this troublesome issue. But while you are biding your time, your disgruntled workers may be hard at work, and not necessarily at their jobs, but at making their concerns heard—and not just in the boardroom alone, but out there in the community. It would be a shame—perhaps even a career-limiting move for you—if your board learned about the employee unrest at a dinner party or from the local newspaper.

A labor dispute is just one example of the type of in-house information you want to think long and hard about *not* sharing with your board. As a rule, we recommend that you ask yourself the following questions when deciding if the issue you are dealing with is one that the board should hear about:

- Does the issue have the potential to become explosive?
- Is the board likely to learn about the issue from others—others on my staff or others in the community?
- Will resolving the issue effectively possibly require policy changes?
- Has the issue surfaced before, and has it benefited from board attention in the past?
- Am I reluctant to bring the issue to the board's attention because it is an issue that may reflect badly on me?

If you answer "yes" to all or most of these questions, think long and hard before *not* putting the issue on the board agenda.

Obviously we are strong proponents of the "no-surprises school of leadership." No CEO ever lost his job—at least, not that we are aware of—for sharing too much information with his or her board. In contrast, plenty of former CEOs had to move on because their boards were surprised one-too-many times.

WHO'S THE BOSS?

Don't ever lose sight of your place in the pecking order. The vast majority of board members wholeheartedly want to support you, but you don't have carte blanche. Yes, you are paid to lead, but you are also paid to follow the board's lead. You may not always agree with the direction in which the board has you headed and, clearly, you have a right, albeit a responsibility, to speak up in such cases. But ultimately, if the board charts a course and you choose not to follow it, you have only yourself to blame for the potential consequences.

Without exception, all of the CEOs we interviewed seemed to clearly understand the concept of serving at the board's pleasure. And, interestingly, all of the board chairs we interviewed really downplayed their "implicit power" over their CEO. We suggest that in the vast majority of cases, you can depend on your board's support because your board members trust you and believe you want to do the right thing. But cross the line, lose sight of your role in relation to the board, and the dynamics are likely to change quite quickly. Only the lucky few learn from their boards that they have overstepped their bounds before it is too late.

THE VISIONARY CEO

Are you a visionary? As CEO, you had better be. Your board does not expect you to be clairvoyant, but they do expect you to lead them into the future because of your first-hand understanding of the healthcare marketplace. Remember, most of your board members are not intimately familiar with the issues of the day. Even your more senior board members probably have considerably less insight into the complexities of the issues they must address.

Given that you are the resident expert, your responsibility is to try to anticipate the future. Your board is counting on it. Fred Wolf, former chair of the board at Springboat Springs (Colorado) Healthcare Association puts it this way: "You can have the best board in the world, but if they don't have someone in there as CEO that can run the place with an eye on the future, the organization is going to suffer."

YOU CAN'T ALWAYS PLAY IT SAFE

Certainly as CEO, you have a responsibility to keep your organization on a steady course. You want to articulate a vision that your board can embrace and your staff can work to fulfill. Schizophrenic leadership—a vision that constantly fluctuates—breeds confusion and undermines others' confidence in you.

That said, you are also the individual who is best positioned to propose bold new directions for your organization. You are in this unique position for a simple reason. First, as CEO, you obviously understand healthcare and its intricacies—in fact much, much better than your board does. Second, you have a first-hand understanding of the inner workings of your organization— its strengths and weaknesses.

More than anyone else on your board or on your staff, you have—or should have—a "big-picture" understanding of your organization and its needs to flourish in the future. With this knowledge comes responsibility—a responsibility to identify new initiatives that will help fortify your organiza-tion for the future.

The vast majority of healthcare CEOs in the United States have an employment contract, so chances are you do, too. This employment contract is your insurance policy for risk taking. The good news is that in most cases if you have taken your board and your organization down the wrong path, but not because of negligence on your part, no retribution will come about. Your job may not be on the line or, if it is, you have a severance package in place that offers a measure of security.

The flip side is that you can play it safe. Ironically, playing it safe by not taking risks probably puts you in even greater peril. If you perpetuate the status quo, you may be fine for now; but chances are your organization is not going to be positioned well for the future. So even if your current board is satisfied with your leadership, you run the risk that a future board will question why you didn't do more to keep the organization on a forward course.

Taking risks is risky. But we believe that not taking risks is even riskier. Given our view, we recommend that you routinely ask yourself the following questions:

1. Am I aware of national, regional, or local trends that have the potential to affect my organization?
2. How entrenched is my organization in its current way of doing things? Are we flexible enough to respond quickly to changing market forces?
3. In what ways is my organization vulnerable or potentially vulnerable, and what actions could we take to fortify our position?
4. Should I put these issues and potential solutions on the table for board consideration?

If you have trouble answering the last question, you must do some soul searching. You need to explore why you might not want to discuss these issues with the board. If your reluctance comes primarily from the unpleasantness of the topic or if you are concerned that the board won't buy into your proposed solutions, then you probably need to force yourself out of your comfort zone. Do your homework, look at the issue(s) from all sides, and then start broaching the issue with your board chair. Your reluctance may turn out to be a Pandora's Box, but it may be one that had to be opened.

A final word of advice to CEOs: Although your job shouldn't be your life, the city or town where your hospital is located should be your home. In other words, if you take a CEO job with the attitude that you are just "passing through" on the way to bigger and better things, it will be noticed. This word of advice came from Terry Gerber, board chair at Memorial Health Systems in South Bend, Indiana, as he reflected on the system's CEO, Philip Newbold: "When you have a CEO coming and going from different systems—meaning they already think they are going somewhere else—the result will not be nearly as good as if the CEO adopts the community. Maybe they didn't feel this way initially, but I can tell you today that Phil and his wife consider South Bend their home. Because a CEO who sees the community as his or her home wants the organization to reflect the values of the community, it shows."

You may be wondering how boards feel about their CEOs. That is hard to say. We do know, however, that most healthcare system and hospital CEOs *believe* that their governing boards support their work. That's according to a recent survey of 214 CEOs whose hospitals participate in the San Diego-based purchasing alliance. Ninety-five percent of the CEOs believe their boards support them. We hope they are right.

The Meaning of Marketing

Eric N. Berkowitz, Ph.D.

Primary care satellites, integrated delivery systems, managed care plans, and physician-hospital organizations (PHOs) are but a few of the elements that dominate the structure of the health care industry today, as the government, employers, consumers, providers, and health care suppliers deal with a new health care market. This marketplace is typified by massive restructuring in the way health care organizations operate, health care is purchased, and care is delivered. Competing in this new environment will require an effective marketing strategy to deal with these forces of change. This chapter will focus on the essentials for effective marketing and their implementation in this new health care marketplace. This discussion begins with an examination of what marketing is and how it has evolved within health care since first being discussed as a relevant management function in 1976.

MARKETING

For anyone involved in health care during the past ten years, the term *marketing* generates little emotional reaction. Yet, health care marketing—a commonplace concept today—was considered novel and controversial when first introduced to the industry two decades ago. In 1975, Evanston Hospital, in Evanston, Illinois, was one of the first hospitals to establish a formal marketing staff position. Now, more than 20 years later, marketing has diffused throughout health care into hospitals, group practices, rehabilitation facilities,

Editor's Note: Reprinted with permission from Eric N. Berkowitz, *Essentials of Healthcare Marketing*, Chapter 1, pages 3–38, © 1996, Aspen Publishers, Inc.

and other health care organizations. In this book, fundamental marketing concepts and marketing strategies are discussed. Although health care is undergoing significant structural change, the basic elements of marketing will be at the core of any organization's successful position in the marketplace.

The Meaning of Marketing

There are several views and definitions of marketing. The most widely accepted definition is that of the American Marketing Association—the professional organization for marketing practitioners and educators—which defines **marketing** as "the process of planning and executing the conception, pricing, promotion, and distribution of ideas, goods, and services to create exchanges that satisfy individual and organizational objectives."[1]

Central to this definition of marketing is the focus on the consumer, whether that be an individual patient, physician, or organization such as a company contracting for industrial medicine. This definition also contains the key ingredients of marketing that lead to consumer satisfaction. Increasingly in health care, customer satisfaction is the key issue.

The Joint Commission on Accreditation of Health Care Organizations, the industry's major accrediting agency for operating standards of health care facilities, required—in its 1994 accreditation manual—that hospitals improve on nine measures of preformance, one of which is patient satisfaction. This focus on patient satisfaction for hospital accreditation is an overt recognition of the need for health care facilities to be marketing oriented, and, thus, customer responsive.

Prerequisites for Marketing

This book's definition of marketing includes several prerequisite conditions that must exist before marketing occurs. First, there must be two or more parties with unsatisfied needs. One party might be the consumer looking to fulfill certain needs; the second, a company seeking to exchange a service or product for economic gain. A second prerequisite for marketing is the desire or ability of another party to meet those needs. Third, parties must have something to exchange. For example, a physician has the clinical skills that will meet an individual patient's need to have a torn meniscus repaired. A consumer must have the health insurance or financial resources to exchange for the receipt of these medical sevices. Finally, there must be a means to communicate. In order to facilitate an exchange between two parties, each party must learn of the other's existence. It is this last aspect of health care that has formally evolved in recent years.

Until 1975, advertising and promotion really did not exist within health care. Communication to facilitate exchange occurred by word of mouth. One would consult with a physician, and that individual in turn recommended the physician to other consumers who would then seek out that particular doctor. Prior to 1975, the American Medical Association had within its codes of ethics a prohibition against advertising. That very year, the U.S. Supreme Court ruled that professional associations were subject to federal antitrust laws. The American Medical Association revised its code of ethics to be less stringent regarding advertising. Further legal actions between the Federal Trade Commission (FTC) and the American Medical Association had, by 1982, removed even those restrictions. The FTC believed the restriction on advertising deprived consumers of the free flow of information regarding health care alternatives and services. The FTC and the federal courts recognized the value of communications to consumers. Communication is a prerequisite for marketing. It is only in the last two decades that more formal means of communication have evolved within health care and that marketing strategies have become more viable.

Who Does Marketing?

Traditionally, only for-profit commercial businesses in consumer or industrial settings conducted marketing. In this text, they will be referred to as traditional business. Yet, the application of marketing broadened in the late 1960s.

In 1969, two marketing academics—Philip Kotler and Sidney Levey—at Northwestern University in Illinois, published an article about broadening the concept of marketing. Their writing was the first attempt to recognize that for-profit and nonprofit businesses engaged in marketing activities. They recognized that marketing activities occurred in both service and product businesses. At the core of these organizations' activities was the notion of "exchange."[2]

Viewing the concept of exchange as the core of marketing allowed people to consider other areas where marketing might also be useful. Fine arts centers and museums, hospitals, and school districts began to see the relevance of marketing strategies and tactics to their settings. A consumer exchanges time and money for the pleasure of seeing a display of fine art. A patient pays for medical services provided by a free-standing diagnostic clinic, while a school district provides education in exchange for public support through tax levies.

The scope and nature of who markets has broadened considerably. Marketing is conducted by individuals and organizations. Marketing is relevant to for-profit and nonprofit entities. Throughout this chapter, examples of marketing programs at businesses such as General Motors or Johnson & Johnson will be discussed, along with the marketing programs of health care providers such as the Geisinger Health System in Danville, Pennsylvania or the Mayo Clinic in Rochester, Minnesota. While there are distinct aspects within any industry that require the modification of marketing principles to fit particular needs, the core of marketing and the marketing mix is relevant for almost every organization.

THE ELEMENTS OF SUCCESSFUL MARKETING

Marketing Research

Within the definition of marketing is the discussion of a process of planning and executing to meet consumer needs. Marketing requires an understanding of consumer wants and needs. This understanding is derived through an assessment of these needs. **Marketing research** is a process in which there is a systematic gathering of data from customers to identify their needs.

The Four Ps

The heart of marketing strategy is the development of a response to the marketplace. As noted in the definition, marking is the "execution of the conception, pricing, promotion, and distribution of the goods, ideas, and services." To respond to customers, an organization must develop a product, determine the price customers are willing to pay, identify what place is most convenient for customers to purchase the product or access the service, and finally, promote the product to customers to let them know it is available.

Product, price, place, and promotion are referred to as the **four Ps** of marketing strategy.[3] It is these four controllable variables that a firm uses to define its marketing strategy. The mix of these four controllable variables that a business uses to pursue a desired level of sales is referred to as the **marketing mix**. The definitions of the four major elements of marketing as discussed below provide the focus of this chapter.

Product

Product represents goods, services, or ideas offered by a firm. In this text, the term "product" also will be used interchangeably with health care services and ideas. In health care, the nature of the product has changed dramatically. Twenty years ago, one could define the product simply as a medical procedure or as an orthotic device to correct a physical disability. In today's climate, the discussion of the health care product includes not only these traditional products, but also products and services such as prepaid health insurance plans offered by health maintenance organizations (HMOs), or a group purchasing contract such as that offered by the Premier Health Alliance of Westchester, Illinois, a nationwide association of hospitals.

Price

Price focuses on what customers are willing to pay for a service. What price represents is addressed in the definition of marketing in terms of exchanges. A company provides a service and customers exchange dollars for receipt of a service that satisfies their needs. An employee paying an annual premium to an HMO or an insurance company reimbursing a physician's fee are both exchanges involving some determined price.

The issue of pricing for health care services has become a major concern of marketing strategy as the health care environment changes. Several factors are contributing to the greater role that the pricing variable is playing in developing marketing strategy. On one level, more employers are requiring employees to pay a greater percentage of their health care insurance premiums. Many insurance companies also now require consumers to make a co-payment for medical services, whereas in the past, insurance companies paid the full medical bill. Companies that historically have paid the full premium for health care costs have become concerned about the price of medical services. These employers are now looking for ways to become more efficient buyers of their health care coverage. Finally, within the health care system itself, new structural organizations such as HMOs have begun to contract with providers and hospitals for services. These organizations are seeking discounts from providers and hospitals for services. These organizations are seeking discounts from providers in return for their subscribers' business. These same managed care organizations must determine how to price their prepaid health care plans to attract compannies to offer them to their employees, and to stay competitive with other health care plans in the marketplace. For marketers, the issue of price is understanding what level of dollars a customer is willing to exchange for the receipt of some want-satisfying services or products. In the current health care climate, determining the value of these services—represented by the price—is the major challenge facing health care organizations.

Place

Place represents the manner in which goods or services are distributed by a firm for use by consumers. Place might include decisions regarding the location or the hours a medical service can be accessed.

Increasingly, as more health care organizations establish managed care plans to enroll consumers in an insurance option that provides for all their health care needs, the place variable assumes a more critical role. Companies offering prepaid health care plans must consider location and primary care access for potential enrollees. While 40, 20, or even 10 years ago, a physician would establish an office in a location convenient for the doctor, today the consumer dictates this variable element of the marketing mix.

Promotion

The final P represents promotion. For many people this has historically meant advertising, and advertising has meant marketing. Yet, as can be seen in the definition, promotion is just one part of marketing; promotion alone is not marketing. **Promotion** represents any way of informing the marketplace that the organization has developed a response to meet its needs, and that the exchange should be consummated. Promotion itself involves a range of tactics involving publicity, advertising, and personal selling.

As discussed earlier, formal communication in the form of advertising was not allowed as recently as 1975. Yet while the past 20 years has seen a change in terms of the amount of advertising, other promotional tactics such as personal selling have become more relevant to compete effectively in today's marketplace. Health insurance companies and HMOs all employ sales forces. A national health care organization, Continental Medical Systems of Harrisburg, Pennsylvania, has a sales force to generate referrals to its specialized rehabilitation hospitals located around the country. Even local acute-care hospitals now often have physician referral staff who call on physicians to ensure that their needs are being met at the facility where they admit patients.

THE DILEMMA OF NEEDS AND WANTS

One of health care marketing's major concerns pertains to the issues of needs and wants. Health care professionals often speak of the fact that what consumers want may not be what they need. Clinical and professional responsibility demands treatment of the need. A **need** has been defined as a "condition in which there is a deficiency of something, or one requiring relief."[4] A **want** is defined as the "wish or desire for something."[5] A consumer *needs* to have medication for hypertension. A person may *want* medication to suppress the appetite and thus lose weight. To which need or want should the health care marketer respond?

Underlying any response in health care must be whatever constitutes providing quality care for the patient. Meeting medical needs must be the primary purpose of the system. Yet wants should not be ignored. For the health care professional, consider the just-cited dilemma of a pill for weight reduction. Should the system respond to this want? A marketer's response would most likely be yes, but the response must be medically appropriate. In fact, the marketer would try to understand more closely what it is the consumer wants (or is buying). In this instance, it is less likely to be a pill and more probably a more attractive appearance through weight reduction. The request for medication might be met more appropriately with creation of an eating disorders program or a wellness center that helps establish an exercise and fitness regimen. The ultimate want that the customer has can be satisfied, but the methodology must observe appropriate practice standards.

Identifying the Customer

In health care, this need/want dilemma often masks the major question, "Who is the customer?" Consider recent trends in the field of obstetrics. For many years, the consumer—the expectant mother—wanted to have her significant other with her in the delivery room. The medical community responded by claiming that this want was inappropriate. It would compromise good standards of care. In fact, the issue had less to do with standards of care and more with standards of convenience for the provider. Now, in most delivery rooms in the United States, a woman in labor will be accompanied by her significant other, a nurse midwife, and possibly, the obstetrician.

The medical community argued that the need to restrict access to the labor suite was for "good standards in obstetrical care." In reality, medicine lost sight of who the customer was and how her needs and wants could be met. In the delivery process, the physician may be viewed as part of the production line, not as the customer. Medical needs are not compromised in modern labor rooms, but customer needs are being more closely addressed.

While the composition of people present in the labor and delivery room has been resolved, a new conflict between needs and wants has arisen within obstetrics again as organizations try to control costs. Many managed care plans have moved to a 24-hour discharge practice for mothers who have an uncomplicated delivery. Plans like Maryland's Blue Cross & Blue Shield follow up with a home visit by a nurse the next day. The health insurers want more cost-effective deliveries. Yet the American College of Obstetricians and Gynecologists (ACOG) does not believe this policy meets the needs of the patients and the newborn babies. In May 1995, the ACOG called for a moratorium on such discharge practices until further study. The college recommends stays of 48 hours for routine deliveries and 96 hours for Caesarian sections. Here, the wants of one group and the needs of another are in conflict and still to be resolved.[6]

In our current health care marketplace, most health care organizations have multiple markets or customers to whom they must be attentive. Figure 12.1 shows an array (but probably not all-encompassing) of potential markets for a health care organization. An organization offering a mental health or substance abuse program for adolescents might have to accommodate the needs of judges, probation officers, or social workers. Schools might be the market for a sports medicine program. Long-term care facilities might be the market for a geriatric assessment program. Also included are the more traditional markets represented by physicians, nurses, patients, referral physicians, employee assistance personnel at companies, managed care plans, and regulators. One increasingly important market includes employers. For many years, this segment was considered of secondary importance, since companies paid the full insurance premiums for their labor force. Now, however, companies are controlling rising health care costs by dealing directly with providers to meet their employees' health care needs.

Figure 12.1   Multiple Healthcare Organization Markets

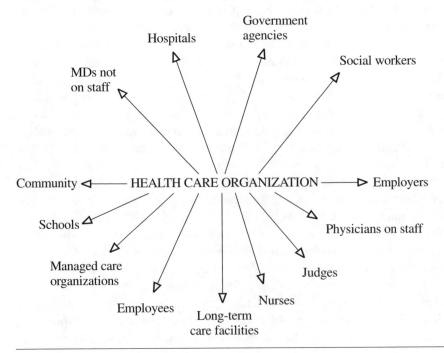

As the topic of markets is discussed in this book, it is important to be aware that health care organizations have multiple markets—the importance of each one is a function of the program or issue being addressed.

THE EVOLUTION OF MARKETING

In both traditional businesses and in health care the marketing concept has taken several decades to evolve. In health care this evolution has occurred in a relatively short time period. As previously noted, the first hospital to hire a person with a marketing title was Evanston Hospital in Illinois in 1975. In traditional product businesses, the evolution of the marketing concept took longer.

Production Era

To understand how marketing has evolved, let's consider its development in a corporation such as Pillsbury Company of Minneapolis-St. Paul, long known as a manufacturer of flour, baking goods, and other food products. Let's also trace this same evolution in the typical hospital.

Pillsbury located itself in the Minneapolis-St. Paul, Minnesota, market in the 1800s. The location, along the Mississippi River, offered the company a source of water power. (In that era, the Mississippi River had waterfalls that far north.) This location was also close to the raw materials needed for the production of Pillsbury's product. Robert Keith, a former Pillsbury president, described the company at this stage of its development. "We are professional flour millers. Blessed with a supply of the finest North American wheat, plenty of water power, and excellent milling machinery, we produce flour of the highest quality. Our basic function is to mill high-quality flour, and of course we must hire salesmen to sell it, just as we hire accountants to keep the books."[7]

At this stage of the company's evolution, the primary focus of the business was producing a high-quality product—flour. The sales and even the consumption or purchase of the product were incidental to the firm's focus—it was assumed that people would buy Pillsbury flour because it was high quality.

Many hospitals were and are at this stage in their own evolution. One might rewrite Keith's statements for a production-oriented hospital to say, "Our basic function is to provide high-quality medicine. Accompanied by the highest forms of technology, we have physicians, nurses, and allied health personnel to provide this service. And, we have administrators to keep the books." For a production-oriented hospital or health care organization, the focus is on providing high-quality medicine. As can be seen in Table 12.1, the health care organization's focus is on delivering clinical quality.

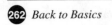

Sales Era

For many traditional businesses such as Pillsbury, the production orientation worked well until the early 1900s. By 1920, the automobile became part of our way of life and changed the world for consumers and companies. The federal government began to finance the construction of a roadway system in the United States. Consumers became more mobile in the everyday life of work, shopping, and recreation. For companies, the strategic change was in the hiring of traveling salespeople. Competition heightened as competing sales forces fought for customers who formerly were the domain of manufacturers in their particular region. Robert Keith so characterized Pillsbury's business focus at this stage: "We are a flour-milling company, manufacturing a number of products for the consumer market. We must have a first-rate sales organization which can dispose of all the products we make at a favorable price."[8]

For hospitals, the sales era occurred in the mid-1970s with the change in reimbursement. Under cost-based reimbursement, competition with other hospitals was not a major concern. Hospitals had patients, lengths of stay were not an issue, and occupancy rates were high. Hospitals treated patients and passed along the actual cost, along with an appropriate profit margin, for reimbursement by the third-party payers. The focus for a hospital administrator in the sales stage was twofold. The first and top priority was to get as many patients as possible. Traditionally, this goal was accomplished by attracting as many physicians as possible to admit patients to the hospital. Since this era preceded the days of utilization reviews, hospitals had no concerns about attracting efficient physicians who could care for patients in some limited time period. The hospital wanted to ensure that as many patients as possible wanted to be admitted into the facility who were so directed by their doctors.

Changing Mr. Keith's statement, one might characteize the focus of a sales-oriented hospital as: "We are a high-quality hospital providing numerous medical services to the market. We must attract physicians in the

Table 12.1 The Evolution of Marketing

Business Orientation	Pillsbury	Hospital
Production	Product quality focus	Clinical quality focus
Sales	Generating volume	Filling beds
Marketing	Satisfying needs and wants	Identifying health care needs and meeting them

community to want to admit to our facility. And, we must encourage patients to want to come here." This stage of marketing evolution focused on sales. Hospitals tried to entice doctors to admit to a particular facility. Hospitals built medical office buildings attached to their facilities offering doctors the convenience of admitting patients at the hospital contiguous to their offices. Hospitals developed physician relations programs to bond with the providers. They sponsored seminars for physicians, or provided valet parking and attractive doctors' lounges. All these were attempts to build the census, fill the beds.

At this time, hospitals also recognized that the patient might play a role in the hospital selection decision.[9] A second, concurrent strategy of selling to the public also occurred. In the mid-1970s, many hospitals adopted mass advertising strategies to promote their programs, including the use of billboard displays and television and radio commercials touting a particular service. The advertising goal was to encourage patients to use the hospital facilities when the doctor presented a choice, or to self-refer if necessary. In health care, this was the evolution to sales.

Marketing Era

The evolution to marketing occurred after World War II. In the late 1940s, many companies found that their level of technological sophistication had increased dramatically as a result of their wartime efforts. Moreover, consumers were returning from the war and establishing households, escalating the demand for products and services. For many companies the major question became one of deciding which products or services to offer. Pillsbury's perspective changed to: "We are in the business of satisfying the wants and needs of consumers." With this focus, it is the customer who drives the production process and directs the organization's efforts.

So, too, in health care, a similar perspective can and is being achieved. Health care providers can offer any number of services by reallocating their financial resources. The underlying question, however, becomes, which service to offer? This is where a marketing-oriented perspective is valuable. In health care, the focus of a marketing-oriented institution can be viewed as "We address the health care needs of the markeplace." Such a marketing-oriented focus might lead to a product or service line that includes home health care, geriatric medicine, after-hours care, or wellness centers. The trend toward integrated delivery systems is a response to a marketplace that does not want to deal with a fractionated health care system of providers, free-standing medical centers, a hospital, and an insurance firm. The integrated system formation can deliver a seamless health care product to the buyer that

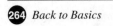

involves not only delivering the clinical care, but also accepting the risk for the cost of that care through a managed care product. It is a focus that begins with the consumer; the organization responds to this demand.

THE MARKETING CULTURE

Some organizations achieve a final level of evolution, where marketing becomes part of the corporate culture, diffused throughout all levels of the organization. The focus of marketing no longer lies solely under the responsibility of the marketing department. Rather, in the health care setting, marketing is peformed by the clinical nurse administrator for the neurology program. The admitting desk clerks and the house maintenance staff understand and appreciate the need to maintain a customer orientation.

The evolution to this stage may be seen in organizations that have adopted a patient-focused system. Sentara, an integrated delivery system in Hampton, Virginia, and Lakeland Regional Medical Center, a large tertiary hospital in Lakeland, Florida, are two such institutions. These organizations have made the customer the central focus of all their activities. Admitting is accomplished on the floor where the patient is assigned a bed, employees cross-train for skills that allow them to be the most patient-responsive possible without compromsing the quality of care delivered. Whenever possible, certain diagnostic equipment is brought to the patient rather than having the patient move through the hospital. It is the primary responsibility of each employee to respond to customer needs first. The development of patient-focused care in such organizations is the transference of a marketing culture throughout the organization. Rather than having the patient (customer) go to the provider (such as when the patient moves through the delivery system for treatment or clinical testing), the provider goes to the patient whenever possible to administer the necessary clinical interventions.

For organizations at this stage, the concept of a marketing orientation has taken hold. A **marketing orientation** has five distinct elements:

1. Customer orientation: having a sufficient understanding of the target buyers to be able to create superior value for them continuously
2. Competitor orientation: recognizing competitors' (and potential competitors') strengths, weaknesses, and strategies
3. Interfunctional coordination: coordinating and deploying company resources in a manner that focuses on creating value for the customer
4. Long-term focus: adopting a perspective that includes a continuous search for ways to add value by making appropriate business investments

5. Profitability: earning revenues sufficient to cover long-term expenses and satisfy key constituencies.[10]

THE NON-MARKETING-DRIVEN PLANNING PROCESS

While the patient-focused health care approach represents the diffusion of a marketing orientation throughout a health care institution, such an approach has not always been the perspective taken by health care providers. Most health care organizations have been characterized by a non-market-driven culture and planning process. In no place is the difference between being marketing-oriented and non-marketing-oriened more apparent than when a health care organization goes about its long-range planning process.

To understand the difference between a marketing-driven and non-marketing-driven process, it is important to recognize the implications of the difference between the two concepts on long-range planning.[11]

Figure 12.2 shows the sequence involved when a non-marketing-driven organization conducts long-range planning. In most health care organizations, long-range planning is assigned to a committee comprising administrators, key members of the hospital's board of directors, and a few influential physicians. Typically, the first step involves a review of the organization's mission and goals. A hospital might reaffirm its mission "to provide high-quality health care regardless of race, creed, religion, and [in small print] ability to pay."

The second step of the planning process—strategy formulation—is often difficult and time-consuming. At this point, members of the long-range planning committee debate what objectives should be included in the hospital's five-year plan. Now, the real implications of the non-marketing-driven approach become evident. Often, a senior physician stands up at the strategy formulation stage and makes a speech such as the following: "I've been at this hospital since the day I entered the medical profession. This hospital is my life and I never even admitted a patient to another facility. Of course, I'm also being recognized as an expert in the future of medicine. I've been invited to conferences to speak on the futgure of medicine and I've just published an article in the *New England Journal of Medicine*. As I think about what services we need to provide in the new ambulatory care wing of the hospital, it's clear to me that we need a sports medicine program." Usually, the physician making this recommendation appears to be a self-serving orthopedic surgeon.

At this stage in the planning process, several committee members become dismayed. Some think the hospital should, instead, offer an expanded geriatric medicine program; other committee members want to get into rehabilitative

Figure 12.2   Non-Marketing-Based Planning Sequence

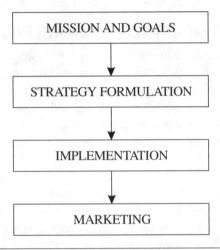

medicine. Yet this physician is very influential and has lined up committee votes in favor of a sports medicine program before the committee met. The vote is taken and the final tally is seven to five in favor of a sports medicine program, which becomes part of the strategic plan.

The next stage of the long-range planning process—implementation—is more difficult. The hospital realizes it has no staff members trained in sports medicine. The hospital hires a physician recruiting firm to find a new medical director for sports medicine. The position is filled and it is at this stage of the process where conflict often occurs within the organization. Many committee members opposed opening a sports medicine program, yet now, the new director and new program require resources. Other services within the hospital find their budgets for the coming fiscal year are reduced in order to reallocate dollars to sports medicine. Other program directors are upset because they lose space in the new ambulatory care wing due to the needs of the sports medicine service. The new sports medicine director has an aggressive agenda. She has hired her staff, purchased the necessary equipment, and is setting up shop.

A state of anxiety soon takes hold of the hospital's administrators. As the date moves closer to the grand opening of the sports medicine program, they ask, "Who is really going to use the service?" Recognizing the need for patient volume, they attempt to market the program. But what happens is not marketing but sales. The hospital administrator typically places a frantic call to the public relations director requesting an open house for the new sports medicine program. Advertisements are placed in the local community paper. Invitations to tour the facility are distributed to influential people. The goal is to attract visitors to the new program. On the day of the open house, attendance is disappointing. Four months later the finance committee convenes to review the performance of the sports medicine program. It is a failure. Why?

The first repsonse is to blame public relations; the PR director didn't promote the service well. This may be a possible explanation. A second hypothesis suggests the failure is the fault of the new sports medicine director, whose interpersonal style is discouraging other physicians from referring patients to the program. Yet, there may be a third, more viable explanation— the sports medicine program wasn't needed. The program differed little from the competition's offering, hence, patients had no reason to switch facilities.

This scenario is a common result of non-marketing-driven planning process. The problem with a non-marketing-driven process is that it requires a group of people (or one powerfully persuasive committee member) to have insight into what kinds of health care service the marketplace wants, how it wants that service configured, and what it is willing to pay for it. This approach to delivering a service or health care product to the market is an internal-to-external development process. The product is sold first. The challenge then is to find enough buyers willing to use the service or product at a level sufficient to make a profit. This approach is risky at best in that it relies on the market forecasting ability of a few people within the organization.

It is this limitation of the internal-to-external perspective of the non-marketing-driven approach, as well as overcoming the political power of a few people within the organization, that are addressed by taking a marketing-driven approach to planning.

A MARKETING-DRIVEN PLANNING SEQUENCE

A marketing-driven planning sequence is dramatically different from a non-marketing-driven process, as illustrated in Figure 12.3. The first step is the same; every organization has the right to determine its mission and goals. Yet the marketing-driven approach is substantially different at step two. It is at this stage of needs assessment where market research begins to make its contribution. The hospital conducts a survey to determine which services are most needed. Should sports medicine, geriatric medicine, or women's health services be offered in the new ambulatory care wing of the hospital?

When determing the most needed service, it is essential to examine the competition. If there are existing competing services in the market, the necessary differential advantage for these new offerings must be identified.

Figure 12.3   Marketing-Driven Planning Sequence

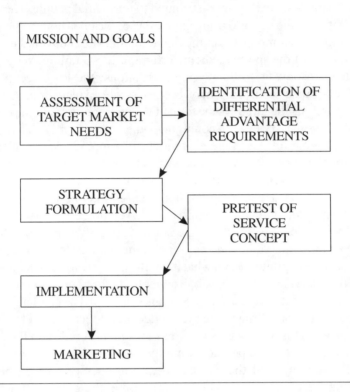

While the sources of a differential advantage are discused later in this chapter, a **differential advantage** is the incremental benefits of a product relative to competing products that are important to the buyer and perceived by the buyer. In our example, the hospital's survey reveals that 20 percent of the market wants sports medicine, 25 percent would like to see a new geriatric program, and 50 percent wants women's health. Further research shows that the major differential advantages that would lead women to use this service over their existing providers are convenient location and hours.

With the market research completed, the strategy is clear. A conveniently located, accessible women's health program is written into the hospital's long-range plan. Prior to full-scale implementation, however, market research is employed again in the form of a pretest. Pretesting involves returning to the market with a product sample to ensure that the specifications meet customer expectations. In a service business such as health care, the pretesting stage is particularly difficult. Unlike many product businesses that can manufacture a prototype without incurring major fixed costs, a new health program might require a redesign of physical space, the hiring of trained personnel, and acquisition of new technologies. Pretesting must still be done, however, without the addition of all these costs.

To pretest a service in health care effectively, the personnel involved with the program and with customer relations must develop a detailed concept description of the service. They then assemble a sample of potential female patients similar to those in the target market and walk them through a concept test of the service. Consumers can be questioned about hours, service location, and appointment procedure. Reactions to the concept generate appropraite modifications. Full-scale implementation then begins. At this point, the hospital needs to market—not sell—the program. Market reseach has determined the product, the price customers are willing to pay, and how the service should be distributed (i.e., locations, hours). All that remains for the hospital is to inform the target market about the availability of the desired new service through the appropriate promotions.

Is a Marketing Planning Approach Needed?

A comparison of Figures 12.2 and 12.3 shows that using market research can lead to a dramatically different result in long-range planning. Yet, is a marketing-driven planning process needed in health care? Twenty or 30 years ago, a non-marketing-driven process was sufficient. Competition wasn't a prime factor. In most communities, including major metropolitan areas, demand exceeded supply. A hospital would offer a new service and the major issue was how to meet demand for it. Twenty or 30 years ago most health care organizations were in a reasonably strong financial position due to cost-based reimbursement and unrestricted lengths of stay. Efficiency and financial prudence were nonissues.

The present competitive health care environment has prompted many organizations to adopt a maketing-driven planning approach. Health care providers find themselves facing significant competition. In many instances, and for many subspecialties, the problem is one of supply exceeding demand. The challenge is to encourage demand for your service at the expense of yor competitors. Organizations must find a differential advantage to encourage buyers to use their services. Health care organizations today must be fiscally astute. Few have the excess financial resources to afford the mistake of offering a service that is not needed in the marketplace. A marketing-driven planning process is one tool to help minimize such mistakes.

We have described a non-marketing-driven approach to planning as an internal-to-external methodology.[12] That is, members inside the organization try to foretell or dictate what the market wants and how the service should best be configured to meet those wants. In comparison, a marketing-driven approach follows an external-to-internal methodology. First, there is an assessment of what the market wants, then the organization's response. Health care providers must realize that a marketing-driven planning process does not guarantee success; but it does, however, minimize the probability of failure.

THE STRATEGIC MARKETING PROCESS

The marketing-driven planning model just discussed is devised within the context of a more macro setting. Figure 12.4 shows the setting in which marketing occurs. An organization must develop a marketing strategy that is sensitive to three factors: (1) important stakeholders, (2) environmental factors, and (3) society at large.

Stakeholders

Stakeholders represent any group with which the company has, or wants to develop, a relationship. As seen in Figure 12.4 the stakeholders can represent

Figure 12.4 Environment and Marketing Strategy

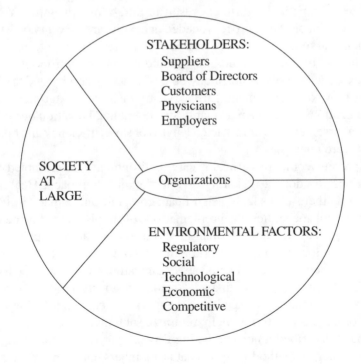

customers. For health care organizations, these customers might be patients, physicians who refer to the organization, social workers for an adolescent chemical dependency program, payers, managed care providers with whom contracts are developed, or companies that contract for an industrial medicine program.

Many organizations such as hospitals or proprietary chains also have boards of directors that serve an oversight function. Organizations develop their marketing strategy in light of the direction and values provided and communicated by this constituency. A third major stakeholder group includes suppliers. In health care, suppliers can represent companies that provide laboratory testing or maintenance services, or they again can represent physicians. For many hospitals, physicians are customers. In a group practice setting, physicians represent the shareholders or owners. In other organizations, physicians, by providing coverage of the emergency room, might actually be suppliers.

Uncontrollable Environment

Any marketing strategy is developed within the context of a braoder environmental perspective. The **environment** pertains to regulatory, social, technological, economic, and competitive factors to which the organization must be sensitive when developing a strategy. These elements, which are briefly described below, are uncontrollable, but impact marketing strategy. For example, a company cannot change the uncontrollable trend that society is aging. Yet a company can develop a strategy to respond to marketplace needs resulting from this trend. Between 1990 and 1993, the number of adult day-care centers nationwide increased almost 50 percent to 3,000 such facilities. Forecasts predict that 10,000 such centers will be needed by the year 2000 in response to an aging marketplace.[13] Building planned retirement communities or developing long-term care facilities are just two strategies for dealing with this trend.

Regulatory Factors

Regulatory factors include legal issues and requirements. In many health care communities, programs cannot be instituted without prior government approval. Some strategies, such as paying physicians for referrals, are illegal.

Social Forces

Social forces include demographic and cultural trends to which organizations must be sensitive. An aging population, a changing work ethic, and a culturally diverse marketplace are some of the issues to consider when developing marketing plans.

Technological Factors

Technological factors affect few industries more dramatically then they do health care. It is these technological forces that can change the viability of any service. Until the 1950s, the treatment of polio victims constituted a major revenue stream for many hospital facilities. As we know, this disease was all but eliminated by the technological achievement of the Salk vaccine in the 1950s.

Ecnomic Factors

Economic factors include changes in income distribution or fiscal conditions such as borrowing rates that can determine any company's investment plans. The rising cost of health care has led one major customer group—corporations—to work more aggressively with their health care providers in seeking solutions to rising costs.

Competitive Forces

Competitive forces are the final uncontrollable element in any marketing plan. Strategies and program must be developed in light of this constraint and should reflect the considerations that exist in the marketplace.

Society

Ultimately, all marketing programs and strategies are developed within the context of a broader societal perspective, a context that requires an ethically responsible decision-making process. For example, many companies have become more keenly aware of and responsible for the impact of their products and programs on the environment. The broader societal market represents all the individuals, groups, businesses, and other entities that affect, are related to, or derive benefit from the health care organization, as seen in Exhibit 12.1

TARGET MARKET

At the core of the marketing program is the **target market**, the group of customers whom the organization wishes to attract. In the development of a marketing strategy, the target market is within an organization's control as a function of the effectiveness of the marketing mix developed by the health care providers.

The notion of controlling the target market, however, is an idea that is often lost on health care providers. Whom a health system attracts to its facilities and whom it targets may be two different populations. Too often in the past, health care organizations have defined their market by simply identifying who walked into their facility or used the emergency room.

Exhibit 12.1 Organizations in the Health Care Environment

Organizations That Plan for and/or Regulate (Primary and Secondary Providers)	Organizations That Provide Health Services (Primary Providers)	Organizations That Provide Resources (Secondary Providers)	Organizations That Represent Primary and Secondary Providers	Individuals and Patients (Consumers)
• Federal Regulating Agencies –Health Systems Agencies (HSAs) –Department of Health and Human Services (DHHS) –Health Care Financing Agency (HCFA) • State Regulating Agencies –Public Health Departments –State Planning Agency (CON) • Voluntary Regulating Groups • Joint Commission On Accreditation of Healthcare Organizations • Other Accrediting Agencies	• Hospitals –Voluntary (Barnes Hospital) –Governmental (VA Hospitals) –Investor Owned (Humana, AMI, NME) • State Public Health Departments • Long-Term Care Facilities –Skilled Nursing Facilities (Beverly Enterprises) –Intermediate Care Facilities • HMOs and IPAs (Care America) • Ambulatory Care Facilities • Hospices (Hospice Care, Inc.) • Physician's Offices • Home Health Care Institutions (VNA, Upjohn Healthcare Services)	• Educational Institutions –Medical Schools (Johns Hopkins) –Nursing Schools –Health Administration Programs • Organizations That Pay for Care –Third-Party Payers –Government (Medicare) –Insurance Companies (Blue Cross) –Social Organizations (Shriners) • Pharmaceutical and Medical Supply –Drug Distributors (McKesson) –Drug & Research (Merck, Eli Lilly) –Medical Products (Johnson & Johnson, Bausch & Lomb)	• American Medical Associaton (AMA) • American Hospital Association (AHA) • State Medical Associations • Individual Professional Associations	• Independent Physicians • Nurses • Allied Health Professionals • Technicians • Patients

Source: Reprinted from Ginter, P. M., Duncan, W.J., Richardson, W. D., and Swayne, L. E., Analyzing the Health Care Environment: You Can't Hit What You Can't See, *Health Care Management Review,* Vol. 16, No. 4, p. 44, Aspen Publishers, Inc., © 1991.

Health care organizations developed profiles of their patients and developed strategies based on the users. Yet the central issue to marketing strategy is to decide whom you want to attract and then determine what this group's needs are. The organization that defines a target market, such as "all consumers with incomes above $75,000 who have private insurance and live in a particular area," can then focus its market research on identification of an appropriate strategy to meet the needs of the targeted group. Sharp Health Care of California has decided that one of its target markets will include Mexican patients. Sharp Health Care, a large health care system that includes various health care subsidiaries and five hospitals in San Diego, California, opened a hospital under the Sharp name in Mazatlan, Mexico in December 1994. Sharp also hopes to capture referrals from this target market by an affiliation agreement with Hospital Notre Dame in Tiajuana, Mexico. To support this effort, Sharp will provide continuing medical education programs for that hospital's medical staff.[14] Determining the target market resulted in several strategies to attract this consumer population.

ORGANIZING FOR MARKETING

Establishing the marketing function within an organization can be accomplished in one of several ways. The two most common organizational structures for marketing are by product and by market.

Product-Oriented Organization

The product management structure has been increasingly common in health care settings, structured as shown in Figure 12.5. In this setting, the responsibility, authority, and accountability rests with the product line manager. Nursing, pharmacy, laboratory, and other departments coordinate their services across, and in support of, the product lines. In the true **product-oriented organization**, each distinct product or related set of products has its own marketing organization.

The product manager is responsible for developing and overseeing the marketing strategy for the product or **strategic business units**, which are businesses operated as separate profit centers within a large organization. In a product management structure, individual managers commonly share staff resources, such as marketing research, as well as operational personnel, such as the sales force. The product manager approach is of value when a product has such unique requirements that it demands the commitment of a separate individual.

Product line management has two major advantages for health care organizations. First, having someone responsible for all aspects of a product line helps to refine the service area and to meet needs more easily. This struc-

Figure 12.5 Product-Oriented Organization

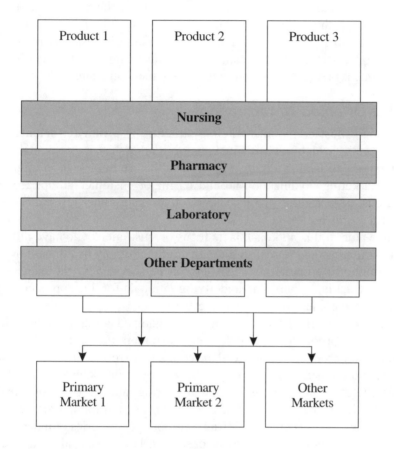

Source: Reprinted from Zelman, W. N. and Parham, D. L., Strategic, Operational, and Marketing Concerns of Product-Line Management in Health Care, *Health Care Management Review*, Vol. 15, No. 1, p. 32. Aspen Publishers, Inc., © 1990.

ture helps combine services and benefits for customers. Second, packaging related services into product lines helps contribute to continuous, rather than sporadic, planning.[15]

A disadvantage with the product management structure in traditional businesses has been the fact that the product manager has no direct control over many operational details—the product manager must negotiate for sales force time or marketing research resources. This same limitation holds in health care. While the product manager has the focus to develop program plans, there is no direct operational control over how the service is delivered within the facility. Often, in many health care organizations, the product manager acts as the salesperson for the program. For health care organizations, there is another consideration that may limit the value of a product organization. If the same customer is targeted for more than one product line, it could lead to significant marketing inefficiencies or customer resistance. For example, a referral physician may be unwilling to see four different product line representatives from one tertiary medical center.

Market-Oriented Organization

The second most common marketing structure is a **market-oriented organization** in which each distinct major market has its own marketing organization, as seen in Figure 12.6. A health care organization might design a marketing organization around its major customer groups (referral physicians, corporations, managed care buyers, and other referral sources) as shown in this figure.

The value of this approach is its focus on customers who have different buying structures and purchasing requirements. For any health care organization, supporting marketing activities can be serviced by the manager of each major market group. The underlying rationale for this approach is that each major customer group has distinct needs.

For decades, IBM Corporation was organized around product lines. In 1994, the corporation concluded that customers demanded solutions to problems, not products. This forced the company to restructure around major markets and industries. In this way, IBM can develop expertise in financial services, telecommunications, or manufacturing and meet the information needs of these respective industries. Whether the solution is provided by a local area newtork system, a mainframe computer, or a series of independent desktop computers is irrelevant to the customer. This same analogy applies to the health care setting. Corporate expectations and demands differ from the requirements and concerns of a second major market of referral physicians. In each instance, solutions to problems are sought rather than the purchase of a specific clinical program.

REQUIREMENTS FOR ORGANIZATIONAL MARKETING SUCCESS

Many hospitals and medical groups have problems making the transition to becoming a market-oriented organization. Often, marketing has not met the expectations of filling hospital beds or generating substantial numbers of new subscribers into the HMO. The disappointment in marketing is due to a lack of appreciation of what it means to be marketing driven, and of what

Figure 12.6 Market-Oriented Organization

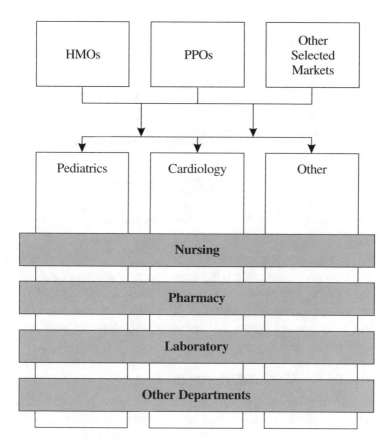

Source: Reprinted from Zelman, W. N. and Parham, D. L., Strategic, Operational, and Marketing Concerns of Product-Line Management in Health Care, *Health Care Management Review*, Vol. 15, No. 1, pp. 29–35, Aspen Publishers, Inc., © 1990.

marketing alone can accomplish. There are for prerequisites for successful marketing, as shown in Figure 12.7.

Pressure To Be Market-Oriented

First, there must be pressure to be market-oriented. There must be a shared view that is accepted throughout the organization concerning the need for an improved marketing program. To some extent, this represents the fourth stage in the evolution of marketing that is appearing in organizations previously

Figure 12.7 Prerequisites to Marketing Success

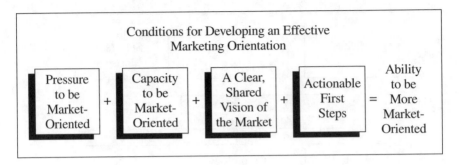

Source: Reprinted from Diamond, S. L. and Berkowitz, E. N., Effective Marketing for Health Care Providers, *Journal of Medical Practice Management*, Vol. 5, No. 3, p. 198, with permission of Williams & Wilkins, © 1990.

mentioned, such as Sentara. Not only must senior management want to become more market-oriented, but peer pressure to understand and to respond to customer needs must be strong throughout the organization. Information and reward systems must recognize the value of a customer orientation, and department program objectives and measurement systems must be tied to progress on this goal.

Capacity To Be Market-Oriented

A second criterion for organizational marketing success is the capacity to be market-oriented. The health care organization must have enough staff members who are not only experienced and adequately trained, but also devoted to improving the organization's marketing effort. Management, staff, and clinical personnel must be receptive to ideas on how to become more market-oriented and have a marketing budget to support their efforts. Although Figure 12.8 shows a recent drop in hospital spending for marketing, overall, hospital marketing budgets have nearly quadrupled since 1984.

Besides financial support, significant time must be devoted to improving marketing efforts and to developing an understanding of how these efforts integrate with other organizational priorities.

Shared Vision of Market

A clear, shared vision of the market is a third prerequisite to success. Many questions must be answered when developing an understanding of the marketplace: Who are the key customers and stakeholders? What are their needs? What change must the organization make in terms of its marketing

Figure 12.8   Hospital Marketing Budgets: Rising Again

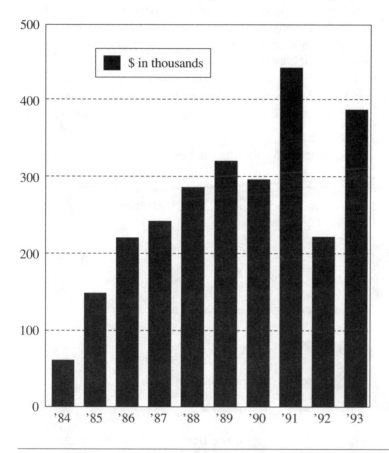

Source: Data from *Marketing News*, Vol. 28, No. 1, p. 1, American Marketing Association, 1994.

mix to meet the needs of these core constituencies? How will this organization differentiate itself from other providers?

Action Plan To Respond to Market

Last, the organization must develop a clear set of actionable steps to respond to market needs. It will need a detailed marketing plan that includes the necessary strategies and tactics along each of the four Ps. This also requires well-defined mechanisms to track the progress of and address minor difficulties in implementation before they become major customer problems.

Missing any one of these elements can lead to marketing ineffectiveness. Figure 12.9 reveals the results of these prerequisite gaps. Without the pressure to be market-oriented, there is a "bottom of the In box" feeling toward marketing. The words are mouthed but there is no pressure to change. Lacking the capacity to be marketing-oriented leads to frustration and anxiety. Attempting to be efficient, many health care providers have pared resources. Yet, marketing personnel and programs must be viewed as an investment to generate additional revenue, not solely as an expense item.

Many health care organizations' marketing efforts have suffered from a fast start that quickly fizzled because of the absence of a clear, shared vision of the market. Well-designed, effective marketing programs require an in-

Figure 12.9   Prerequisites to Marketing Success

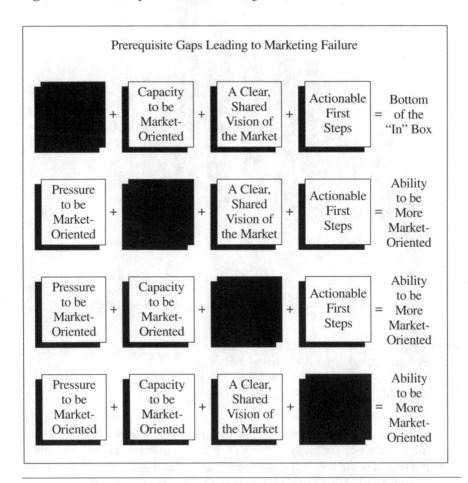

Source: Reprinted from Diamond, S. L. and Berkowitz, E. N., Effective Marketing for Health Care Providers, *Journal of Medical Practice Management*, Vol. 5, No. 3, p. 203, with permission of Williams & Wilkins, © 1990.

depth understanding of the marketplace. Many hospitals, in the 1980s, began to advertise programs before they even knew what they were advertising.[17] This same problem seems to be reoccurring now as many health organizations rush to promote their integrated delivery systems with little understanding of system definition or market requirements.

False starts, another pitfall for marketing, occur when there are no actionable, first steps in place. Effective marketing requires detailed plans that specify the tactics to be implemented within each of the four Ps. Allocated responsibilities, benchmarks for measuring performance, and timetables are specified at the planning process. With all four components in place, the contributions of the marketing function and resultant strategy to any health care organization's success increase dramatically.

THE CHANGING HEALTH CARE MARKETPLACE

No discussion of marketing in health care can begin without an overview of the dramatic restructuring occurring in the industry today. As this chapter began, it mentioned terms that any reader of health care literature or practitioner in the field faces daily—integration, satellites, managed care. What are the implications of these changes for marketing? To appreciate the impact on marketing of the restructuring occurring within health care today, it is instructive to reexamine the traditional industry structure from which we are rapidly moving away.[18]

The Traditional Industry Structure

In communities that have not truly experienced the formation of an integrated delivery system, the health care marketplace can be considered fractionated, in that such entity operates independently. Figure 12.10 shows the major components of this traditional health care structure. At the top of the figure is the hospital, then physicians, followed by the community-at-large.

The focus of the hospital's marketing efforts are twofold, represented by the solid arrows. The focus primarily has been on physicians. The key to maintaining a census within the facility is by encouraging doctors to admit to one's own particular facility as opposed to a competitor's. Consider, then, what has been the typical marketing efforts by hospitals in this regard.

Most hospitals today have a physician relations staff who call on physicians to ensure they are satisfied with the facility and to determine whether the hospital can provide any additional services to meet their needs. Other hospitals have built connecting medical office buildings and rented space at attractive rates for doctors' offices, on the premise that physicians will admit

Figure 12.10   The Traditional Industry Structure

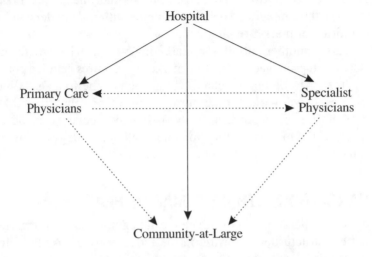

to the hospital most convenient to their offices. In any case, physicians are a major focus of marketing efforts.

A second market for the hospital in the traditional industry structure is the community-at-large. Since 1975, hospitals have targeted their advertising efforts at building name recognition within the community for the facility and its programs. The rationale for this strategy is that patients may ask their doctors to refer them to a specific hospital, or they may self-select the facility when they need medical treatment.

The second level of this chart involves physicians and their marketing focus, represented by the dotted lines. Here, too, there have been two markets—other doctors and the community-at-large. Specialists focus their efforts on generating referrals from primary care doctors, although in some specialties, such as plastic surgery and dermatology, it's common to see direct appeals to the community-at-large through advertisements. Primary care physicians have historically attracted new patients in the community either through word-of-mouth, or through more formal communication strategies including advertisements or detailed telephone directory listings. This type of market structure is very similar to that faced by consumer product companies. That is, the decision to buy the service is typically made by one individual or a small group of individuals. A doctor decides to admit to a particular hospital, or a family decides to become regular patients at a particular medical clinic. In this type of consumer market, mass communication is vital since there are so many people within the community who could, at any point of time, avail themselves of the medical provider's service. Similarly for the specialist, there is always a large number of primary care doctors who could refer patients to them. The comfort of this world is knowing that individual buyers only represent their own volume of business.

This is a somewhat simplified but macro view of the traditional health care market structure that has existed for many years, and still does in communities with little managed care or little pressure from employers to control health care costs. This world, however, is rapidly disappearing. The health care marketplace of the next decade will be defined as more of an industrial marketplace.

The Evolving Industry Structure

In communities such as Minneapolis-St. Paul, San Francisco, and Phoenix, the health care marketplace is undergoing a massive restructing. Hospitals and physicians are banding together in new structures in which they will operate as a single entity in the management of health care delivery. These entities are either contracting with HMOs or offering their own prepaid health care plans to provide medical care to the community. In this new health care environment, the structure of the industry has changed and is more typical of that shown in Figure 12.11.

Figure 12.11   The Evolving Industry Structure

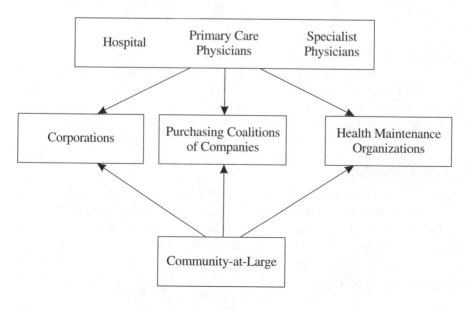

These changes carry tremendous marketing implications. The hospital is still at the top of the figure, but is now joined by physicians. They are one organizational entity that can bring to bear all the necessary resources to meet the health care needs of the community. In a sense, this box can be viewed as the integrated delivery system, representing the hard assets (inpatient beds, surgery centers, laboratory, rehabilitation facility, and long-term care beds), and the personnel (skilled clinicians) that can deliver the expertise, the appropriate technologies, and the setting for needed care.

At the bottom of the chart is still the community-at-large. These people represent the individuals who will need the services of the integrated delivery system. Yet, access to this care is now affected by a new intermediary shown in the middle of the figure. The community-at-large now goes through the new intermediaries to gain access to a particular health care provider.

The doctors who used to be the market have been replaced by corporations or HMOs. These entities decide which facilities can be used by their employees or by their subscribers. Employers are contracting directly with some providers for particular aspects of care. Many HMOs contract with a particular health care facility, which means that health plan subscribers can only use the contracted provider.

From a marketing perspective, the implications of this restructuring are dramatic. While the traditional health care structure was a consumer market with a large number of potential buyers (doctors who could use the facility or patients who could access the hospital), this new structure is more typical of an industrial marketing setting in which there are a restricted set of buyers for a company's products. Pratt & Whitney in Hartford, Connecticut, for example, is a manufacturer of engines for jet aircraft. There are a limited number of buyers for jet engines. So, too, a hospital in any community may find there are only a handful of HMO plans with which it can obtain a contract, or one or two corporate purchasing coalitions that will contract directly for the care of the employees they represent. In this world, effective marketing becomes essential because each buyer now represents a significant amount of business and potential revenue.

CONCLUSIONS

As the health care industry restructures, so too must the perspective regarding marketing's challenges. Historically, the customer has been either the individual doctor who was free to choose where to admit a patient and send a referral, or the individual patient free to choose where to go for treatment. In the evolving health care marketplace, the customer will be an organization responsible for buying or contracting for the health care coverage of a large group of people. In the traditional marketplace, health care was purchased on an episodic basis. When an individual was sick and received medical treatment, payment for that treatment came from the government or from an insurance company. In the evolving marketplace, health care will be delivered for a contractual amount agreed upon between buyer and provider. It will then be the provider's responsibility to deliver the medically necessary care at that predetemined price for a particular length of time. Buyers are increasingly concerned about the value they receive for their health care dollar.

The restructuring of health care only serves to underscore the importance of marketing. In the traditional industry setting, if one doctor is unhappy and no longer admits to a particular hospital, the hospital suffers from the loss of only one doctor. In this traditional environment, if one patient is unhappy with service received at the medical clinic or in the emergency room and decides never to return to that facility, the loss to the organization is the future revenue from one patient.

The new environment of health care, however, requires that marketing be at the core of the organization's strategy. With only a few major buyers in a marketplace that will be contracting for service, the challenge is clear. A health care provider or supplier cannot afford to lose a customer. That customer—be it the corporation, HMO, or group purchasing alliance—represents significant revenue through its contract agreement. It is important also to recognize that the buyer represents users who must also be satisfied. Dissatisfaction among users can lead the buyers to change providers or suppliers rather than face continual dissatisfaction from their employees or subscribers. As the health care industry restructures, marketing is moving into an age where it will be a functional area of major importance for an organization's survival. Knowing the needs and wants of a smaller core of buyers who hold greater economic influence will be the primary requirement to obtaining new business.

KEY TERMS

Marketing	Want
Marketing Research	Market Orientation
Four Ps	Differential Advantage
Marketing Mix	Stakeholders
Product	Environment
Price	Target Market
Place	Product-Oriented Organization
Promotion	Strategic Business Units
Need	Market-Oriented Organization

CHAPTER SUMMARY

1. Marketing is a process that involves planning and execution of the four marketing mix variables: product, price, place, and promotion.

2. Effective marketing for health care organizations involves the recognition of multiple customers or markets who often have a diverse array of needs and wants.

3. A non-market-based approach to planning is one in which the conception of the service begins internally within the organization. Marketing-based planning is an external-to-internal process.

4. The strategic marketing process must consider the broad macro environment consisting of stakeholders, environmental factors, and society at large.

5. Health care marketing planning requires identification of the target market, which may differ from the organization's present customer base.

6. In a product-oriented organization, services are managed as separate profit centers, or strategic business units.

7. In a market-oriented organizational structure, major markets or customer groups are the focus.

8. Marketing success has four prerequisites: pressure, capacity, vision, and actionable steps.

9. The structure of the health care industry is evolving from a consumer market to an industrial market.

10. In the evolving health care industry, the focus of marketing efforts will also change. In the consumer market, marketing efforts were directed at physicians and consumers. In the new marketplace, intermediaries like HMOs, employers, and buying coalitions that will control access to patients will be the important target for marketing activities.

NOTES

1. AMA Board Approves New Definition, *American Medical News* 15, no. 5 (March 1, 1985): 1.

2. P. Kotler and S. J. Levy, Broadening the Concept of Marketing, *Journal of Marketing* 33, no. 1 (1969): 10–15.

3. This conceptualization of the four Ps was first proposed by J. McCarthy, *Basic Marketing: A Managerial Approach* (Homewood, Ill.: Richard D. Irwin, Inc., 1960).

4. *Webster's New World Dictionary* (New York, N.Y.: Simon and Schuster, Inc., 3rd College Edition, 1994), 906.

5. Ibid., 1504.

6. K. Pallarito, State Legislatures Enter Debate on Mom, Newborn Hospital Stays, *Modern Healthcare* 25, no. 24 (1995): 22.

7. R. F. Keith, The Marketing Revolution, *Journal of Marketing* 24 no. 3 (January 1960): 36.

8. Ibid.

9. E. N. Berkowitz and W. Flexner, The Market for Health Services: Is There a Non-Traditional Consumer?, *Journal of Health Care Marketing* 1, no. 1 (Winter 1980–81): 25–34.

10. J. Narver and S. Slater, The Effect of a Market Orientation on Business Profitability, *Journal of Marketing* 53, no. 4 (October 1990): 20–22.

11. This discussion is based on E. N. Berkowitz, Marketing as a Necessary Function in Health Care Management: A Philosophical Approach, in *The Physician Executive*, ed. W. Curry (Tampa, Fla.: American College of Physician Executives, 1994), 221–228.

12. W. A. Flexner and E. N. Berkowitz, Marketing Research in Health Services Planning, *Public Health Reports* 94, no. 6 (November–December 1979): 503–513.

13. Adult Day Care Is Worth Looking Into, *Briefings on Long Term Care* 2, no. 5 (May 1994): 1–3.

14. L. Kertesz, California-Based Sharp Taps Mexican Market, *Modern Healthcare* 24, no. 35 (1994): 28.

15. E. M. Robertson, Product Line Management Focuses on the Customer, *Health Care Competition Week* 8, no. 23 (1991): 1–2.

16. S. L. Diamond and E. N. Berkowitz, Effective Marketing: A Road Map for Health Care Providers, *The Journal of Medical Practice Management* 5, no. 3 (Winter 1990): 197–204.

17. S. Powills, Hospitals Calling a Marketing Time-Out, *Hospitals* 60, no. 11 (June 5, 1986): 50–55.

18. This discussion is drawn from an unpublished working paper, E. N. Berkowitz and M. Guthrie, The New Health Care Paradigm (November 1994).

Strategic Alliances:
A Worldwide Phenomenon
Comes to Healthcare

Howard S. Zuckerman, Ph.D.; Arnold D. Kaluzny, Ph.D.;
and Thomas C. Ricketts III, Ph.D.

I n an increasingly turbulent environment, companies around the globe and
across a multitude of industries are turning to alliances as a cooperative, interorganizational mechanism for adaptation. Such alliances are designed to
achieve strategic purposes not attainable by a single organization, providing
flexibility and responsiveness while retaining the basic fabric of participating
organizations. The purpose of this chapter is to assess the development and
operation of alliances in other industries and healthcare. To achieve this
purpose, we begin with a detailed analysis of other industries and then follow
with an analysis of healthcare, addressing questions such as the following:

- What are alliances designed to achieve?
- How do they achieve their objectives?
- What problems do they face and how are they resolved?
- How have they performed?

ALLIANCES AS A VEHICLE FOR INTERORGANIZATIONAL RELATIONS

Alliances are legion. In the airline industry, for example, Air Canada—a midsize airline—has formed alliances with carriers in the United States, Europe,

Editor's Note: This chapter is from Chapter 1 of *Partners for the Dance* by Howard S.
Zuckerman, Arnold D. Kaluzny, and Thomas C. Ricketts III, 1995, HAP

and Asia (Chipello 1992). To cut costs and increase market position, Air Canada provides maintenance services for Continental and shares schedules, reservation codes, and frequent-flyer benefits with United. Sabena, to secure needed capital, has allied with Air France. The two airlines will coordinate schedules to feed each other's flights, exchange technical and maintenance service, and jointly purchase fuel.

Several approaches to cooperation are evident in the automobile industry. For example, Jaguar–Ford and Saab–Scania–General Motors have formed alliances to ward off Japanese competition in Great Britain. Daimler–Benz is beginning joint activities to build busses with companies in China, providing the Chinese with needed production technology while enabling Daimler–Benz to expand its presence in Asia (*Wall Street Journal* 1993). Chrysler's alliance with Mitsubishi seeks to gain both product and production technology (McClenahen 1987). In planning to bring a new sports coupe to the market, Chrysler sought to gain a new product and expose its personnel to Japanese work practices and management, while Mitsubishi sought new manufacturing technologies. General Motors, Ford, and Chrysler, in a significant policy departure, are exploring an alliance to design pollution free, technologically advanced cars, building on research links among the three automobile companies and governmental laboratories (Behr and Brown 1993).

The communication and media industries likewise may be characterized by a wave of alliances as telephone, cable, and computer hardware/software companies seek to be at the forefront of rapidly developing technological breakthroughs. Pushed by changing technology, rising competition, and an EEC deadline for ending all state monopolies, European telephone companies are forming international partnerships (Hudson 1993). Alliances are emerging linking British Telecommunications with MCI, France Telecom with Deutsche Bundespost Telekom (Eunetcom), and Dutch, Swedish, and Swiss companies (Unisource). AT&T is considering allying with major cable companies to bring its customers into one interactive multimedia network, tying the current disparate cable systems into an integrated network of common switching and transmission functions (Keller 1993a). AT&T has already formed alliances with Japanese and U.S. companies—Matsushita, NEC, Toshiba, McCaw Cellular—to promote its wireless data services (Keller 1993b). Major competitors, notably the "Baby Bells" and MCI, are likewise forming alliances to develop and market cellular services. Motorola's wireless telecommunications venture involves aligning with 11 other partners in a complex consortium to provide geographic representation, telecommunications expertise, and access to markets (Grant 1993). Among the partners are Sony, Mitsubishi, Bell Canada, and Sprint, plus several Russian and Chinese groups. Time Warner and US West also plan an alliance to put both companies at the forefront of the interactive television and telecommunications market, combining resources to develop an electronic superhighway (Roberts 1993). An alliance of 11 companies, including such giants as IBM, Apple, US West, Bell Communications Research, Eastman Kodak, Southwestern Bell, and Phillips Electronics, have formed a strategic alliance to develop and market multimedia technology for the home (Pope 1992).

The evidence is clear that many companies in many industries, including former and present competitors, are entering into a variety of alliances.

What Are Alliances Designed to Achieve?

As the examples above suggest, alliances seek to achieve sharply focused, swiftly attained goals, relying on the complementary strengths of the partners involved. The number of alliances is likely to increase for the following reasons:

- Accelerated pace of technological change
- Broader range of technological capabilities
- Industry and economic maturation
- Shorter product lives
- Larger capital requirements
- Higher risk ventures
- Entry by new firms (especially those with government support)
- Multiple proficiencies required by customers that no single firm can possess
- Deregulation and trade agreements opening previously closed markets, promoting globalization of industry (Harrigan 1987).

Alliances arise out of mutual need and a willingness among and between organizations to share risks and costs, to share knowledge and capabilities, and to take advantage of interdependencies to reach common objectives (Lewis 1990). The basic aim of alliances is to gain competitive advantage, leverage critical capabilities, increase the flow of innovation, and improve flexibility in responding to market and technology changes. For example, alliances allow participation in highly volatile industries, where knowledge spreads rapidly, at substantially lower investment and risk than would be the case for a single organization (Badaracco 1991). Alliances also enable partners to enhance flexibility and accelerate getting to the market by taking advantage of complementary strengths and capabilities in areas such as production, marketing and distribution, and technology. These characteristics are especially shared by the actors in the healthcare industry.

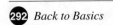

The influence of new knowledge and new technologies on interorganizational structures, coupled with the need for new ways to coordinate the complexity that comes with alliances, will be continuing themes in organizational relations. Alter and Hage (1993) propose the following outline to summarize the benefits and costs of interorganizational cooperation:

Benefits

- Opportunities to learn and adapt new competencies
- Gain resources
- Share risks
- Share cost of product and technology development
- Gain influence over domain
- Access to new markets
- Enhance ability to manage uncertainty and solve complex problems
- Gain mutual support and group synergy
- Respond rapidly to market demands and technological opportunities
- Gain acceptance of foreign governments
- Strengthen competitive position

Costs

- Loss of technical superiority
- Loss of resources
- Sharing the costs of failure
- Loss of autonomy and control
- Loss of stability and certainty
- Conflict over domain, goals, methods
- Delays in solutions due to coordination problems
- Government intrusion and regulation

These benefits and costs apply across industries and include service industries like healthcare.

How Do Alliances Seek to Achieve Their Goals?

Alliances are established along a variety of lines—joint ventures, marketing and distribution agreements, consortia, or licensing arrangements. Alliances require thinking in terms of "combinations" of firms. For example, Japanese firms often cooperate in order to penetrate new markets, which has often proven to be a key step to market dominance (Lewis 1990). International companies often ally with local companies to yield successful entry into new markets, drawing on the knowledge and customer base of the local company in conjunction with the capital and technological resources of the international firm. Working with competitors is often the basis for an alliance against a common enemy. Newspapers often share facilities to compete with television, Ford dealers compete yet share advertising, and pharmaceutical companies use each other's sales forces (Lewis 1990). Joining forces is further desirable in the face of difficult economic conditions or the combined power of other alliances. Alliances may also be useful in enhancing flexibility, innovation, and performance in customer/supplier relationships. Captive supply units, not subject to market pressures, tend to develop cost, quality, and technology gaps. Alliances may thus be able to secure the benefits of vertical integration, without the drawbacks associated with ownership.

Successful alliances appear to have several key ingredients, beginning with shared objectives among the participants. Commitment is based on mutual need; the alliance will endure only so long as mutual need exists (Henderson 1990). Risk sharing completes the bond, creating a powerful incentive to cooperate for mutual gain. It is important to note, however, that mutual reliability means mutual vulnerability. Relationships matter a great deal in alliances, and success requires mutual trust, cooperation, and understanding (Badaracco 1991).

Alliances have been labeled as "virtual corporations," seen as temporary networks of companies that come together to exploit fast changing opportunities (Byrne 1993). Such corporations share costs, skills, and access to global markets. Their key attributes are identified as (1) technology and information networks, (2) excellence as each partner brings distinctive competencies, (3) opportunism in meeting specific market opportunities, (4) trust as partners share a destiny, and (5) a borderless market where suppliers, competitors, and customers cooperate. The key is flexibility—absent hierarchies and vertical structures—as alliances enable companies to broaden offerings or produce sophisticated products less expensively.

What Problems Face Alliances and How Are They Managed?

Alliances must be carefully entered into, with clear objectives, a realistic appraisal of an organization's skills and resources, and knowledge of the strengths of each partner (Wysocki 1990). Alliances should be approached carefully and systematically, often involving consideration of several potential partners with common or compatible culture and similar approaches to issues and problems is critical. Partners must understand their motivation in entering an alliance. Alliances are designed to create competitive strength or augment a strategic position, not hide weaknesses (Hamel, Doz, and Prahalad 1989). As such, they are seen by many as anticipating long-term relationships, established for strategic purposes. Further, alliances must generate tangible value, leading to win-win relationships. It has been found useful in organizations to have a "champion", or "boundary spanner" (Alter and Hage 1993), whose personal objective it is to see the alliance succeed. In many ways, the notion of alliances and the underlying premise of strength through cooperation, is hard for American companies and managers to accept. The sense of individualism, the desire for control, and the "not invented here" syndrome often makes American companies uncomfortable with alliances (Modic 1988). The close bonds required by alliances are inconsistent with traditional American business practices. For example, the IBM–Apple alliance will be successful only if the two companies are willing to place their need for this alliance above other priorities (Lewis 1991). They must learn to appreciate and adjust to each other's views, to rely on each other's information, and respect each other's need to maintain their own internal cultures.

How Have Alliances Performed?

Surveys indicate that CEOs of American companies tend to be much less positive about the results of alliances as compared to their European and Asian counterparts (Modic 1988). Especially problematic appear to be joint ventures. In examining why alliances are seen as unsuccessful, the following reasons have been suggested:

- Judging the alliance by short-term financial results rather than long-term strategic objectives
- Lack of trust among the partners
- Uneven commitment and imbalance of power
- Lower operating levels (who must make it work) not informed about or involved in the alliance
- Absence of clear understanding of partners' respective motivations and expectations
- Lack of mutually accepted performance measures (Sherman 1992; Bowersox 1990)

Thus, lessons from other industries and other countries would suggest that alliances provide the opportunity and the potential to add value to organizations but that there are many challenges to be addressed in their development and operation. At issue now is how the concept of alliances applies in healthcare.

ALLIANCES IN HEALTHCARE

> Healthcare reform is obviously driven by costs, access, and quality, but it seems the only thing we hear about today is cost . . . Let us not in our zeal to reform destroy the best healthcare system in the world.
>
> *Monroe Trout, 1993*

> I think the Clinton plan is like a mule. A mule has no pride of ancestry and no hope of progeny. It has no sense of ancestry since it is a strange hybrid of capitation and fee for service. It has no hope of progeny because I don't see any way that this can work its way through the Congressional process and have any rebirth in the structure in which it was presented. However, the mule does some useful things. The mule has focused in a very political way on the advantages of capitation. Second, this has taken healthcare reform outside of Washington. The real activity is underway in lots of places across the country . . . The message to all of you here, alliance providers and researchers, for God's sake, get on board. The world is changing and you'd better get with it because that's the way it's going to go.
>
> *Alexander McMahon, 1993*

Alliances in healthcare function in a larger environment, and that larger environment is likely to be influenced by the advent of healthcare reform, whether federal, state, local, or privately initiated. As illustrated by the comments of Monroe Trout and Alex McMahon, healthcare reform is a complex undertaking involving different perspectives reflecting different degrees of urgency and levels of involvement. Yet, the underlying bases for alliances in healthcare are fundamentally the same as those in other industries. As stated by Zuckerman and Kaluzny (1991):

> In healthcare, much of the development of alliances can be traced to changes in the environment. As access to needed resources is threatened and new challenges are presented to health services providers, organizations seek to reduce their dependencies on and their uncertainty about the environment by banding together. . . . While there is clearly a growing degree of interdependency, there also remains a substantial amount of organizational independence and autonomy not possible under other interorganizational arrangements such as horizontal and vertical integration. Alliances appear to offer flexibility and responsiveness, with limited effects on the structure of participating organizations. In recent years, we have seen these new organizations become institutionalized as a form of organizational cooperation involving organizations heretofore considered autonomous, if not competitive, entities.

These conditions apply to all parts of the American healthcare industry but are amplified in rural communities which are faced with the further need to find a way to keep their healthcare systems alive. Healthcare providers enter into alliances in order to gain economies of scale and scope, enhance the acquisition and the retention of key resources, expand their revenue and service base, increase their influence, and improve market position (Zuckerman and D'Aunno 1990). Alliances, transcending existing organizational arrangements, permit activities not otherwise possible, link organizations through shared strategic purpose, provide access to technologies previously unavailable, and capitalize on the growing need for organizational interdependence (Kaluzny et al. 1993; Luke, Begun, and Pointer 1989). Alliances make it possible to gain access to resources without owning them, encouraging organizations to look outward as well as inward as they struggle with how to do more with less. These issues of access and the need to look beyond immediate borders and boundaries is especially important in the rural context.

What Are the Types of Strategic Alliances in Healthcare?

Alliances in healthcare may be categorized into two general types. The first may be described as "lateral," where similar types of organizations, often with similar needs or dependencies, come together to achieve benefits such as economies of scale, enhanced access to scarce resources, and increased collective power (Zuckerman and D'Aunno 1990). For example, strategic alliances have formed among hospitals based on common religious preferences, particular types of hospitals, or geographic distribution. These alliances serve to take advantage of pooled resources, thereby expanding the strength and capabilities of any single members to benefit the entire membership. Their domain can be extensive, including group purchasing, insurance, information sharing, and human resource management among the array of programs and services. Such alliances—defined by Kanter (1989) as "service alliances," and capturing elements of Alter and Hage's (1993) "obligational" and "promotional" networks—will receive substantial attention throughout this book.

The second type may be described as "integrative," where organizations come together for purposes largely related to market and strategic position and securing competitive advantage. Many of the attributes of such alliances are incorporated in Kanter's (1989) formulation of "stakeholder alliances," emphasizing linkages among buyers, suppliers, and customers, Johnston and Lawrence's (1988) "value-adding partnerships," and Alter and Hage's (1993) notion of "systemic networks." These alliances may be illustrated by the emergence of "corporate partnerships," linking providers and suppliers through long-term agreements and close relationships. Of particular interest will be the role of alliances as a mechanism to build integrated delivery and financing systems. Such systems are defined as regional, market-based organizations, serving the healthcare needs of a defined population (Shortell et al. 1993). These systems are being developed to achieve vertical as well as horizontal integration, clinical as well as administrative integration, and integration of financing as well as delivery. How such systems achieve integration is a key issue. There is reason to believe that alliances will play an important role in their evolution, representing a mechanism to achieve integration without the necessity of ownership and/or control of each of the key components. These integrative alliances will likely prove especially important in the context of an already changing environment and healthcare reform.

There are no geographic limitations to alliances, but rural organizations often seek alliances with urban organizations for different reasons than they would with other rural providers or companies. The geography of rural America does have an influence along with the factors we have described so far. We will consider them in more depth as we look more closely at healthcare.

How Do Alliances Form?

The formation of healthcare alliances may be described in terms of stages of development or a life cycle model. Each of the stages or each step in the life cycle has important implications for successful development of the alliance. For example, the Kanter (1994) formulation, which appears quite applicable, proposes that alliance formation moves through stages defined as (1) selection or courtship, (2) engagement, (3) setting up housekeeping, (4) learning to collaborate, and (5) changing within. The first stage requires each organization to undertake a realistic appraisal of itself as well as of each of the potential partners. After developing the basic agreement in the engagement stage, partners next begin to experience the difficulties making the transition to a new form and relationship. They experience problems with coordinating resources, cultural differences, opposition to the alliance, lack of understanding, and dissimilarities in operating styles. Thus, the learning stage calls for building mechanisms—strategic, tactical, cultural, interpersonal, and operational—to bridge these gaps and overcome the barriers, while the final stage involves the internal changes needed to sustain the relationship over time. In a comparable approach, Forrest (1992) proposes three stages: (1) pre-alliance, (2) agreement, and (3) implementation. Like Kanter, Forrest emphasizes the importance of careful appraisal and selection of an appropriate partner, calling for a close fit in terms of expectations, values, goals, interdependence, trust, and commitment. The agreement stage serves to specify the terms and conditions of the alliance—its scope, objectives, resource requirements, management structure, mechanisms for conflict resolution, exit terms, and performance measures. In the implementation stage, emphasis is on open communication, timely decision making, ongoing review of objectives to ensure consistency with a changing environment, and strengthened mutual commitment.

Viewing the development of alliances in terms of a life cycle, steps along the way may be portrayed as (1) emergence, (2) transition, (3) maturity, and (4) critical crossroads (D'Aunno and Zuckerman 1987b). Perhaps most applicable to the "lateral" alliances noted earlier, alliances among organizations which share ideology or resource dependencies emerge in response to environmental threats or uncertainty. Members early on develop purposes, expectations, and criteria for participation, because these steps are seen as less costly organizational alternatives and providing an opportunity to reduce dependency. In the transition, mechanisms for control, coordination, and decision making are established, and trust and commitment are heightened, setting the foundation to enable the members to secure anticipated benefits as the alliance matures and grows. In reaching the critical crossroads, members face demands for greater commitment, more centralization in decision making, and more dependence upon the alliance for needed resources, which are, to some extent, counter to the reasons for initially forming the alliance and thereby raising the specter of withdrawal or creating a more hierarchical type of organization.

Moreover, public policy is likely to greatly influence the stages of the life cycle (Longest 1994). For the past decade, public policies have stimulated the growth of alliances as they have forced a healthcare system into greater efficiency, or at least into imposing lower costs on public and private sector purchases of their environment. These policies have presented serious threats to some healthcare organizations, as illustrated by the efforts of the federal prospective payment system for reimbursing Medicare services as well as state policies restricting capitation expansion in the industry.

Much of the alliance activity of recent years may have been stimulated by threats to the continued success of organizations, or at least by the perception that these threats existed or would soon exist within their environments. These policy initiatives may change over time from an essentially negative to a more positive effect. This shift will likely stimulate even faster growth of alliance phenomena in the next few years. One clear example of a policy shift toward such supportive effort is found in the possible changes in antitrust laws. The Clinton proposal for healthcare reform, for example, included specific attention to the effect of existing antitrust laws on the shift to vertically integrated delivery systems. As these systems move into place, initially conforming to the cooperative spirit characterizing alliances other forces pushing for stability and accountability will influence the nature of these relationships moving toward a more permanent interorganizational relationship based on ownership among former alliance participants. As such, we may well witness the influence of public policy shifting focus from "lateral" to "integrative" arrangement.

How Are Alliances Operated?

Sustaining strategic alliances over time requires constant vigilance. It is clear that the relationships within alliances are fragile and characterized by constant change. The belief that members are stronger together than they would be separately is required, and securing the anticipated benefits calls for ongoing commitment of time, energy, and resources. Indeed, in contrast with the long-standing control model of organizations, alliances are more appropriately defined in terms of a commitment model. As Kanter (1989) suggests, "If an increasing amount of economic activity continues to occur across, rather than within, the boundaries defined by the formal ownership of one firm, managers will have to understand how to work with partners rather than subordinates . . ." Such a model underscores the importance of designing and communicating common purposes, developing realistic expectations, and clearly framing the domain, scope, and activities of an alliance. As the purposes of an alliance may shift over time, the operating domain and the membership may also need to be reassessed. For example, as many hospital alliances evolved from "association" type efforts toward a "business" focus, areas of activity and criteria for members had to be reassessed. Likewise, as noted by Weinstein (1993), as member organizations address their attention to building vertically integrated healthcare systems, the role and contribution of their national alliances (lateral) will likely be reassessed. Managing these potentially profound changes and balancing the interests of multiple constituencies is a delicate and difficult task testing the commitment, openness, and willingness to share resources and information among the members, and challenging the alliance to continually add value and provide strategic benefit.

In a major review of the research literature on factors influencing successful collaboration among organizations, Mattessich and Monsey (undated) summarized their findings into the following six categories, suggesting *membership, communications*, and *resources* are most important:

1. Environment
   - History of cooperation or collaboration
   - Cooperating groups seen as leaders
   - Political/social climate is favorable
2. Membership
   - Mutual respect, understanding, trust
   - Appropriate cross section of members
   - Members see collaboration as in their self-interest
   - Ability to compromise
3. Process/Structure
   - Members share stake in both process and outcome
   - Multiple layers of integrated decision making
   - Flexibility in structure and methods
   - Development of clear roles, responsibilities, rights, policy guidelines
   - Adaptability to change
4. Communications
   - Open and frequent communications
   - Established formal and informal communication links
5. Purpose
   - Concrete, attainable long-term and short-term goals and objectives
   - Shared vision with agreed upon mission, objectives, strategy
   - Unique purpose
6. Resources
   - Sufficient funds
   - Skilled conveners

Several key themes emerge in the formation and evolution of alliances over time. First is the critical nature of the selection of an appropriate partner(s). It is seen as essential that participating members or partners of an alliance are rigorous in analyzing themselves and each other as to compatibility of goals, purposes, vision, and values, and clear indications of interdependency and complementary. Next is the underlying "glue" of alliances—trust and commitment. Partners must be candid, open, and fair in the workings of the alliance, and able to recognize that maintaining the alliance over time requires continuous nurturing. In fact, the fragile nature of alliances leaves open the question of whether they will prove to be a temporary or permanent organizational phenomenon. In large part, the willingness of members to remain will depend on their perception of how crucial the alliance is to the long-term viability of their organization. Third, the terms and terrain of the alliance must be clear, the operating rules explicit, and expectations mutually understood and agreed upon. Fourth, partners must learn from—and be strengthened by—the alliance. Alliances are seen by many as mechanisms to supplement and complement the core capabilities and knowledge of an organization, not as substitutes for internal development (Montgomery 1991). Indeed, as Lewis (1990) notes, "There is no reason to cooperate unless you grow stronger by the effort."

How Effective Are Healthcare Alliances?

As is the case with healthcare organizations in general, defining and assessing the effectiveness or performance of alliances is now a subject of serious attention in many organizations. The performance of alliances may be viewed along either or both of two dimensions: performance as seen by those who are key internal stakeholders within the alliance, and as seen by those who are external stakeholders, outside but affected by or otherwise interested in the alliance and its impact. To date, attention has been devoted primarily to performance or effectiveness as perceived by those within the alliance. For example, Kanter (1989) suggests that effective alliances are those characterized by the following "six I's:"

1. The alliance is seen as *Important*, with strategic significance, and getting adequate resources and management attention.
2. The alliance is seen as a long-term *Investment* from which members will be rewarded relatively equally over time.
3. The partners in the alliance are *Interdependent*, maintaining an appropriate balance of power.
4. The alliance is *Integrated* in order to manage communication and appropriate points of contact.
5. Each alliance member is *Informed* about plans for the alliance and for each other.
6. The alliance is *Institutionalized*, with supporting mechanisms that permeate interorganizational activities and facilitate the requisite trust relationships among the members.

It has been proposed that the effectiveness of healthcare alliances should be considered in terms of both a variance and process perspective (Kaluzny and Zuckerman 1992). The variance perspective focuses on outcomes, seeking to identify variables that explain variation in alliance performance. For example, are there identifiable changes in market share or financial performance attributable to alliance membership? This perspective is appropriate for analyzing the effects of an alliance on various indicators of performance and/or factors that account for specific stages of the adoption process. The process perspective, on the other hand, focuses on particular conditions, events, or stages in the overall development process. For example, are problems faced in the early stages of alliance development different from those experienced in later stages? This perspective is appropriate in considering the interaction among various factors as alliances and participating organizations adapt over time. Further, application of both the variance and process perspectives occurs at two levels, the first being the alliance as a whole and the second being the organizations comprising the alliance. A related approach views performance in terms of an alliance's ability to achieve stated objectives, acquire needed resources, satisfy key stakeholders, and add value to the membership (Zuckerman and D'Aunno 1990). Performance would be judged in the context of an economic dimension (e.g., economies of scale, new sources of revenue and capital), an organizational dimension (e.g., market position, human resource management), and a social/political dimension (e.g., access to care, availability of services).

In the future, we may expect the issue of effectiveness to take on greater meaning and impact. With healthcare reform looming on the horizon, and major structural and strategic changes already underway in the marketplace, the role of alliances as a key component in the development of integrated healthcare systems will be scrutinized carefully. These emerging integrated systems will be held broadly accountable for their performance, not only internally but externally as well. Such organizations will continue to evaluate themselves in order to enhance operating performance, so they will continue to assess areas such as financial performance, changes in market share, and employee satisfaction. However, they will also find increased accountability in the context of public and social demands, and will be assessed in terms of such factors as access to care, availability of services, and improvements in the health status of a defined population. Further, the unit of analysis will shift to a broader perspective, centering on episodes of care and indicators defined on a per capita basis. A new era of defining and assessing organizational performance has begun.

CONCLUSIONS

We have briefly identified an array of issues about strategic alliances in general and within healthcare in particular. While it is a beginning, it is not sufficient. Managers and researchers alike face an unrelenting flow of challenges that require attention. For example, alliances have been operationalized in a variety of industrial areas; what is the applicability to healthcare? Are there distinct structural characteristics associated with performance, and do these make any difference?

REFERENCES

Alter, C., and J. Hage. 1993. *Organizations Working Together*. Newbury Park, CA: Sage Publications.

Badaracco, Jr., J. L. 1991. *The Knowledge Link: How Firms Compete Through Alliances.* Boston: Harvard Business School Press.

Behr, P., and W. Brown. 1993. "In Policy Departure, United States Joins Detroit in Industrial Alliance." Washington Post Service, *Washington Post* (29 September): F1.

Bowersox, D. J. 1990. "The Strategic Benefits of Logistics Alliances." *Harvard Business Review* 90 (July–August): 36–45.

Browning, E. S. 1990. "Renault, Volvo Agree to Enter Into Alliance. Japanese Expansion, Costs of Developing Products Lead to a Near Merger." *The Wall Street Journal* (27 February): A3, A12.

Byrne, J. A. 1993. "The Virtual Corporation." *Business Week* (8 February): 98–103.

Chipello, C. J. 1992. "Midsize Air Canada Plots Survival in Industry of Giants: Continental Bid Is Example of Alliances Sought to Secure Carrier's Future." *The Wall Street Journal* (12 November): B4.

D'Aunno, T. A., and H. S. Zuckerman. 1987a. "The Emergence of Hospital Federations: An Integration of Perspectives from Organizational Theory." *Medical Care Review* 44 (Fall): 323–43.

————. 1987b. "A Life-Cycle Model of Organizational Federations: The Case of Hospitals." *The Academy of Management Review* 12 (July): 534–45.

Forrest, J. E. 1992. "Management Aspects of Strategic Partnering." *Journal of General Management* 17 (Summer): 25–40.

Grant, L. "Partners in Profit." 1993. *U.S. News and World Report* 115 (20 September): 65–66.

Hamel, G., Y. L. Doz, and C. K. Prahalad. 1989. "Collaborate With Your Competitors—And Win." *Harvard Business Review* 89 (January–February): 133–39.

Harrigan, K. R. 1987. "Alliances: Their New Role in Global Competition." *Columbia Journal of World Business* (Summer): 67–69.

Henderson, J. C. 1990. "Plugging Into Strategic Partnerships: The Critical IS Connection." *Sloan Management Review* (Spring): 7–18.

Hudson, R. L. 1993. "European Phone Companies Reach Out for Partners." *The Wall Street Journal* (30 September): B4.

Johnston, R., and P. R. Lawrence. 1988. "Beyond Vertical Integration—The Rise of Value-Added Partnerships." *Harvard Business Review* 88 (July–August): 94–101.

Kaluzny, A. D., and H. S. Zuckerman. 1992. "Alliances: Two Perspectives for Understanding Their Effects on Health Services." *Hospital & Health Services Administration* 37 (Winter): 477–90.

Kaluzny, A. D., L. Lacey, R. Warnecke, D. Hynes, J. Morrissey, L. Ford, and E. Sondik. 1993. "Predicting the Performance of a Strategic Alliance: An Analysis of the Community Clinical Oncology Program." *Health Services Research* 28 (June): 159–82.

Kanter, R. M. 1994. "Collaborative Advantage: The Art of Alliances." *Harvard Business Review* 72 (July–August): 96–108.

Kanter, R. M. 1989. "Becoming PALs: Pooling, Allying, and Linking Across Companies." *Academy of Management Executives* 3 (August): 183–93.

Keller, J. J. 1993a. "AT&T, Cable-TV Firms Discuss Linking Their Customers in Multimedia Network." *The Wall Street Journal* (27 August): A3.

———. 1993b. "AT&T, Rivals Face Off in Wireless Wars." *The Wall Street Journal* (19 August): B1, B6.

Lewis, J. D. 1991. "Manager's Journal—IBM and Apple: Will They Break the Mold?" *The Wall Street Journal* (31 July): A10.

Lewis, J. D. 1990. *Partnerships in Profit: Structuring and Managing Alliances.* New York: The Free Press.

Longest, B. B. 1994. "Strategic Alliances in Health Care." Presentation at Association of University Programs in Health Administration, San Diego, CA, 11 June.

Luke, R. D., J. Begun, and D. Pointer. 1989. "Quasi-Firms: Strategic Inter-Organizational Forms in the Healthcare Industry." *Academy of Management Review* 14 (January): 9–19.

Mattessich, P. W., and B. R. Monsey. "Collaboration: What Makes It Work. A Review of Research Literature on Factors Influencing Successful Collaboration." Unpublished paper, Amherst H. Wilder Foundation, St. Paul, Minnesota.

McClenahen, J. S. 1987. "Alliances for Competitive Advantage." *Industry Week* (24 August): 33–36.

McMahon, A. 1993a. Comments at the National Invitational Conference on Alliances, Chapel Hill, NC, November 11–12.

Modic, S. 1988. "Alliances: A Global Economy Demands Global Partnerships." *Industry Week* (3 October): 46–52.

Montgomery, R. L. 1991. "Alliances—No Substitute for Core Strategy." *Frontiers of Health Services Management* 7 (3): 25–28.

Ohmae, K. 1989. "The Global Logic of Alliances." *Harvard Business Review* 89 (March–April): 143–54.

Pope, K. 1992. "Multimedia Alliance Is Formed By 11 Big Computer, Phone Firms." *The Wall Street Journal* (7 October): B4.

Roberts, J. L., L. Landro, and M. L. Carnevale. 1993. "Time Warner and U.S. West Plan Alliance. Investment of $2.5 Billion Aims at Melding Phone and TV Technologies." *The Wall Street Journal* (17 May): A3, A6.

Sherman, S. 1992. "Are Strategic Alliances Working?" *Fortune* (21 September): 77–78.

Shortell, S. M., D. A. Anderson, R. R. Gillies, J. B. Mitchell, and K. L. Morgan. 1993. "Building Integrated Systems: The Holographic Organization." *Healthcare Forum Journal* (March–April): 20–26.

Trout, M. 1993. Comments at the National Invitational Conference on Strategic Alliances, Chapel Hill, NC.

The Wall Street Journal. 1993. "Daimler–Benz Sets Plan to Expand Asia Presence." *The Wall Street Journal* (27 August): A3, B5.

Weinstein, A. 1993. Comments at the National Invitational Conference on Strategic Alliances, Chapel Hill, NC, November 11–12.

Wysocki, Jr., B. 1990. "Cross-Border Alliances Become Favorite Way To Crack New Markets: Mitsubishi and Daimler Are Just the Latest to See Gain In Swapping Know-How." *The Wall Street Journal* (26 March): A1, A12.

Zuckerman, H. S., and A. D. Kaluzny. 1991. "Strategic Alliances in Health Care: The Challenges of Cooperation." *Frontiers of Health Services Management* 7 (3): 3–23.

Zuckerman, H. S., and T. A. D'Aunno. 1990. "Hospital Alliances: Cooperative Strategy in a Competitive Environment." *Health Care Management Review* 15 (Spring): 21–30.

Human Resources System

John R. Griffith, FACHE

In 1996, healthcare organizations had nearly ten million employees, reflecting a steady increase throughout the preceding two decades.[1] The number of professions and job categories had also increased. A typical medium-sized healthcare organization employs persons in more than three dozen licensed or certified job classifications, including building trades and stationary engineers as well as clinical professions. Many of the positions are held by part-time personnel. The number of individuals employed is about 30 percent larger than the full-time equivalents (FTE) count.

In addition to **employees**, the human resources of a healthcare organization include doctors and others whose services are contracted through arrangements other than employment, and volunteers. The employed healthcare work force supports a physician group of nearly 500,000 in more than two dozen specialties.[2] Finally, healthcare organizations also use contract labor services, via long-term management contracts for whole departments and shorter contracts for specific temporary assistance. Long-term contracts are common for housekeeping, food service, and data processing. Among the shorter are consultation contracts with accounting firms and planning firms, as well as shift-by-shift requests for nurses, clerks, and other hourly workers. In total, a medium-sized healthcare organization requires more than 1,500 persons working at about 1,000 full-time jobs in about 100 different skills.

This group, referred to here as the "members" of the organization, constitutes the most important asset, its human resource. Regardless of the specific relationship, each member joins the organization in a voluntary exchange

---

Editor's Note: This chapter is from Chapter 16 of *The Well-Managed Healthcare Organization, Fourth Edition,* by John R. Griffith, 1999, HAP

transaction. The member is seeking some combination of income, rewarding activity, society, and recognition. The organization is seeking services that support other exchanges. Some aspects of the exchange relationship with members deserve emphasis.

1. The members are absolutely essential to continued operation. Members' motivation and satisfaction directly affect both quality and efficiency. Unusually high motivation can provide a margin of excellence, while a few highly dissatisfied members can temporarily or occasionally disrupt operations.[3]

2. Membership, like the seeking of care, is a free choice for most people. Even those whose skills can be employed only in specific settings, like operating rooms, usually have some choice of which institution they will work at and how much work they will seek. Success in attracting and keeping members tends to be self-sustaining; the organization with a satisfied, well-qualified member group attracts more capable and enthusiastic people. The well-run organization markets itself to its members almost as much as it markets itself to its customers.

3. The members represent only about 3 percent of the community served, but because of their close affiliation and their frequent contact with patients, they are unusually influential.

    • As a promotional force, members—both those who come into direct contact with patients and those whose unseen services determine patients' safety and satisfaction—are powerful. What they say and do for patients and visitors will have more influence on competitive standing than any media campaign the organization might contemplate.

    • As an economic force, members are also significant. Healthcare organizations are always important employers in a community. Healthcare organizations are often the largest employers in a community, even without including their affiliated physicians and their employees. Furthermore, about half the payroll represents income from outside the community, largely Social Security payments for Medicare. Finally, most of the employment opportunities are in unskilled and semi-skilled jobs. The economic impact is weighted to lower-middle-class females, a group presenting serious employment problems for many communities.

    • As a political force, members can command increased respect for the healthcare institution among elected officials of government and labor unions by demonstrating their support of it. While members are only about one-tenth as numerous as patients, their strength can be multiplied when the issue is important enough to motivate their families, as is often the case when substantial numbers of jobs are at stake.

This chapter reviews the purpose of human resources management, the functions that must be performed to sustain an effective workforce, the organization to accomplish the functions, usually called the human resources department, and the measures of success in performing the functions.

PURPOSE OF THE HUMAN RESOURCES SYSTEM

The purpose of the **human resources system** is to plan, acquire, and maintain the skills, quality, and motivation of members consistent with fulfillment of the organization's mission. Because a properly worded mission defines community, service, and cost, this purpose accommodates both the profile of skill levels and the needs for economy defined by the governing board. Motivation and quality reflect the exchange nature of membership contracts; the human resources system manages all of the monetary transactions and many of the nonmonetary rewards.

The human resources department is a major logistic support unit that provides most human resource functions for nonprofessional employees and a large share of those for professional employees. The department is a central element of a human resources system, but not all of it. The department emphasizes recruitment, training, and compensation services; other parts of the organization affect the system with workplace environments and job definitions. Doctors and volunteers are least likely to be directly affected by the human resources department, but well-run organizations are increasingly placing key functions of these groups under the department. In the well-run organization, the human resources department advises on all human resource issues, contributing technical expertise and reinforcing the workplace culture.

FUNCTIONS OF HUMAN RESOURCE MANAGEMENT

Levine and Tyson, reviewing the empirical literature on employee participation, noted that participation produces at least short-run gains in productivity and sometimes produces substantial long-term improvements.[4] The four characteristics that emerge from the literature as promoting productivity are:

1. some form of profit sharing or gain sharing;
2. job security and long-term employment;
3. measures to build group cohesiveness; and
4. guaranteed individual rights.[5]

These characteristics are similar to the empowerment and measurement goals of continuous quality improvement; they depend on the overall performance and culture of the organization. But given sound performance by other parts of the organization, the human resource system must accomplish six functions to support a productive workforce. As shown in Figure 14.1, these functions recruit, train, compensate, and support the member group and support continuous improvement in human resource management generally.

Work Force Planning

Work force planning allows the organization adequate time to respond to changes in the exchange environment with replacement, increases, or decreases in the numbers of members. The work force plan is a subsection of the long-range plan. It develops forecasts of the number of persons required in each skill level by year for the length of time covered by the long-range plan. It also projects available human resources including additions and attrition, even to specifying the planned retirement of key individuals.

Development of plan

The initial proposal for the work force plan should be developed using forecasts of activity from the services plan. The services plan is developed from the epidemiologic needs of the community and the long-range financial plans. The work force plan technically includes, and is always coordinated with, the medical staff plan. As shown in Figure 14.2, the plan should include:

- the anticipated size of the member and employee groups, by skill category, major site, and department;
- the schedule of adjustments through recruitment, retraining, attrition, and termination;
- wage and benefit cost forecasts from national projections tailored to local conditions;
- planned changes in employment or compensation policy, such as the development of incentive payments or the increased use of temporary or part-time employees; and
- preliminary estimates of the cost of operating the human resources department and fulfilling the plan.

The plan is often prepared by a task force including representatives from human resources, planning, finance, nursing, and one or two other CSSs likely to undergo extensive change. The draft is reviewed by the major medical staff specialties and employer departments, and their concerns are resolved. The revised plan is coordinated with the facilities plan because the number and location of employees determine the requirements for many plant services. The final package must be consistent with the long-range financial plan. It is recommended to the governing board through the planning committee.

Figure 14.1 Functions of Human Resources

Function	Description	Example
Work force planning	Development of employment needs by job category	RNs required and available by year
	Comparison with existing work force and identification of changes	Strategy for recruitment, retention, and complement reduction
Work force maintenance	Advertising, school visits, and other promotion	RN recruitment program
	Selection, orientation, and training	Credentials review
	Record of skill levels and performance	Orientation and continuous improvement courses
	Survey of satisfaction and analysis of dissatisfaction	Personnel record of RNs including special competencies
	Grievance management	Satisfaction survey and analysis
		Employee counseling and grievance mediation
Management education	Programs of supervisory training, human relations skills, continuous improvement skills	Head nurse programs in personnel policies, supervision, participation on cross-functional teams
Compensation management	Market surveys of base pay, benefits allowance, and incentives	RN pay scales, payment method, RN benefit selection, benefit cost, compensation, incentives, absenteeism records
	Record of hours worked and earnings	
	Maintenance of benefits eligibility, use, and cost	
Collective bargaining	Response to organizing drives, contract negotiation, and administration	Management of RN labor contract if any
Continuous improvement and budgeting	Analysis of employment markets, benefit trends, and work conditions	Identification of potential shortage situations, of competitive recruitment difficulties
	Development of improvement proposals for general working conditions	Proposals for improvement of benefits or work conditions
	Development of department budget and budget for fringe benefit costs	Human resources department budget and detail for benefits, costs, budgets

Figure 14.2   Illustration of Work Force Plan Content

Category	Current Supply (1999)	Need (FTE) 2000	Need (FTE) 2001	Need (FTE) 2002	Attrition per Year	Recruitment (Reduction) 2000	Recruitment (Reduction) 2001	Recruitment (Reduction) 2002
RN, Inpatient	250 FTE, 300 persons	230	210	200	50	30	30	40
RN, Outpatient	45 FTE, 60 persons	55	60	60	15	25	20	15

RN Strategy: Recruit from three local associate degree schools. Advertise in national and state journals. Offer training to facilitate transfer from inpatient to outpatient. Starting salary 10 percent below nearby metropolitan area. Emphasize health and child care, maintain education and retirement benefits. Encourage LPNs to seek further training.

Costs (2000):

Activity	Cost per Unit	Cost per Employed FTE
Recruitment/orientation	$1,250/recruit	$ 241/FTE
Personnel records, benefits management and counseling	$450/employee	$ 550/FTE
Health benefits	$2,400/employee over 20 hours/week	$ 1,627/FTE
Child care benefits	$100,000 per year*	$ 3,351/FTE
Social Security and Medicare	$ 1,950/FTE	$ 1,950/FTE
Retirement benefits	$ 1,500/FTE	$ 1,500/FTE
Vacation and absenteeism replacements	$900/employee	$ 1,102/FTE
Training programs	$700/FTE	$ 700/FTE
Total cost per FTE		**$11,021**

*Subsidy to Child Care Center. The Center is used by 30 percent of the nurses.

Using the work force plan

The work force plan must be reviewed annually as part of the environmental assessment, along with other parts of the long-range plan. The amended plan and the annual budget guidelines direct the development of even more detailed plans for the coming year. The human resources department works closely with the employing departments to specify individual compensation changes and work force adjustment. The financial implications of these actions are incorporated into the departmental budgets, which set precise expectations for the number of employees, the number of hours worked, the wage and salary costs, and the benefit costs.

Well-run organizations also use the work force plan to guide human resources policies. Among these are the timing of recruitment campaigns; guidelines for the use of temporary labor such as overtime, part-time, and contract labor; and incentive, compensation, and employee benefit design. The plan may be useful in making decisions about new programs and capital, as when the existence of a surplus work force becomes a resource for expanded services. Even such strategic decisions as mergers or vertical integration can be affected by human resource shortages and surpluses. All of these applications of the plan call for close collaboration with other executives and clinical departments. Collaboration is also desirable on short-term work force management issues, particularly training, motivation, lost time, and turnover. Improvements in these areas reduce the cost of the human resources department and can be translated into direct gains in productivity and quality by line managers.

The penalty for inadequate work force planning is loss of the time and flexibility needed to adjust to environmental changes. Many management difficulties are simpler if adequate time is available to deal with them. Inadequate warning causes hasty and disruptive action. Layoffs may be required. Recruitment is hurried and poor selections may be made. Retraining may be incomplete. Each of these actions takes its toll on workers' morale and often directly affects quality and efficiency. Although the effect of each individual case may be modest, it is long lasting and cumulative. The organization that makes repeated hasty and expedient decisions erodes its ability to compete.

Maintenance of the Work Force

Building and maintaining the best possible work force requires continuing attention to exchange relationships between the organization and its members. The organization cannot remain passive. The best people must be recruited, and they are more likely to remain with an organization that actively meets their personal needs. Investments in recruitment, retention, employee services, and programs for training supervisors in human relations become a part of the intangible benefits as perceived by the employee or member. The additional cost of well-designed programs in these areas is relatively small, but the return is very high.

Recruitment and selection

Retention of proven members is generally preferable to recruitment because the risk of dissatisfaction is lower on both sides. However, expansions, changes in services, and employee life cycles result in continuing recruitment needs at all skill levels. Equal opportunity and affirmative action laws, sound medical staff bylaws, and union contracts all require consistency in recruitment practices. A uniform protocol for recruitment establishes policies for the following activities:

1. *Position control.* Documentation of the number of FTEs approved, the identity and hours of persons hired for them, and the number of vacancies controls paychecks authorized and approval of recruitment requests, and keeps the work force at expectations established in the annual budget.

2. *Job description.* Each position must be described in enough detail to identify training, licensure, and experience requirements and to determine compensation. Descriptions are developed by the line, approved and recorded by human resources.

3. *Classification and compensation.* Wage, salary, incentive, and benefit levels must be assigned to each recruited position. These must be kept consistent with other internal positions, collective bargaining contracts, and the external market. Human resources maintains the classification and associates classes with pay scales and incentives.

4. *Job requirements.* The job description is translated to specific skills and knowledge sought with enough precision to permit equitable evaluation of applicants. Human resources assists line managers in making the translation and assessing skills.

5. *Applicant pool priorities and advertising.* Policies covering affirmative action and priority consideration of current and former employees and employees' relatives for job openings. Policies also cover the design, placement, and frequency of media advertising, including use of the organization's own newsletters and publications. Human resources generally develops and administers the policies.

6. *Initial screening.* Screening normally includes review and verification of data on the application. It may or may not include interviews. It includes a brief physical examination and may include drug testing.[6] Particularly for high-volume recruitment, screening takes place in the human resources department so that it will be uniform and inexpensive.

7. *Final selection.* Applicants who pass the initial screening are subjected to more intensive review, usually involving the immediate supervisor of the position and other line personnel. The final selection must be consistent with state and federal equal opportunity and affirmative action requirements and with the job description and requirements. Human resources monitors compliance with these criteria.

8. *Orientation.* New employees need a variety of assistance, ranging from maps showing their work place to counseling on selecting benefit

options. They should be given a mentor who can help them fit into their work group. They should learn appropriate information about the organization's mission, services, and policies to encourage their contribution and to make them spokesmen for the institution in their social group. The mentor is assigned by line personnel, but human resources usually provides the training and counseling.

9. *Probationary review.* Employees begin work with a probationary period, which concludes with a review of performance and usually an offer to join the organization on a long-term basis. Often, increased benefits and other incentives are included in the long-term offer. Line supervisors conduct the probationary review, with advice from human resources.

Modifications of the basic protocol are usually made for professional personnel and for temporary employees. Modifications for temporary employees and volunteers greatly simplify the process to reduce cost and delay, while those for professional personnel recognize that recruitment is usually from national or regional labor markets and that future colleagues should undertake most of the recruitment.

For the medical staff leaders and higher supervisory levels, search committees are frequently formed to establish the job description and requirements, encourage qualified applicants, carry out screening and selection, and assist in convincing desirable candidates to accept employment. The human resources department acts as staff for the search committee while ensuring that the intent of organization policies has been met. Well-run organizations now use human resources personnel to conduct initial reference checks and to verify licensure status and educational achievement for doctors and other professional personnel. This provides both consistency and a clearer legal record.

Healthcare organizations are subject to various regulatory and civil restrictions affecting recruitment. Federal regulations regarding equal opportunity require that there be no discrimination on the basis of sex, age, race, creed, national origin, or handicaps that do not incapacitate the individual for the specific job. Those covering affirmative action require special recruitment efforts and priority for equally qualified women, African Americans, and Hispanics. (Religious organizations may give priority to members of their faith under certain circumstances.) In addition to these constraints, organizations must follow due process, that is, fair, reasonable, and uniform rules, in judging the qualifications of attending physicians. Medical staff appointments are also subject to tests under antitrust laws. Healthcare organizations are required to be able to document compliance with these rules and may be subject to civil suits by dissatisfied applicants. Monitoring and documenting compliance with these obligations is a function of the human resources department.

Workplace diversity

Most healthcare organizations strive to promote diversity in their work force.[7] They pursue affirmative action vigorously and make a deliberate effort to represent the ethnic and gender makeup of their community in their medical staff, management group, and work force.[8] They make a deliberate effort to promote women in management.[9] While this may be driven in part by law or a belief in the need for justice, it is also supported by sound marketing theories. Many people seek healthcare from caregivers who resemble them. African American doctors, nurses, and managers are important to African American patients. Increasing attention to the needs of female workers have clearly influenced the structure of employment benefits and the rules of the workplace.

Work force satisfaction and retention

Healthcare organizations now routinely survey personnel at all levels to assess general satisfaction with the work environment. The surveys must be carefully worded and administered in ways that protect the worker's anonymity. "360-degree" reviews have become popular; these surveys combine elements of satisfaction and evaluation. They allow evaluation by supervisors, subordinates, and both internal and external customers. Special problems identified from the surveys and other monitoring mechanisms are often pursued in focus groups or cross-functional groups. Well-run organizations make an effort to interview persons who are leaving. Their candid comments can be useful to eliminate or correct negative factors in the work environment. They often serve to improve the departing worker's view of the organization as well.

Human resources conducts surveys, interviews, and focus groups, and staffs cross-functional teams working on workplace problems. It analyzes and reports data and seeks benchmarks to guide line managers. It frequently counsels line managers on individual improvement opportunities.

Policies for promotion, retirement, and voluntary and involuntary termination must be similar in fairness and consistency to those for recruitment. For motivational purposes, they should be designed to make work life as attractive as possible, and they should permit selective retention of the best workers. This means that all collective actions should be planned as far in the future as possible and be announced well ahead of time. Criteria for promotion or dismissal should be clear and equitable, and loyal and able employees should be rewarded by priority in promotion and protection against termination.

It also means that all policies are administered uniformly and that there is always a clear route of appeal against actions the employee views as arbitrary. Human resources participates directly in major reductions, designing actions and communications that minimize the impact. It provides counseling and appeals services in individual cases.

Employee services

Most healthcare organizations provide personal services to their employees through their human resources department on the theory that such services improve loyalty and morale and, therefore, efficiency and quality. Evidence to support the theory is limited, but the services are often required if competing employers provide them. Specific offerings are often tailored to the employees' responses. Popular programs are allowed to grow, while others are curtailed. Charges are sometimes imposed to defray the costs, but some subsidization is usual. Those commonly found include:

- Health education, health promotion, and access to personal counseling for substance abuse problems. Employee assistance programs, formally structured counseling to assist with stress management and alcohol and drug abuse, have been popular in recent years.[10] Many large companies have nurses or physicians on site to handle workplace injuries and illness;
- Infant and child care;
- Social events, often recognizing major holidays or corporate events, but also used to recognize employee contributions;
- Recreational sports; and
- Credit unions and payroll deduction for various purposes.

One theme of these activities is to build an attitude of caring and mutual support among healthcare workers, on the theory that a generally caring environment will encourage a caring response to patient and visitor needs.

Occupational safety and health

The hospital and some outpatient care sites are moderately dangerous environments for workers. The hospital contains unique or rare hazards, such as repeated exposure to low levels of radioactivity or small quantities of anesthesia gases and increased risk of infection. In practice, however, accident rates are low. Illness and injury arising from hospital work are kept to low levels by constant attention to safety.[11] The organization's dedication to personal and public health encourages this vigilance. For those who might be complacent or forgetful, two laws reinforce its importance. Workers' compensation is governed by state law. Premiums are based on settlements but also on process evidence of attention to safety. The federal **Occupational Safety and Health Act (OSHA)** establishes standards for safety in the workplace and supports inspections. Fines are levied for noncompliance.

Much of the direct control of hazards is the responsibility of the clinical and plant departments. Infection control, for example, is an important collaborative effort of housekeeping, facility maintenance, nursing, and medicine to protect the patient. Employee protection in well-run organizations stems from procedures developed for patient safety. The human resources department is usually assigned the following functions:

- monitoring federal and state regulations and professional literature on occupational safety for areas in which the organization may have hazards;
- identifying the department or group accountable for safety and compliance on each specific risk;
- keeping records and performing risk analysis, and leading improvement efforts for general or widespread exposures;
- maintaining records demonstrating compliance and responding to visits and inquiries from official agencies;
- providing or assisting training in and promotion of safe procedures; and
- negotiating contracts for workers' compensation insurance, reviewing appropriate language where the insurance is negotiated as part of broader coverage, or managing settlements where the organization self-insures.

Educational services

Human resources departments provide significant educational opportunities for employees and supervisors. In-service education is offered on topics where uniformity of understanding is desired.[12] On issues to be handled uniformly among relatively large groups, human resources personnel provide the entire program. Routine offerings are usually less than two hours long, with multiple sessions when more time is needed. Classes are limited in size, and offerings are repeated to provide greater access. Topics include:

- *Orientation.* Review of the organization's mission, history, major assets, and marketing claims, as well as policies and benefits of employment.
- *Continuous improvement and performance measurement.* Basic education in continuous improvement offered to all employees, including the

reason for, meaning of, and application of concepts, including several basic tools and description of improvement team procedures.

- *Work policy changes.* Reviews covering the objectives and implications in major changes in compensation, benefits, or work rules.
- *Major new programs.* Permanent or temporary actions that affect habits and lifestyles of current workers. (New buildings, relocations, and construction dislocation are often topics.)
- *Retirement planning.* Offered to older workers to understand their retirement benefits and also to adjust to retirement lifestyles.
- *Outplacement.* To assist persons being involuntarily terminated through reductions in work force.
- *Benefits management.* Selection of options and procedures for using benefits, including efforts to minimize misuse.[13]

Clinical departments often use their own supervisors or consultants for professional topics, but human resources in larger organizations provides facilities, promotion, and logistic assistance. Human resources can collaborate with planning and finance units on organization-wide concerns such as the annual budget and continuous improvement.

Guest relations has become a prominent educational offering for human resources departments. These programs use roleplaying, games, and group discussion techniques to reinforce attitudes of caring and responsiveness to patients and visitors. Well-run organizations use the guest relations educational programs as part of a comprehensive effort; workers will respond more effectively to customer needs when their own needs are met by responsive supervision, adequate facilities and equipment, and organization policies that encourage flexibility toward customer needs.

Work force reduction

Rapid change in the healthcare industry has forced many organizations to make substantial involuntary reductions in their work forces. Because job security is an important recruitment and retention incentive, it is imperative that such reductions be handled well. Good practice pursues the following rules:

- Work force planning is used to foresee reductions as far in advance as possible, allowing natural turnover and retraining to provide much of the reduction.
- Temporary and part-time workers are reduced first.
- Personnel in supernumerary jobs are offered priority for retraining programs and positions arising in needed areas.
- Early retirement programs are used to encourage older (and often more highly compensated) employees to leave voluntarily.

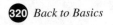

- Terminations are based on seniority or well-understood rules, judiciously applied.

Using this approach has allowed many healthcare organizations to limit involuntary terminations to a level that does not seriously impair the attractiveness of the organization to others.

Grievance administration

Well-run healthcare organizations provide an authority independent of the normal accountability for employees who feel, for whatever reason, that their complaint or question has not been fully answered. Larger human resources departments often offer ombudsman-type programs providing an unbiased counselor for concerns of any kind. Personnel in these units are equipped to handle a variety of problems, from health-related issues they refer to employee assistance programs or occupational health services, to complaints about supervision or work conditions, to sexual harassment and discrimination. Most of the approaches are concerns rather than grievances when they are first presented. The function of the office is to settle them fairly and quickly, and if possible identify corrections that will prevent reoccurrence. The office's success depends on its ability to meet worker needs. It must remain flexible and independent in its orientation, yet management must heed its advice.

A few of the matters presented to ombudsman offices and line officers become formal grievances or complaints. Under collective bargaining, the union contract includes a formal grievance process that is often adversarial in nature, assuming a dispute to be resolved between worker and management. Under non-union arrangements, a grievance procedure is still necessary.

Good grievance administration begins with sound employment policies, effective education for workers and supervisors, and systems that emphasize rewards over sanctions.[14] Effective supervisory training emphasizes the importance of responding promptly to workers' questions and problems. Good supervisors have substantially fewer grievances than poor ones.

When disagreements arise, good grievance administration stimulates the following informal reactions:

- documentation of issue, location, and positions of the two parties to provide guides to preventive or corrective action;
- credible, unbiased, informal review to identify constructive solutions;
- informal negotiations that encourage flexibility and innovation in seeking a mutually satisfactory solution;

- counseling for the supervisor involved aimed at improvement of future human relations;
- settlement without formal review, either by mutual agreement or by concession on the part of the organization; and
- implementation of changes designed to prevent recurrences.

These processes are appropriate in both union and non-union environments. They should make the formal review process typically found in union contracts, leading to resolution by an outside arbitrator, unnecessary in the vast majority of cases. Grievances that go to formal review encourage an adversarial environment. Even if the concession appears relatively expensive, the organization is better off avoiding review and making an appropriate investment in the prevention of future difficulties.

Management Education

Human resources is responsible for training most line managers in three areas: facts about relevant policies and procedures, skills in human relations and supervision, and tools for budgeting and continuous improvement. Under continuous improvement approaches, more than simply mastery of tools is required. Non-health companies report substantial investments in managerial training, up to 80 hours per manager per year.[15] At least one large integrated system also makes a large investment.[16] Employees at all levels must think of themselves and the organization as continuously learning.[17] Many of these skills are delivered by other technical support units, on a "just-in-time" basis. Planning, marketing, finance, and information services personnel provide direct assistance to improvement teams when they need it. Human resources efforts may focus on the most commonly used tools and serve to emphasize the importance of the concept.

Facts about policies and procedures

Effective line supervisors are expected to answer a wide variety of questions from their workers. Many of these will be factual issues about the employment contract and the work environment. Examples are questions about compensation and benefits, incentive programs, and policies on leaves. An educational program to support the supervisors might include:

- Modern theories of human relations and supervision. Learning the supervisor's role and the importance of sound human relations. Policies and goals for the workforce, including the promotion of diversity and the elimination of sexual harassment;[18]

- In-service courses in major policies, important changes, and how to use the procedure manuals. (Leading organizations now have procedures in electronic files that can be quickly searched for the topic. The relevant policy can be quickly printed for the employee, and explained to ensure full comprehension); and
- Telephone and electronic mail access for specific questions, and personal consultation to the employee or supervisor where indicated.

Skills in human relations and supervision

Supervisory training and counseling is a particularly important human resources function. Promising workers are identified well before they are promoted and are trained in methods of supervision and effective motivation. Much of the folklore of American industry runs counter to the realities of sound first-line supervision.[19] Thus, even promising personnel need repeated reinforcement of the proper role and style. Multiple presentations using a variety of approaches and media are used to establish and reinforce basic notions: the use of rewards rather than sanctions, the importance of fairness and candor, the role of the supervisor in responding to workers' questions, and the importance of clear instructions and appropriate work environments.[20] Typical topics cover skills in orienting new people, training new skills, motivating workers, answering worker questions, disciplining, and identifying problem workers. Cases, roleplaying, recordings, films, and individual counseling are helpful in maintaining supervisor's performance.

Tools for budgeting and continuous improvement

Supervisors in continuous improvement programs need a variety of skills to identify opportunities, evaluate them, motivate their personnel, and implement the PDCA cycle. These tools are usually taught in several courses of a day or two each.[21] Budgets and capital budgets have now become complex enough that sessions on how the guidelines are generated, what sorts of improvements and proposals are appropriate, and how to handle the mechanics of preparation and submission are useful.

Human resources often organizes these programs using faculty from planning, marketing, finance, and information services. It is important to tie the mechanical skills of budgeting and continuous improvement projects to the human relations skills necessary to sustain motivation.

Compensation

Employee compensation includes direct wages and salaries, cash differentials and premiums, bonuses, retirement pensions, and a substantial number of specific benefits supported by payroll deduction or supplement. Federal law defines employment status and requires withholding of social security and income taxes from the employee and contributions by the employer.[22] Other employment benefits are automatically purchased on behalf of the employee via the payroll mechanism. Compensation constitutes more than half the expenditures of most healthcare organizations. From the organization's perspective, such a large sum of money must be protected against both fraud and waste. From the employee's perspective, accuracy regarding amount, timing, and benefit coverage should be perfect.

The growing complexity of compensation has been supported by highly sophisticated computer software, with each advance in computer capability soon translated into expanded flexibility of the compensation package. The latest developments in payroll have been increased use of bonuses and incentive compensation, as well as "cafeteria" benefits, which allow more employee choice. Well-run organizations now use payroll programs that process both pay and benefit data for three purposes: payment, monitoring and reporting, and budgeting. This software permits active management of compensation issues in the human resources department through position control, wage and salary administration, benefit administration, and pension administration.

Job analysis

Compensation programs require a description and classification of each job in the organization. The job description used to establish recruiting criteria also serves as a basis for classifying the position in a pay category. Human resources classifies the job in relation to others and establishes a pay scale for it.

Position control

The organization must protect itself against accidental or fraudulent violation of employment procedures and standards and must ensure that only duly employed persons or retirees receive compensation. This is done through a central review of the number of positions created and the persons hired to fill them, called **position control**. Creation of a position generally requires multiple approvals, ending near the level of the chief operating officer. Positions created are monitored by the human resources department to ensure compliance with recruitment, promotion, and compensation procedures and to ensure that each individual employed is assigned to a unique position.

It is important to understand the limitation of this activity; it controls the number of people employed rather than the total hours worked. The number of hours worked outside position control accountability is significant. Position control protects only against paying the wrong person, hiring in violation of established policies, and issuing double checks. It does not protect against overspending the labor budget or against errors in hours, rates, or benefit coverage.

Wage and salary administration

Most healthcare organizations operate at least two payrolls and a pension disbursement system. One payroll covers personnel hired on an hourly basis, requiring reporting of actual compensable hours for each pay period, usually two weeks. The other covers salaried, usually supervisory, personnel paid a fixed amount per period, often monthly. Contract workers, such as clinical support service physicians, are often compensated through non-payroll systems. (Benefits, withholding, and payroll deduction are usually omitted from contract compensation, although certain reporting requirements still apply.)

Wage and salary administration covers all of these disbursements for personnel costs, and includes the following activities:

- *Verification of compensable hours and compensation due.* This is applicable only to hourly personnel. The accountable department is responsible for the accuracy of hours reported, and for keeping hours within budget agreements. The task of the human resources department is to verify line authorization, the base rate, and the application of policies establishing differentials. Modern systems also identify other elements, such as location or activity, to support cost-finding activities. The data become an important resource for further analysis.

- *Compensation scales.* The well-run organization strives to be competitive in each position where comparison can be made to other employers and to treat other positions equitably. To achieve this goal, each job classification is assigned a compensation grade. The human resources department conducts or purchases periodic salary and wage surveys to establish competitive prices for representative grades. At supervisory and professional levels, these surveys cover national and regional markets. For most hourly grades the local market is surveyed.

- *Seniority, merit, and cost-of-living adjustments.* Beginning around World War II wages and salaries were adjusted annually to reflect changes in cost of living and the experience and loyalty reflected by job seniority. Calculating the amount or value of these factors and translating that into compensation at the appropriate time is the task of the human resources department. Well-run healthcare organizations are rapidly diminishing the importance of these compensation factors. Seniority and cost-of-living raises are not directly related either to the market for employment or the success of the organization. Merit raises, increases in the base pay reflecting the individual employee's skill improvements, are difficult to administer objectively[23] and tend to become automatic. Leading organizations are moving to replace all three adjustments with improved compensation scaling and performance-oriented incentive payments.

Incentive compensation

The market demand for competitive performance has made tangible reward for individual achievement desirable, and improving information systems have made it possible.[24] An organization built on rewards and the search for continued improvement is strengthened by a system of compensation that supplements personal satisfaction and professional recognition.[25] Healthcare organizations have advanced significantly toward this goal,[26,27,28] although few reports appear in published literature.

One approach is to recognize that wages and salaries should be based on market conditions, but that adjustments in compensation are most appropriately based on the employee's contribution to organizational goals. Certain constraints must be recognized in designing a system of this type:

- The resources available will depend more on the organization's overall performance than on any individual's contribution. They may be severely limited through factors outside the organization's control. The incentives must recognize this reality, emphasizing overall performance over unit or individual performance.
- Equity and objectivity will be expected in the distribution of the rewards.
- The individual's contribution will be difficult to measure.
- Group rewards attenuate the incentives to individuals. The larger the group, the greater the attenuation.
- The incentive program must avoid becoming a routine or expected part of compensation.

Well-run healthcare organizations are beginning to experiment with incentive compensation. It is likely that successful designs will have the following characteristics:

- The use of incentive compensation will begin at top executive levels and be extended to lower ranks with experience.
- Annual longevity increases will disappear as incentive pay increases.
- Incentives will be limited by difficulties in measurement and administration, but will provide a substantial portion of compensation, particularly for senior management.
- Incentives will be related to overall performance, but will be awarded to individuals based on their perceived contribution.
- Assessment of contribution will be retrospective, but will be based on achievement of improvements in expectations set in the preceding budget negotiation.

A bolder scenario is possible under continuous improvement. Where comprehensive measures covering all six dimensions of performance are available, and workers are comfortable with continuous improvement, work groups can set specific expectations and anticipate incentive payment for meeting them. "Gain sharing" approaches suggest that primary worker groups can effectively set expectations consistent with the needs of the larger organization and that the effort to do so will lead to measurable improvement in achievement. Those gains can then be used in part to reward the workers. At least one healthcare organization has followed that general model for a few years with some success.[29]

Benefits administration

Many of the social programs of Western nations are related directly or indirectly to work, through programs of payroll taxes, deductions, and entitlements. These programs are fixed in place by a combination of market forces, direct legal obligation, and tax-related incentives. Non-wage benefits are generally exempt from income and Social Security taxes, providing an automatic gain of at least 18 percent in the benefits that can be purchased for a given amount of after-tax money. Further gains stem from insurance characteristics. Life, health, accident, and disability insurance are substantially less costly when purchased on a group basis.

As a result, healthcare organizations and other employers in the United States support extensive programs of benefits, which add as much as 40 percent beyond salaries and wages to the costs of employment. (The term "fringe benefits" was common until the total cost of these programs made it obsolete.) The exact participation of each employee differs, with major differences depending on full-time or part-time status, grade, and seniority. In general, there are five major classes of employee benefits and employer obligations beyond wage compensation:

1. *Payroll taxes and deductions.* The employer is legally obligated to contribute premium taxes to Social Security for pension and Medicare benefits, as well as to collect a portion of the employee's pay for Social Security and withholding on various income taxes. Most employers also collect payroll deductions for union dues, various privileges like parking, and contributions to charities such as the United Way. Certain funds, such as uninsured healthcare expenses and child care expenses, can be exempt from income taxes by the use of pre-tax accounts. While the deductions represent only a small handling cost to the employer, they are an important convenience to the employee.

2. *Vacations, holidays, and sick leave.* Employers pay full-time and permanent employees for legal holidays, additional holidays, vacations,

sick leave, and certain other time such as educational leaves, jury duty, and military reserves duty. They grant unpaid leaves for family needs, in accordance with the Family and Medical Leave Act of 1993,[30] and for other purposes as they see fit. As a result, only about 85 percent of the 2,080 hours per year nominally constituting full-time employment is actually worked by hourly workers. The non-worked time becomes a direct cost to the organization when the employee must be replaced by part-time workers or by premium pay. It also is an important factor in the cost of full-time versus part-time employees. Part-time positions often share in employment benefits only on a drastically reduced basis. On a per-hour-worked basis, they can be significantly less costly.

3. *Voluntary insurance programs.* Health insurance is a widespread and popular entitlement of full-time employment. Retirement programs must be funded according to rules similar to those for insurance. Life insurance and travel and accident insurance are also common. Various tax advantages are available for these protections, and they are paid for by combinations of employee and employer contributions. The employer obtains a group rate that is much lower than that offered to individuals. Some employer options for these programs are not technically insurance. They are generally subject to state laws or the federal Employee Retirement Insurance Security Act (ERISA). Direct employer contributions add about 10 percent to the cost of full-time employees. They are rarely offered to employees working fewer than 20 hours per week and may be graduated to those working between half and full time.

4. *Mandatory insurance.* Employers are obligated to provide workers' compensation for injuries received at work, including both full health-care and compensation for lost wages. They are also obligated to provide unemployment insurance, covering a portion of wages for several months following involuntary termination.

5. *Other perquisites.* A wide variety of other benefits of employment can be offered, particularly for higher professional and supervisory grades. These generally are shaped by a combination of tax and job per-formance considerations. Educational programs, professional society dues, and journal subscriptions are commonly included. Cars, homes, club memberships, and expense accounts are used to assist executives to participate fully in the social life of their community. The theory is that such participation increases the executives' ability to understand community desires and identify influential citizens. Added retirement benefits, actually income deferred for tax purposes, and termination settlements are used to defray the risks of leadership positions.

In managing employment benefits, the human resources department strives to maximize the ratio of gains to expenditure. Four courses of action to achieve this are characteristic of well-run departments; three of them relate to program design and one to program administration.

1. *Program design for competitive impact.* The value of a given benefit is in the eye of the employee, and demographics affect perceived value. A married mother might prefer child care to health insurance because her husband's employer already provides health insurance. A single person whose children are grown might prefer retirement benefits to life insurance. Young employees often (perhaps unwisely) prefer cash to deferred or insured benefits. Employee surveys help predict the most attractive design of the benefit package. Flexibility is becoming more desirable as workers' needs become more diverse. Recent trends have emphasized cafeteria benefits, where each employee can select preset combinations.

2. *Program design for cost-effectiveness.* Several benefits have an insurance characteristic such that actual cost is determined by exposure to claims. Health insurance, accident insurance, and sick benefits are particularly susceptible to cost reduction by benefit design. Health insurance, by far the largest of these costs, is minimized by the use of managed care approaches, including copayments, premium sharing, and selected provider arrangements. Accident insurance premiums are reduced by limiting benefits to larger, more catastrophic events. Duplicate coverage, where the employee and the spouse who is employed elsewhere are both covered by insurance, can be eliminated to reduce cost. Costs of sick benefits can be reduced by eliminating coverage for short illnesses and by requiring certification from a physician early in the episode of coverage.

3. *Program design for tax implications.* Income tax advantages are a major factor in program design. Many advantages, such as the exemption of health insurance premiums, are deliberate legislative policy, while others appear almost accidental. Details are subject to constant adjustment through both legislation and administrative interpretations. As a result, it is necessary to review the benefit program periodically for changing tax implications, both in terms of current offerings and in terms of the desirability of additions or substitutions.

4. *Program administration.* Almost all of the benefits can be administered in ways that minimize their costs. It is necessary to provide actual benefits equitably to all employees; careless review of use may lead to widespread expansion of interpretation and benefit cost. Strict interpretation can be received well by employees if it is prompt, courteous, and accompanied by documentation in the benefit literature initially given employees. Health insurance is probably the most susceptible to poor administration. Careful claims review, enforcement of copay

provisions, and coordination of spouse's coverage are known to be cost-effective. Prevention of insured perils is also fruitful. Absenteeism and on-the-job injuries are reduced by effective supervision. Accidents and health insurance usage are reduced by effective health promotion, particularly in cases of substance abuse.[31] Counseling is also believed to reduce health insurance use. Workers' compensation is reduced by improved safety on the job site and case management of expensive disabilities. Unemployment liability is reduced by better planning and use of attrition for work force reduction. Human resources management affects all these activities through employee services, supervisory training, work force planning, and occupational safety programs.

Pensions and retirement administration

Pensions and retirement benefits pose different management problems from other benefits because they are used only after the employee retires. Nonpension benefits are principally health insurance supplementing Medicare. Recent developments have led healthcare organizations to offer bonuses for early retirement as a way of adjusting the work force.

Pension design and retirement program management involve questions of benefit design and administration that are directly analogous to those of other insured benefits. Because the benefit is often not used for many years and represents a multi-decade commitment when use begins, pensions are funded by cash reserves and retiree's health insurance premiums are shown as a liability on the organization's balance sheet. As a result, pension issues also include the definition of suitable funding investments, that is, to what extent they should be divided between fixed-dollar returns and those responsive to inflation, and the management of the funds, including investment of them in the organization's own bonds or stock. Finally, pension-related issues include the motivational impact of the design on the tendency of employees to retire.

The pension itself, but not necessarily other retirement benefits, is regulated under ERISA. Regulations for ERISA specify the employer's obligation to offer pensions, to contribute to them if offered, to vest those contributions, and to fund pension liabilities through trust arrangements. These regulations leave several elements of a sound pension and retirement policy to the organization:

- the amount of pension supplementing Social Security;
- the amount, kind, and design of Medicare supplementation (capitation and other programs encouraging economical use of benefits have become more common);
- opportunities for additional contribution by employees;

- accounting for unvested liabilities (benefits not paid if the employee leaves the organization before the time required for vesting);
- funding of unvested pension liabilities;
- use of unvested funds to finance the organization's needs;
- division of investments between equity and fixed-dollar obligations and selection of those investments; and
- incentives to encourage or discourage retirement (Age 65 is an arbitrary and increasingly irrelevant standard. Federal law allows most older workers, including healthcare workers, the right to continue work without a mandatory retirement age.).

Many of these issues can be and frequently are delegated to pension management firms or fund trustees. Others are important parts of a well-planned work force management program that must be handled by the human resources system. In addition to these financial, technical, and motivational concerns, most organizations accept an obligation to provide retirement counseling, including education to help the employee manage pensions and health insurance benefits.

Retired workers represent large future liabilities. At the time of a female employee's retirement, the organization typically commits itself to pension payments and support of Medicare supplementary health insurance for a period averaging nearly 15 years. ERISA requires a trust fund to support pension payments, and the health insurance supplement payment is represented as a liability on the balance sheet. In past times of high inflation, many hospitals felt obligated to adjust pensions for very old workers because inflation has eroded their buying power below subsistence levels. Such adjustments are, by definition, not funded.

Although healthcare organizations are currently using retirement bonuses as a method of work force reduction, at other times it may pay to retain older workers. In general, they are more amenable to reduced hours, have reliable work habits, and are less likely to have unpredictable absences.

Economic, legal, and social considerations in compensation

Employment compensation, including benefits, is an exchange transaction governed primarily by an economic marketplace. It follows then, that the market is the best and usual source of information on compensation. Healthcare organizations depart from the market price for labor at their peril: a lower price may not attract enough qualified personnel, and a higher one may waste the owners' funds. Wage and salary surveys to determine market prices are available for purchase, particularly for national markets; however, continuing contact with appropriate markets is one of the important functions of the human resources system.

Legal restrictions are also important. Healthcare organizations are subject to federal and state laws governing wages, hours, and working conditions. As noted, they are also obligated to follow equal opportunity and affirmative action regulations. The human resources department is usually accountable for compliance with most of these regulations and for all records and documentation in support of compliance.

Social considerations are more complex. Many people who are concerned with healthcare are also concerned with related issues of a good society, such as the availability of meaningful work, the adequacy of low wages and pensions, the equity of payment for equivalent work, and the avoidance of exploitation of minorities or subgroups of the society. These questions are rarely straightforwardly addressed. In particular, efforts to improve compensation are often associated with reductions in the number of jobs available, possibly by reducing the competitiveness of the organization. Well-run organizations tend to do the following:

- comply with market trends;
- comply with applicable laws and regulations;
- take advantage of indirect ways to increase employment or compensation to disadvantaged groups; and
- advocate as an organization more significant redress of these important social problems.

This posture allows large healthcare organizations to play a limited role in resolving social problems. They can increase work available in inner-city areas by locating facilities there. They can provide scholarships for disadvantaged persons seeking education in health professions. They can promote the use of local contractors who employ from disadvantaged groups.

Collective Bargaining Agreements

Extent and trends in collective bargaining

Healthcare organizations are subject to both state and federal legislation governing the right of workers to organize a union for their collective representation on economic and other work-related matters. Federal legislation generally supports the existence of unions; state laws vary. As a result of the extension of federal law to hospitals and of the increased availability of funds, hospital organizing drives became more common and more successful around 1970. By 1980, 20 percent of all hospital employees were unionized. The likelihood of unionization differed significantly by state, with the northeastern states and California most likely, and was far more common in urban areas. The overall percentage unionized held stable throughout the decade, although unionization in general declined.[32] The number of certification elections (the initial step of union recognition) in healthcare organizations declined steadily throughout the 1980s, although the percentage of successful elections increased slightly, to just over 50 percent in 1991. The decline was particularly noticeable in hospitals. There were 90 successful elections per year in 1980–1982, and 40 per year in 1989–1991. A small number of decertification elections offset these.[33]

By 1990, union members were only 15 percent of the U.S. work force, down from 25 percent shortly after World War II. In hospitals, unskilled workers and building trades were the most likely to be organized. Nurses were next most likely; other clinical professionals were rarely organized. Hospitals that were organized were more likely to remain organized for several years.[34] Small and declining numbers of house officers were union members.[35] Periodic efforts to organize attending physicians gained little headway.[36]

A 1989 Supreme Court decision upheld rules by the National Labor Relations Board establishing eight job classes for unionization in all hospitals. The classes are physicians, registered nurses, all professional personnel other than doctors and nurses, technical personnel (including practical nurses and internally trained aides, assistants and technicians), skilled maintenance employees, business office clerical employees, guards, and all other employees. Any organizing vote must gain support of a majority of all the members of a given class.[37] The ruling stimulated interest in unions among most of the groups identified by the ruling, including physicians, and renewed organization efforts by unions.[38,39,40] The efforts led to more successful organizing activity in healthcare than in other industries,[41] but it did not cause major changes in the overall importance of unions.[42]

Most healthcare organizations are likely to seek a position that discourages unionization or diminishes the influence of existing unions. Such a strategy is actualized through the organization's response to work-related concerns of employees.

Work-related employee concerns

Union organization drives and collective bargaining tend to be strong where employees perceive a substantial advantage to collective representation. This perception is stimulated by evidence of careless, inconsiderate, or inequitable behavior on the part of management in any of the key concerns of the workplace: response to workers' questions, output expectations, working conditions, and pay.

It is possible to diminish both the perceived advantage and the real advantage of unionization by consistently good management. Many companies have existed for decades in highly unionized environments without ever having a significant union organization. The first step is to make certain there is little room for complaint about the key concerns of the workplace and no obvious opportunity for improvement. The union then has nothing to offer in return for its dues, and its strength is diminished. The first task of the human resources department in this regard is to achieve high-quality performance on its functions. The second is to assist other systems of the organization to do the same, and the third is to present the organization so that its performance is recognized by workers.

Organization drives and responses

Organization drives are regulated by law and have become highly formal activities. The union, the employees, and management all have rights that must be scrupulously observed. The regulatory environment presumes an adversarial proceeding. Under this presumption, management is obligated to present arguments against joining the union and to take legal actions that limit the organizers to the framework of the law. If management fails in this duty, the rights of owners and employees who do not wish union representation are not properly protected. Well-run organizations respond to organizing drives by hiring competent counsel specifically to fulfill their adversarial rights and obligations. They act on advice of counsel to the extent that it is consistent with their general strategy of fair and reasonable employee relations.

Negotiations and contract administration

Collective bargaining is usually an adversarial procedure, although collaboration with unions can and should occur. The management position should avoid confrontation as much as possible, and seek collaboration. Well-run organizations use experienced bargainers and have counsel available for the more complex formalities. Once again, management is obligated to represent owners and employees who are not represented at the bargaining table. Healthcare organizations with existing unions pursue a strategy of contract negotiation that attempts to minimize or eliminate dissent. They will accept a strike on issues that depart significantly from the current exchange environment for workers or patients, but as a strategy they avoid strikes whenever possible.

Under certain circumstances, management must pursue contracts that reduce income or employment for union members. Two rules govern such a case: it must apply equally to nonunion workers, and it must be well justified by external forces in the exchange environment.

Contract administration is approached in a similar vein, but the adversarial characteristic of organizing and bargaining should not carry over into the workplace. The objective is to comply fully with the contract but to minimize an adversarial environment that uses the contract as a source of controversy. Considerable supervisory education is necessary to implement this policy. Supervisors should know the contract and abide by it, but whenever possible their actions should be governed by fundamental concerns of human relations and personnel management. Any distinction between unionized and nonunionized groups should be minimized.

Continuous Improvement and Budgeting

The human resources department is obligated to support continuous improvement in its own unit and throughout the organization, and to prepare a budget for its own activities consistent with collective needs. Its customers are both employees and employing units. Leading thought in human resources management places great emphasis on this function; it is regarded as the central contribution of the unit.[43]

Continuous improvement

The competitive environment will demand extraordinary efforts to improve human relations.[44] Most healthcare organizations must make major improvements in labor efficiency and cost. The best will understand that the loyalty, skill, and motivation of the work force are also critical and that any effort to address the problems of costs must involve increasing the contribution and the compensation of many workers. Pursuing these concepts will improve efficiency while simultaneously making workers more valuable to themselves and to the organization. At the other extreme, badly managed organizations will take hasty, ill-considered actions devastating those persons who are terminated and demoralizing those who remain. The demoralization will generate problems of cost, quality, and attractiveness to patients and qualified professionals.

Continuous improvement of human relations begins with competency in each of the functions of the human resources system. It includes information systems for retrieval and analysis of human resources data and measures of performance for the human resources department itself, emphasizing service to other systems and outcomes quality. As shown in Figure 14.3, there are usually several opportunities to expand human resources services. When the indicator directly measures the workforce, as in the employee satisfaction and labor cost illustration in Figure 14.3, the human resources opportunity is clear. Even if the opportunity is in operational performance improvement, training and motivational issues may be the underlying cause.

Figure 14.3   Typical External Improvements for Human Resources
Services

Indicator	Opportunity	Example
Employee satisfaction variance	Identify special causes and address each individually	Improve employee amenities Special training for supervisors with low employee satisfaction
Inadequate operational performance improvement	Support line review of causes	Focus groups on motivation Seek evidence of worker dissatisfaction Review incentive programs
High health insurance costs	Promote more cost-effective program	Revise health insurance benefits Install managed care Promote healthy lifestyles
Labor costs over benchmark	Support orderly employment reduction	Curtail hiring in surplus categories Design and offer early retirement program Start cross-training and retraining programs

Human resources has extensive obligations to support continuous improvement in other units. These include advising on personnel requirements and recruiting, resetting wage and salary levels, and assisting with training programs. Most important, they include continuous reinforcement of the motivating factors for improvement, particularly empowerment. Empowerment is easily destroyed by authoritarian supervisory practices.[45] Motivation drops quickly when these develop. Human resources must monitor, counsel, and train constantly to support an effective program.

The internal continuous improvement of human resources is designed to anticipate line needs and be ready for them as they arise. Improving internal information systems, particularly those associated with work force planning and management, are examples. Recruitment, benefits, regular and incentive compensation, and outcomes measures of work force maintenance can be benchmarked against competitors and non-healthcare service organizations. Programs for special work groups can be redesigned or invented. Because these programs should be anticipatory, there may be no direct measure of need for them. Figure 14.4 gives some common examples.

Figure 14.4 Typical Internal Improvements for Human Resources Services

Indicator	Opportunity	Example
Potential RN shortage	Expand RN recruitment program	Install expanded part-time RN program, emphasizing retraining, child care, flexible hours
High benefits cost	Redesign benefit package	Cafeteria benefits with elimination of extremely high cost elements
Low incentive payments	Redesign incentive pay program	Expand eligibility for incentives, improve measurement of contribution

Budget development

Human resources is responsible for its own budget covering all six dimensions of performance. Figure 14.5 indicates the measures and some likely management questions to be reviewed in the budget for each dimension.

It is important to establish realistic constraints on cost. The department almost never generates revenue. Its costs and services can sometimes be benchmarked against similar institutions, but one benchmark is the price

Figure 14.5 Issues in Human Resources Budget Development

Dimension	Possible Issues
Demand	Hours of training provided per employee Adequacy of coverage of training programs, counseling, recruitment assistance
Cost	Comparison of costs with history and similar organizations
Human Resources	Satisfaction and performance of department's own employees
Output/ Efficiency	Comparison of output to demand Comparison of cost per hire, cost/employee to competitors and similar organizations
Quality	Comparison to competition, other service organizations
Customer Satisfaction	Employee satisfaction with benefits, training programs, etc. Supervisor satisfaction with department

of outside contracts. It is possible to purchase human resources individual services from commercial vendors. Some companies provide complete work force management. Thus, many of the discussions of appropriate levels of quality and unit cost revolve around competitive sources for equivalent services. It is possible to sell human resources services to line departments on a scheme of transfer pricing. While this approach may result in economies, it may also unduly dampen demand for services. The costs of inadequate training and counseling to line departments may be unreasonably high. Even so, demands, outputs, and unit costs of specific human resources services are important and should be studied as part of the budget.

ORGANIZATION AND PERSONNEL
Human Resources Management as a Profession

Human resources management emerged as a profession after World War II, in response to the complexities created by union contracts, wage and hour laws, and benefits management. Healthcare organizations were sheltered from these developments for several years, but as the need arose healthcare organizations moved to establish an identifiable human resources system and to hire specially trained leadership for it. Although there is no public certification for the profession, there is an identifiable curriculum of formal education and a recognizable pattern of professional experience. Healthcare practitioners have an association, the American Society for Healthcare Human Resources, a unit of the American Hospital Association. Well-run organizations now recruit their human resources director or vice president from persons with experience in the profession generally and preferably with experience in healthcare. Larger organizations often have several professionals. Professional training and experience contribute to mastery of the several areas in which laws, precedents, specialized skills, or unique knowledge define appropriate actions.

Organization of the Human Resources Department
Internal organization

The human resources department is organized by function, in order to take advantage of the specialized skills applicable to its more time-consuming activities. Figure 14.6 shows a typical accountability hierarchy for a larger organization with labor union contracts. Smaller organizations must accomplish the same functions with fewer people. They do so by combining the responsibility centers shown on the lower row. (Collective bargaining is less common in smaller institutions.)

In very large organizations, human resources tends to be decentralized by work site. While some activities, such as information processing, can be centrally managed, others require frequent contact with employees and supervisors. A central office can monitor planning, support more elaborate educational programs, and maintain uniformity of compensation, benefits, and collective bargaining. Decentralized representatives available in each site concentrate on implementation of these programs and issues of work force maintenance and continuous improvement. Work force planning is generally handled by an ad hoc team led by the vice president for human resources. While various sites must participate as well as various work groups, a centralized approach maximizes the opportunities for promotion and relocation without layoff.

Division of responsibility with other systems

The more controversial organizational problems relate to the division of human resources functions between the department and the unit accountable for the member's costs and output. Whether the human resources department is involved or not, the functions of the human resources system must be performed for all organization members. By the same token, all members require supervision by and assistance from their accountable unit. Thus, the

Figure 14.6   Organization of a Large Human Resources Department

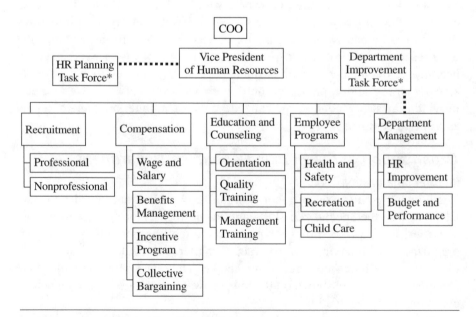

*Task forces draw on department members and outsiders as indicated.
Dotted lines show chairs.

question of the exact domain of the human resources department is inevitably a matter of judgment.

Well-run organizations have identified the question as one of appropriate joint contribution to the needs of the member. They seek the solution not in the assignment of functions to either the line or the human resources department, but rather in the identification of the amount and kind of contribution each unit can make in completing each function. This approach recognizes that the goal is to perform each function well for each member of the work force and that the human resources system must be a collaboration between the department and the line unit involved. In judging the assignment of specific functions, one bears in mind the human resources department's contributions: uniformity, economy, and specialized human resources skills. The operating unit's contributions are professional and technical knowledge of the specific tasks.

MEASURES AND INFORMATION SYSTEMS

Quantitative assessment of human resources must address the state and performance of the member group as well as the human resources department. The human resources department is the "source of truth" on human resources measures.[46]

Measurement of Human Resource

It is possible to measure many characteristics of the workforce using sophisticated accounting, personnel record keeping, and satisfaction surveys. Precise definitions of the concepts being measured are easily obtained from accounting practice and standard definitions. Figure 14.7 lists many of the commonly used measures for assessing the membership.

Membership assessment is a routine part of the annual environmental assessment. The values for measures in the four dimensions can be compared with benchmarks and comparable organizations and with their own history.

Measurement of the human resources department obviously begins with the measures shown in Figure 14.7. The level of achievement on these measures is an outcomes quality measure for the department; the state of the workforce is its principal product. An additional set of measures is important in assessing the department itself, as shown in Figure 14.8.

Cost measurement of the human resources activity and its components is relatively straightforward. Concerns are sometimes raised about the cost of time spent in human resources activity by personnel not in the human resources department, an amount that would not normally be captured by the accounting system. Examples are time spent in training or participating in task forces with a direct human resources goal. These concerns assume that

Figure 14.7 Measures of the Human Resources Department

Dimension	*Measure*
Demand	New hires per year Unfilled positions
Costs and Efficiency	Number of workers Full- and part-time hours paid Overtime, differential, and incentive payments Benefits costs by benefit Human resources department costs
Quality	Skill levels and cross-training Recruitment of chosen candidates Examination scores Analysis of voluntary terminations
Satisfaction	Employee satisfaction Turnover and absenteeism Grievances

time spent on these activities results in lost production elsewhere. In fact, the premise may be false; the morale or skills improvement resulting from participation may cause production increases rather than decreases.

Customer satisfaction measures are easily obtained in conjunction with other member surveys. Focus groups or task forces may provide supplementary information. Quality measures can be developed for specific activities, such as benefit administration and paycheck errors. Recruitment is often measured by the time to fill positions, and the percentage of top-ranked candidates actually recruited. Process measures, such as the percentage of eligible members participating in various programs, or the content and presentation of educational materials can be developed.

Most of the measures of departmental performance can be benchmarked. It is useful to compare performance with other service industries, rather than strictly within healthcare.

Information Systems

Structure

The information systems of human resources management are built around seven core files of information, as shown in Figure 14.9. These files record the status of the human resource—personnel counts, qualifications, compensation, and vacancies—and the activity—unit costs, satisfaction, turnover, absenteeism, grievances, and training. Many of the files are automated.

Figure 14.8 Measures of Human Resources' Functional Effectiveness

Dimension	Concept	Representative Measures
Demand	Request for human resources department service	Requests for training and counseling services Requests for recruitment Delay in filling positions Number of employees
Cost	Resources consumed in department operation	Department costs by functional account Physical resources used by department
Human resources	The work force in the department	Satisfaction, turnover, absenteeism within the department
Output/ efficiency	Cost/unit of service	Cost per hire, employee, training hour, paychecks issued, etc.
Quality	Quality of department services	Time to fill open positions Results of training Audit of services Service error rates
Customer satisfaction	Services as viewed by employees and supervisors	Surveys of member satisfaction with human resources

Actions such as employment, training, anniversary reviews, promotion, or termination are electronically captured, along with data generated by payroll systems.

Ethical issues

Important ethical questions are raised in connection with the information in these files. The records involved are usually viewed as confidential. At the simplest ethical level, human resources files, like patient records, must be guarded against unauthorized access and misuse.

More serious questions arise when basic concerns have been met. Reduction of dissatisfaction, turnover, absenteeism, grievances, accidents, and illness is a socially useful goal of human resources management. It is clearly proper, even desirable, to study variations as measures of supervisory effectiveness that can be improved by systems redesign, counseling, and education. Yet, actions based on worker characteristics such as age, sex, or race or

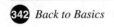

Figure 14.9 Core Files of the Human Resources Information System

File	Uses
Position Control (list of approved full-time and part-time positions by location, classification)	Provides a basic check on number and kinds of people employed
Personnel Record (personal data, training, employment record, hearings record, benefits use)	Provides tax and employment data aggregated for descriptions
Work Force Plan (record of future positions and expected personnel)	Shows changes needed in work force
Payroll (current work hours or status, wage or salary level)	Generates paychecks Provides labor cost accounting
Employee Satisfaction (results of surveys by location, class)	Assesses employee satisfaction
Training Schedules and Participation (record of training programs and attendance)	Generates training output statistics and individual records
Benefits Selection and Utilization (record of employee selection and use of services)	Benefits management and cost control

records such as illness and grievances can be illegal and are often ethically questionable. Some facts, such as drug test data, are potentially destructive, and the database cannot be made error free. Some companies have attempted to deny employment opportunities in situations in which there was high risk of occupational injury. For example, such an approach would deny employment in operating rooms to female nurses in their childbearing years because there are known pregnancy risks related to exposure to anesthesia.

One must note that in almost all cases harm results from the misuse of information rather than the acquisition of it. In fact, knowledge of age-, sex-, and race-related hazards can only be deduced from studies of their specific impact. Thus, denial of the value of all or part of the information potential is also unethical—it permits the organization to do less than it should on behalf of all workers. A sound policy must balance the advantages of investigation against its dangers. These rules help:

- Information access is limited to a necessary minimum group. Those with access are taught the importance of confidentiality and the organization's expectation that individuals' rights will be protected.

- Formal approval must be sought for studies of individual characteristics affecting personnel performance. Often a specific committee including members of the organization's ethics committee reviews each study. Criteria for approval include protection of individual rights, scientific reliability, and evidence of potential benefit.
- Actions taken to improve performance are reward oriented rather than sanction oriented. Considerable effort is made to find nonrestrictive solutions. (In the operating room example, avoidance of the more dangerous gases would be one such solution, improved air handling another, and concentrating use in one location a third. While none of these may be practical, all should be considered before a restrictive employment policy is established.)
- When used, sanctions or restrictions offer the individual the greatest possible freedom of choice. The right of the individual to take an informed risk should be respected, although it may not reduce the organization's ultimate liability. (In the operating room example, a nurse may accept employment with a full explanation of the risks as they are currently known. The complex probabilities of pregnancy, stillbirth, and infant deformity clearly depend on her personal lifestyle and intentions. Weighing them would be the nurse's moral obligation. Legally, the organization's liability for later injury might be reduced by evidence that full information was supplied about the hazards involved, although such an outcome is uncertain.)

SUGGESTED READINGS

Carter, C. C. 1994. *Human Resources Management and the Total Quality Imperative.* New York: American Management Association.

Dreachslin, J. 1996. *Diversity Leadership.* Chicago: Health Administration Press.

Fottler, M. D., S. R. Hernandez, and C. L. Joiner (eds.). 1994. *Strategic Management of Human Resources in Health Services Organizations,* 2nd ed. Albany, NY: Delmar Publishers.

Jackson, S. E., and Associates (eds.). 1992. *Diversity in the Workplace: Human Resources Initiatives.* New York: Guilford Press.

Pfeffer, J. 1994. *Competitive Advantage Through People: Unleashing the Power of the Work Force.* Boston: Harvard Business School Press.

Sibson, R. E. 1998. *Compensation,* 5th ed. NY: AMACOM Books.

U.S. Department of Labor. 1993. *Framework for a Comprehensive Health and Safety Program in the Hospital Environment.* Washington, DC: U.S. Department of Labor, Occupational Safety and Health Administration, Directorate of Technical Support, Office of Occupational Health Nursing.

NOTES

1. U.S. Bureau of the Census, *Statistical Abstracts of the U.S., 1997,* 117th ed. Washington, DC: U.S. Bureau of the Census, Table 662 (1997).

2. J. P. Weiner, "Forecasting the Effects of Health Reform on U.S. Physician Workforce Requirement: Evidence from HMO Staffing Patterns." *Journal of the American Medical Association* 272(3), pp. 222–30 (July 20, 1994).

3. J. Pfeffer, *Competitive Advantage Through People: Unleashing the Power of the Work Force.* Boston: Harvard Business School Press, Ch. 2 pp. 27–65 (1994).

4. D. I. Levine and L. D. Tyson, "Participation, Productivity, and the Firm's Environment." In A. S. Blinder, ed., *Paying for Productivity.* Washington, DC: The Brookings Institution pp. 183–243 (1990).

5. *Ibid*, p. 205.

6. J. W. Fenton, Jr., and J. L. Kinard, "A Study of Substance Abuse Testing in Patient Care Facilities." *Health Care Management Review* 18(4), pp. 87–95 (Fall, 1993).

7. S. Cejka, "The Changing Healthcare Workforce: A Call for Managing Diversity." *Healthcare Executive* 8(2), pp. 20–3 (March–April, 1993).

8. S. E. Jackson and Associates, eds., *Diversity in the Workplace: Human Resources Initiatives.* New York: Guilford Press (1992).

9. A. M. Rizzo and C. Mendez, *The Integration of Women in Management: A Guide for Human Resources and Management Development Specialists.* New York: Quorum Books (1990).

10. J. C. Howard and D. Szczerbacki, "Employee Assistance Programs in the Hospital Industry." *Health Care Management Review* 13, pp. 73–9 (Spring, 1988).

11. U.S. Department of Labor, "Framework for a Comprehensive Health and Safety Program in the Hospital Environment." Washington, DC: U.S. Dept. of Labor, Occupational Safety and Health Administration, Directorate of Technical Support, Office of Occupational Health Nursing (1993).

12. K. N. Wexley and J. Hinrich, eds., *Developing Human Resources.* Washington, DC: Bureau of National Affairs (1991).

13. M. L. Finkel, "Evaluate and Communicate Health Care Benefits." *Employee Benefits Journal* 22(4), pp. 29–34 (December, 1997).

14. C. R. McConnell, "Behavior Improvement: A Two-Track Program for the Correction of Employee Problems." *Health Care Supervisor* 11(3), pp. 70–80 (March, 1993).

15. E. A. McColgan, "How Fidelity Invests in Service Professionals." *Harvard Business Review* 75(1), pp. 137–43 (January–February, 1997).

16. J. R. Griffith, *Designing 21st Century Healthcare: Leadership in Hospitals and Healthcare Systems.* Chicago: Health Administration Press, pp.183–4 (1998).

17. D. A. Garvin, "Building a Learning Organization." *Harvard Business Review* 71(4), pp. 78–91 (July–August, 1993).

18. R. K. Robinson, G. M. Franklin, and R. L. Fink, "Sexual Harassment at Work: Issues and Answers for Health Care Administrators." *Hospital & Health Services Administration* 38(2), pp. 167–80 (Summer, 1993).

19. E. Jansen, D. Eccles, and G. N. Chandler, "Innovation and Restrictive Conformity Among Hospital Employees: Individual Outcomes and Organizational Considerations." *Hospital & Health Services Administration* 39(1), pp. 63–80 (Spring, 1994).

20. J. F. Manzoni and J. L. Barsoux, "The Set-up-to-Fail Syndrome." *Harvard Business Review* 76(2), pp. 101–13 (March–April, 1998).

21. C. C. Carter, *Human Resources Management and the Total Quality Imperative*. New York: American Management Association (1994).

22. W. B. Moore and C. D. Groth, "Independent Contractors or Employees? Reducing Reclassification Risks." *Healthcare Financial Management* 47(5), pp. 118, 120–4 (May, 1993).

23. M. T. Kane, "The Assessment of Professional Competence." *Evaluation and the Health Professions* 15(2), pp. 63–82 (June, 1992).

24. R. E. Sibson, *Compensation*, 5th ed. New York: AMACOM Books (1998).

25. D.I. Levine and L.D. Tyson, "Participation, Productivity, and the Firm's Environment." In A. S. Blinder, ed., *Paying for Productivity*. Washington, DC: The Brookings Institution, pp. 183–243 (1990).

26. A. Barbusca and M. Cleek, "Measuring Gain-Sharing Dividends in Acute Care Hospitals." *Health Care Management Review* 19(1), pp. 28–33 (Winter, 1994).

27. S. Laverty, B. J. Hogan, and L. A. Lawrence, "Designing an Incentive Compensation Program That Works." *Healthcare Financial Management* 52(1), pp. 56–9 (January, 1998).

28. J. R. Griffith, *Designing 21st Century Healthcare: Leadership in Hospitals and Healthcare Systems*. Chicago: Health Administration Press, pp.111, 184 (1998).

29. J. R. Griffith, *Designing 21st Century Healthcare: Leadership in Hospitals and Healthcare Systems*. Chicago: Health Administration Press, pp.111 (1998).

30. R. W. Luecke, R. J. Wise, and M. S. List, "Ramifications of the Family and Medical Leave Act of 1993." *Healthcare Financial Management* 47(8), pp. 32, 36, 38 (August, 1993).

31. J. W. Fenton, Jr., and J. L. Kinard, "A Study of Substance Abuse Testing in Patient Care Facilities." *Health Care Management Review* 18(4), pp. 87–95 (Fall, 1993).

32. R. Tomsho, "Mounting Sense of Job Malaise Prompts More Healthcare Workers to Join Unions." *Wall Street Journal*, B1 (June 9, 1994).

33. C. Scott and C. M. Lowery, "Union Election Activity in the Health Care Industry." *Health Care Management Review* 19(1), pp. 18–27 (Winter, 1994).

34. C. J. Scott and J. Simpson, "Union Election Activity in the Hospital Industry." *Health Care Management Review* 14(4), pp. 21–8 (Fall, 1989).

35. G. J. Bazzoli, "Changes in Resident Physicians' Collective Bargaining Outcomes as Union Strength Declines." *Medical Care* 26(3), pp. 263–77 (March, 1988).

36. *McGraw-Hill's Washington Report on Medicine & Health* 40 (February 24, 1986).

37. C. R. Gullett and M. J. Kroll, "Rule Making and the National Labor Relations Board: Implications for the Health Care Industry." *Health Care Management Review* 15(2), pp. 61–5 (Spring, 1990).

38. D. Burda, "Service Employees International Union Accelerates Organizing Drives in Wake of Ruling on Bargaining Units." *Modern Healthcare* 21(19), p. 7 (May 13, 1991); L. Perry, "$500,000 Added to Nurses Unionizing Efforts." *Modern Healthcare* 21(14), p. 14 (April, 1991).

39. M. L. Ile, "From the Office of the General Counsel, Collective Negotiation and Physician Unions." *Journal of the American Medical Association* 3: 262(17), p. 2444 (November 3, 1989).

40. L. V. Sobol and J. O. Hepner, "Physician Unions: Any Doctor Can Join, But Who Can Bargain Collectively?" *Hospital & Health Services Administration* 35(3), pp. 327–40 (Fall, 1990).

41. C. Scott and C. M. Lowery, "Union Election Activity in the Health Care Industry." *Health Care Management Review* 19, pp. 18–27 (Winter, 1994).

42. M. H. Cimini and C. J. Muhl, "Labor-Management Bargaining in 1994." *Monthly Labor Review* 118, pp. 23–39 (January, 1995).

43. D. Ulrich, "A New Mandate for Human Resources." *Harvard Business Review* 76(1), pp. 124–34 (January–February, 1998).

44. J. Barnsley, L. Lemieux-Charles, and M. M. McKinney, "Integrating Learning into Integrated Delivery Systems." *Health Care Management Review* 23(1), pp. 18–28 (Winter, 1998).

45. C. Argyris, "Empowerment: The Emperor's New Clothes." *Harvard Business Review* 76(3), pp. 98–105 (May–June, 1998).

46. R. Galford, "Why Doesn't This HR Department Get Any Respect?" *Harvard Business Review* 76(2), pp. 24–6 (March–April, 1998).

Managing Change

Thomas A. Atchison, Ed.D.

Why is change management so important today? The answer cannot be easily explained. Some historical perspective shows why the demand for better change management has become increasingly critical. The evolution of healthcare in the United States is, for the most part, a function of the various payment mechanisms. Since the 1965 Medicare law, healthcare delivery models have developed a pattern of redefining themselves to preserve their existence. Survival today is further complicated because of the relatively new demands for compliance, the critical importance of improved physician integration, and the ever-growing need to enhance information capabilities. The key component in all of these attempts to survive is the staff who manages and serves the patients and other customer groups.

Personal costs always attend the structural accommodation to marketplace survival. The challenge of leadership, and the purpose of this article, is to minimize personal cost and to balance the corporate need to survive and thrive with the human need to feel valued in the process. Successful healthcare leaders spend as much time on the return on human capital as they do on the return on financial capital.

TANGIBLES AND INTANGIBLES

All of the above anticipated changes can be easy or hard according to the degree of alignment between personal and organizational dynamics. The potential for alignment or misalignment is a function of perception and

Editor's Note: This chapter is the lead article of *Frontiers* 16:1 by Thomas A. Atchison, Fall 1999, HAP exists within two complementary domains: the tangible and the intangible elements of an organization (see Figure 15.1). Many stories of failed mergers are surfacing in the healthcare press. In each case, the failure is a result of the intangibles. Organizational changes do not fail because they are badly designed, they fail because the values of the people who must make the change work clash with the purpose of the plan.

The tangibles are those elements that can be measured easily using common statistical techniques. Tangibles typically are associated with the business and clinical elements of the delivery system. These factors consume a great deal of time because of the current focus on payment and measured quality outcomes. Often trustees are drawn from commercial businesses and therefore feel more comfortable discussing financials than such things as values-behaviors alignment and the effect on patient sat-

Figure 15.1   Tangible and Intangible Elements of an Organization

TANGIBLE INPUTS	TANGIBLE OUTPUTS
Cash People Policy/Procedures Strategy Plant Information Systems Communications	Profit Market Share Products Customer Satisfaction Growth Productivity Quality

INTANGIBLE INPUTS	INTANGIBLE OUTPUTS
Mission Values Vision Inspiration Leadership Style Recognition Motivation	Culture Commitment Morale Job Satisfaction Team spirit Pride/Joy/Trust Quality

isfaction. Too often the tangible elements become the targets for change, with little regard to the interdependent outcomes largely controlled by the intangibles.

The intangibles are more elusive to common measurement and often elicit comments about "the soft side" or "the touchy-feely stuff." Such comments discount the fundamentals of organizational dynamics in healthcare delivery. Whereas the Frederick Taylor–based models of linear programming may be helpful for manufacturing, they fall very short of helping healthcare leaders deal with the complexities in our "humans helping humans" business.

The basic tenet of this article is that change management is only successful to the degree that healthcare leaders are able to measure and manage the intangibles. We must learn to measure and manage the intangibles with the same rigor and intensity that we currently use with the tangibles.

The elements in these two domains can be classified as either inputs or outputs (see Figure 15.1). Leaders need to understand that such behaviors as teamwork, morale, and trust are outcomes of a complex mix of inputs. Profit, for example, is not something a leader can "do," but is the result of a complex of good business practices.

Measurement of Progress

The main importance of the interaction of inputs and outputs is in the measurement of progress. Most reports that deal with tangible outcome elements list data on such business outcomes as profit, market share, length of stay, cost per discharge, and other measures of clinical quality. The goal is to have these outcome measures fall within some predetermined range of acceptable limits. Variation on these outcome measures stimulate discussions about which input variables need to be changed to improve the outcome measures—Do we need to review the Community Image Plan, review the number of FTE's per occupied bed, or look at the MSO practice patterns? Discussions about the tangible inputs and how they affect the business outcomes of healthcare typically result in the use of basic gap analysis and problem-solving techniques. This same process—collecting baseline data on the outcomes, comparing the data to some desired benchmarks, discussing the reasons for any variation, targeting appropriate interventions, and remeasuring to determine progress—is the basis for effective change management of the intangibles as well.

Effective change management always includes measuring the intangibles as a priority. The alignment of the tangibles with the intangibles is the most essential factor that determines success or failure, and the process of alignment of these two domains begins with data. Healthcare leaders who understand how change is managed always collect baseline data on those tangible and intangible outcomes that most influence alignment of the human motivational values and organizational priorities.

CORPORATE CULTURE

The key ingredient of any successful change management attempt is the strength of the corporate culture. Culture is the infrastructure upon which all change is managed. Schein (1995, 9) defines culture as "a pattern of basic assumptions—invented, discovered, or developed by a given group as it learns to cope with its problems of external adaptation and integration—that has worked well enough to be considered valid and therefore has to be taught to new members as the correct way to perceive, think, and feel in relation to their problems." I presented another definition in *Trustee* (Atchison 1996, 28): "In short, a corporate culture is the company's personality. Culture, like personality, is a consistent way of behaving regardless of the situation." Understanding the dynamics of building, strengthening, or changing a corporate culture is a key factor in defining the difference between successful leaders in today's healthcare environment and those who view change in a more reactive and episodic manner. Change management and cultural alignment must be integrated. Interventions designed to change a behavior that run counter to the dominant culture are doomed to fail. Conversely, those interventions that use the culture as the context for all change efforts will succeed.

The relationship between the intangibles and the tangibles is profound. Kotter and Heskett (1992) make a strong case for the relationship between those companies who focus on culture as a strategic objective and those who ignore culture as an influence in organizational performance. They indicate the difference between firms with performance-enhancing cultures and those without such cultures by demonstrating the significant economic and social cost to low-performance cultures.

Owensboro Mercy Health System

Greg Carlson, the president and CEO of Owensboro Mercy Health System (OMHS) in Owensboro, Kentucky, based a post-merger organizational change process on the formula of "strategic imperatives plus core values equals success." Strategic and tactical plans always constitute the "what" to be done and the corporate values indicate the "how" the plans should be done. Successful change management processes balance what needs to be done with how things are done in the organization. The how factor is represented in Figure 15.1 as the intangible outcome labeled "culture."

Figure 15.2 Owensboro Mercy Health Syatem Corporate Culture, at Baseline (1996)

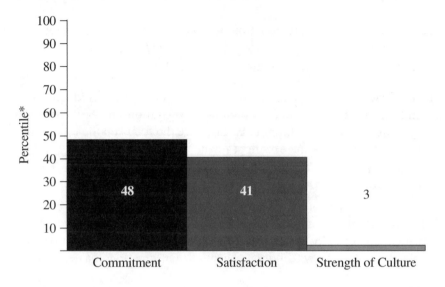

*Comparison based on national database of healthcare providers.

Carlson understands the importance of culture and change management. Shortly after being named CEO he used the *Healthcare Organizational Assessment* (Atchison Consulting Group 1986) to measure the strength of the culture of his newly merged entity.

Figure 15.2 shows the initial baseline of OMHS' corporate culture as compared on a percentile basis to a national database of healthcare providers. The data are very clear. Any significant change efforts in the tangible areas of finance, service mix, and staffing would need to be carefully crafted to the process of culture strengthening. All attempts to alter the tangibles with such a low strength of culture would be met with great resistance and possibly failure.

As a solution, multiple interventions were engaged at OMHS. The executive team was aligned first, and a series of management level processes designed to have all managers understand and live the values followed immediately. The results of this intense and focused 18-month cultural transformation process are shown in Figure 15.3.

Carlson's emphasis on corporate culture as the basis for operational success proved Kotter and Heskett's (1992) argument. The economic gains experienced by OMHS are unique in terms of today's mergers (see Table 15.1). Four rate reductions were put into effect following the merger:

1. Ten percent reduction on room and board on October 1, 1995 (date of merger);
2. Three percent overall reduction on June 1, 1996;
3. One percent overall reduction on June 1, 1997; and
4. Four percent overall reduction on June 1, 1998.

Peat-Marwick, the OMHS auditors, have reported cost reductions at $18.7 million through the first 20 months of operation and $39.8 million in charge reductions to the community. I believe the focus on the intangibles to be the main reason for the excellent financial performance.

Clarian Health Partners

Clarian Health Partners is a much larger merger in the early stages of building a culture to underpin strategic goals. Clarian is the merger of three large and prominent hospitals in Indianapolis—Methodist Hospital, Indiana University Medical School, and Riley Children's Hospital. The creation of a new culture

Figure 15.3 Owensboro Mercy Health Syatem Corporate Culture, After Intervention (1997)

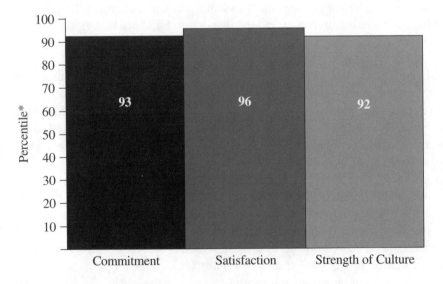

*Comparison based on national database of healthcare providers.

Table 15.1   Status of Owensboro Mercy Health System

	5/31/96	5/31/97	5/31/98*
Gross revenue ($ million)	229,000	231,800	246,044
Net revenue	143,400	142,200	150,988
Profit	13.5	16.7	23.24
Profit as in percentage of net revenue	9.4	11.7	15.89
Number of executives	13	7	8
Number of FTEs (premerger 1,935)	1,710	1,738	1,795[†]
Length of stay (days)	4.6	4.3	4.1

Note: All data are for the 12 months ending at the date shown.

*Projected based on six months annualization.

[†]Increase from volume and new services such as urgent care, community wellness, slep lab, inpatient chemical dependency, and other new or expanded services.

is so important to Clarian that the board of trustees defined the process in an excellent description of the process of managing change through cultural transformation.

> Culture is founded on implicit and explicit value structures (beliefs). Organizational effectiveness will be increased when this value structure is made explicit (avoid cross purposes, misunderstanding, misdirected efforts) and aligned with the operational and strategic requirements of the organization. Making the structure explicit involves both articulating the values and identifying the desired behaviors considered congruent with the values. This provides the basis for cultural alignment" (Clarian 1997).

The Clarian trustees showed insight unusual to healthcare institutions today when they brought the issue of values-behavior alignment to the board. William Loveday, the president and CEO, has lead an ongoing process of measuring and managing the intangibles using several techniques that have been proven effective in the tangibles sphere. Data have been collected and specific targets have been set. Internal accountability for achievement of these targets lies with the Department of Organizational Development headed by Steve Wantz.

The steps being used at Clarian and that were so successful at OMHS will be described later in this article. The important lesson from these cases is that change can best be managed when the values of the organization and the behavior of those people responsible for the work are aligned and drive tangible success—that is, when there is a strong corporate culture.

Development of Corporate Culture

Corporate culture development is critical to change management and especially to long-term business success. Authors have been writing about this most important intangible outcome for years (Deal and Kennedy 1982; Kotter and Heskett 1992; Schein 1995). Industries other than healthcare have embraced the importance of culture as the infrastructure for change. Ford motor company recently announced a cultural transformation as their methodology for change ("Ford Rolls Out New Model" 1999). Jacques Nasser, Ford's CEO, believes that change can best be managed when the cultural context is well understood. The article states that "[Nassar's] goal is to change the nation's No. 2 auto maker from a lumbering bureaucracy to one that responds quickly to consumer needs and is rewarded with the kind of high stock multiples that smart growth companies enjoy." Nasser understands the interdependence of the intangible input of service with the tangible outcome of shareholder value.

The cover story for *Business Week* on May 17, 1999 was "Remaking Microsoft," and the article discusses how Steve Ballman, the president of Microsoft, is shaking the corporate culture. He states that the new culture will drive their future. "We needed to give people a beacon that they could follow when they were having a tough time with prioritization, leadership, where to go, what hills to take" (*Business Week* 1999, 48).

Cognitive and Behavioral Theory

The complex process of change management via values and behavioral alignment is explained best by cognitive and behavioral theory. The view of Thompson and Luthans (1990) regarding organizational change also begins with the intangible construct, *culture*. Culture is a generic term for a host of behaviors that connote general operating norms of conduct for an environment. These behaviors are viewed collectively and are developed into a cognitive construct by the individual. While culture may be articulated in cognitive expressions, its development and maintenance come from behavioral interactions that tend to confirm or create dissonance with the articulated cognition (Thompson and Luthans 1990, 328). The cognitive and behavioral approach to change management requires an understanding of the importance of perception.

Perception. Most failed attempts at change are a function of the disassociation between behavior and the espoused culture. For example, several healthcare systems profess that their employees are their greatest assets, and yet these same companies behave in ways that maximize net operating revenue at the expense of the employees. The popular healthcare press continues to write about failed merger attempts and mergers that are being undone. Behind each of these stories is a culture clash. Change management is successful to the degree that the goals fit within a cultural context that is understood by the people who must actually change. Without such a context, no true long-term change will take place.

Perception is reality when dealing with change processes based on intangibles. The ways individuals view an event determines their position and drives their behavior, and the way individuals view an event is determined by previous experiences with similar events, what an individual focuses on, personal goals, and current environment. No healthcare professional is a tabula rasa. Multiple life experiences form relationships with the outside world, and certain reliable behaviors are produced when the individual is presented with a familiar stimulus pattern. The body of work from Kurt Lewin and B.F. Skinner supports the notion that we are not free from strong relationships with symbols, signals, and stimuli. Skinner called this phenomenon "stimulus control." I use the words "triggers" and "filters" to explain how perception affects the change process.

Triggers are those stimuli in the environment that reliably produce a predictable response. The relationship between the stimuli and the response are conditioned through experience. For example, a manager who is perceived to be critical of new ideas because of her confrontational style will "trigger" compliant, noninnovative behaviors—regardless of how much she says she wants new ideas. The strength of the bonds between the stimuli and the response is a function of the frequency, duration, and outcomes of previous connections. This pattern is one of the main reasons change is difficult with a staff that has had little change over several years. The change leader must try to decode the power of the organizational symbols that control undesirable behaviors. People who change corporate names, titles, work space, pay/benefit systems, and other significantly meaningful connections to work without understanding how these factors affect behavior are begging for resistance and failure. Symbols are very important—especially with our society's emphasis on political correctness and sensitivity to being a victim. For example, the symbolic effects of placing a nurse who has worked for ten years on a medical floor into a service line for community health can have a huge effect on performance.

Filters are cognitive structures that, like triggers, control behavior. Filters determine which data elements individuals consider important. Typically, there are many factors in any change process. Individuals will reliably discount those data elements that run counter to their beliefs and exaggerate the importance of those data elements that support their point of view. This phenomenon is sometimes called "the Pygmalion effect" or "a self-fulfilling prophecy." Those involved in the change process come with significant predeterminations about the outcomes. Too often this dynamic is expressed as skepticism and cynicism.

Motivation. Perceptual alignment is the first critical step to successful change management; the second most important factor is motivation. An interesting relationship exists between perception and motivation. Remember, perception equals reality. All humans are 100 percent motivated 100 percent of the time. Motivation cannot be increased or decreased; however, it can be unleashed, directed, or suppressed. We view the world according to our experiences, which determine the direction of the motivation, which drives behavior. Motivation is directed toward those behaviors that are the most meaningful. Meaning is a function of how we view the world. Change management experts use multiple techniques to assess the ways perception affects motivation.

Braskamp and Maehr (1986) make a scholarly presentation on the importance of collecting baseline data about motivational influences. They posit that adult professionals choose to personally invest time and energy in those behaviors that are most consistent with their internal motivational influences. Braskamp and Maehr highlighted four key influences to motivation: recognition, accomplishment, power, and affiliation. In *Turning Healthcare Leadership Around* (Atchison 1990, 33–36), I define and describe these variables in the context of the healthcare industry.

- *Recognition*. Some workers crave attention. They continually seek feedback on the quality of their work from their bosses and colleagues. To be seen as high-producing winners is all-important to them. They enjoy seeing their names in print, winning awards, and receiving public recognition at special events. For these workers, the emphasis is on external reinforcement for good work through verbal and written plaudits, awards, perks, supplemental benefits, and merit and salary increases.
- *Accomplishment*. Some employees are in their offices by 7:30 and race through project after project. They are eager to get involved in new ventures in the hope of achieving ever greater things. Anchored to their desks, these workers rarely take time out for lunch or routine conversation. In their professional life they emphasize productivity, doing the job right, and exploring new opportunities.
- *Power*. Some staff members just want to win. They enjoy going head-to-head with the president of the medical staff, the chairperson of the city planning council, or anyone else. Instead of feeling intimidated by escalating competition from neighboring hospitals, they are exhilarated by it. Their professional life is driven by competition and conflict and the quest for power.
- *Affiliation*. Finally, some employees want to create a family feeling among their staff members. They invest at least one-third of their

day trying to build an atmosphere of trust and camaraderie among their employees. Birthdays, anniversaries, graduations, and births are celebrated with lunches and receptions. When an employee has a personal or family problem, they take time to talk it through with him and suggest solutions. Their professional life is driven by a desire to respect their employees and to treat them as part of the hospital family.

The relative importance of the two motivational influences of recognition and accomplishment determine whether a person or group is externally or internally motivated. When recognition dominates accomplishment, then the change methodology needs to focus on external rewards and use a more linear, management by objectives (MBO)-type approach. When accomplishment dominates recognition, the MBO-type approach will fail. Change management interventions with persons and groups who rate accomplishment highly are most successful when time is spent engaging the participants in the decision about goals and deadlines, with the ways to achieve these goals left up to the individuals. Linear and highly structured change methods frustrate high achievement individuals, and in fact can run counter to success. Likewise, unstructured interventions with no clear path or end-product rewards will frustrate those with high-recognition needs.

The relationship between power and affiliation determines the way individuals will behave in groups. When power has more motivational influence than affiliation, the individual or group will be characterized as competitive and prone to conflict. Individuals are motivated by the desire to win their position as much or more than to do what is best for the group. Change management interventions with individuals motivated by power can be very difficult. The challenge for the change leader is to try to use such individuals' energy and need to win to move forward. This challenge is further complicated if the power-motivated individual is influenced greatly by recognition. Typically, this motivational pattern performs better in a sales organization than in healthcare. They behave badly in team-oriented change management interventions.

Affiliation-influenced individuals or groups perform best in groups. The need to be with, around, and supported by others is their raison d'etre. Loyalty and caring for others are the most common descriptors of these individuals. Change management strategies must include a great deal of group process work. Their need to be assured and supported can be greater than the need to finish a task. Once again, this problem is further complicated if these individuals have a high need for external recognition. High-affiliation and high-recognition motivational patterns are very common in healthcare, especially in direct care providers. Interventions that are successful with high achievers who may also have high power needs (e.g., senior executives and physician leaders) will not work with those with high affiliation and recognition needs.

Data about motivation and perception should be gathered at the beginning of any structured change process. Because we all view the world through our own eyes and because our motivational influences are different, the only way to match interventions with human complexity is to know the degree of perceptual alignment and the main motivational influences. Too often health-care leaders attempt to manage change without any specific data about the individuals involved in the process. They may purchase an education-based intervention strategy. For example, to increase patient and other customer satisfaction scores, a healthcare leader may purchase a program that contains a series of training modules and expect everyone to attend these modules only to be confronted by unwilling participants. One-size-fits-all, externally driven solutions are not effective change management interventions. In fact, such solutions can erode the very behavior the organization is trying to achieve.

Carlson and Loveday both began their discussions about organizational alignment with data about the motivational influences of the persons re-sponsible for the desired change. The OMHS and Clarian data showed wide variation among the various leadership and management groups. Figures 15.4 and 15.5 show the personal incentive scales for representative groups from both systems.

Figures 15.4 and 15.5 demonstrate the wide variation among just a few of the subgroups in these two systems. Variation of this magnitude is commonplace in all healthcare organizations. Therefore, the belief that one intervention strategy (e.g., educational modules) will be sufficient to manage change is not logical.

The ability to measure the perceptual variation and relative motivational influences and compare responses to a national database is the foundation for all successful change management. The resultant data drive decisions about the most effective interventions for each group. Treatment without data-based diagnosis is malpractice. How many healthcare executives would run their organizations without very precise cost data on each department? How many executives would try to improve tangible business-focused operations without differential data and analysis of the effects of various strategies on the targeted goals? Yet how many executives try to alter the most complex aspect of healthcare systems, human behavior, without differential data on those motivational influences that underpin the behaviors targeted for change? This gross omission explains the high failure rate of most change management attempts. The lack of data-based decisions about change also explains the "magic bullet" dynamic. This is the belief that one program, consultant, speech, or technique will always work for all involved. Magical

Figure 15.4   Personal Incentive Scales for Employees of OMHS

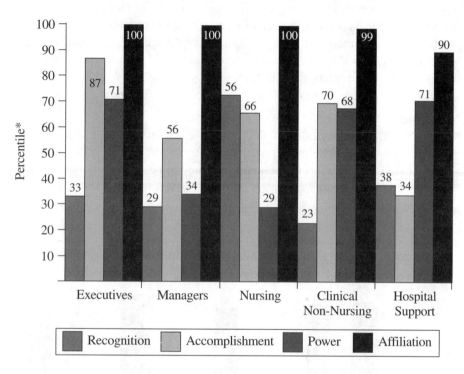

*Comparison based on national database of healthcare providers.

thinking needs to be replaced with precise data about human perception and motivation.

Ego Psychology

Cognitive and behavior theories give change managers powerful tools. To a lesser degree there is some use in understanding a little about ego psychology and need theory. The main issue around the construct of ego has to do with resistence to change. Neither egocentric nor narcissistic individuals respond well to managed change. Each type represents a degree of self-absorption. The egocentric personality displays a way of functioning characterized by an inability to assume the point of view of others. A very small number of personalities exist whose self-absorption achieve a pathological state that Erich Fromm (1964) called "malignant narcissism." These individuals are characterized by an "unsubmitted will." Change management leaders are all too often distracted by the "cynic" or "zealot." Behind these cynical and zealot behaviors is some degree of egocentrism or an unusual degree of self-absorption. These types cannot change; therefore, the change manager can only ignore them or suggest they get some help to better cope with those life experiences that they cannot recognize to be in their best interests. Unfortunately, sometimes these personality types are well positioned in the organization as medical staff leaders, nurse managers, union representatives, or, as I sadly discovered, the CEO.

Need Theory

No article on change management would be complete without some discussion of need theory. The most popular and discussed theory is described by Abraham Maslow (1970). He believes that human behavior is controlled to a large degree by a person's position on one of seven levels. The seven levels

Figure 15.5   Personal Incentive Scales for Employees of Clarian

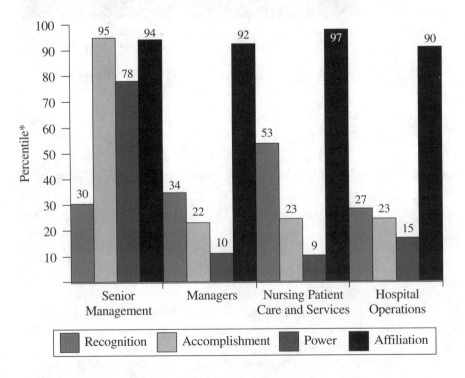

*Comparison based on national database of healthcare providers.

are hierarchical in the sense that higher-level needs will be attended to only after lower-level needs are satisfied. A common example is that if someone is hungry, they are not concerned with cognitive pursuits. Maslow's seven needs are:

1. Physiological (food and drink);
2. Safety (security and psychological safety);
3. Belongingness and love (affiliation, acceptance, and affection);
4. Self-esteem (competence, approval, and recognition);
5. Cognitive (knowledge and symmetry);
6. Aesthetic (goodness, beauty, truth, and justice); and
7. Self-actualization (focus on virtues and a harmonious life).

Maslow's theory informs those involved in change management planning of participants' main concerns. This fact becomes most important if an individual's behavioral pattern changes dramatically. Maslow's theory is helpful in explaining why an individual who historically has performed at levels five and six might perform at levels one, two, and three. For example, a series of atypical behaviors by a nurse executive recently became a concern to the senior executive. An investigation discovered that the nurse executive had been diagnosed with breast cancer (a condition that had taken her mother). Change management interventions that include this individual must incorporate some assistance to meet her current needs.

VARIABLES FOR SUCCESS

These theories are very useful in planning the baseline assessment and differential analyses of the data. The variables that determine whether a change management process will be successful are many. Three environmental factors present the difficulty in precise application of these theories: readiness to change, the ability to change, and the time required to change.

Readiness to Change

Readiness to change is determined to a large degree by motivational influences but also by personal history, degree of control, and perceived desirability. An individual or group that has experienced a number of failed change attempts will view new attempts with the predictable skepticism of "here we go again." The strength of the skepticism determines the degree to which change leaders must develop an improved readiness prior to implementation. One technique to improve readiness is an audit of past programs to assess where they were effective and what did not work. The information from the audit can be used to introduce the new program and minimize the negative effects of the skeptics. Healthcare executives who introduce new change interventions without some sense of the level of readiness will have mixed results at best. In the worst case, skeptics' resistance will be reinforced and make change even more difficult in the future.

Ability to Change

The ability of the individual to change also has a critical influence on the success of any change management process. An irrational but pervasive belief exists that all humans can change in any direction and display a limitless universe of new behaviors. Rarely discussed is the notion of limits to the human capacity to change. For example, the importance of intelligence is seldom included in planning. During a recent engagement, an enlightened healthcare executive stated (after a detailed analysis of the variation in effect of a one-size-fits-all change strategy) that "brains count." In a world of politically correct speech, discussing the fact that all humans have limits of intellectual potency may not be popular; however, to assume differently eliminates an important variable to success. Although measurement of the intellectual capacity of the participants of a change process is unnecessary, common sense must be used and change managers must accept that some participants will perform better because of higher intelligence. A skilled change leader creates interventions that maximize the benefits of intellectual capacity without expecting people to perform beyond their limits.

Timing of Change

A third important variable that influences success is timing. The time necessary to achieve significant change is a difficult variable to predict. In a healthcare world filled with stress and pressure, everything seems to be STAT. Unfortunately, the normal developmental change process cannot be compressed to accommodate the urgency of the moment. John Kotter (1995, 59) speaks to this point: "The most general lesson to be learned from the more successful cases is that the change process goes through a series of phases that, in total, usually require a considerable length of time. Skipping steps creates only the illusion of speed and never produces a satisfying result." The good thing about timing is that it is under the control of the change leader. Assume an institution wanted to change the way patients viewed the hospital. The change leader announces on Monday that their will be measurable change by Friday. Another change leader announces that measurable change is expected in six months. The constant in both cases is the goal of measurable change. The variable is the time given to achieve the goal. Successful change managers understand the developmental nature of change management and set timing parameters that stretch the participants without creating unrealistic and frustrating expectations.

Readiness, capacity, and timing at have the greatest effect on success. A simple model that incorporates these three helps in deciding the best interventions and timing. Change is easy and even enthusiastically pursued when the person involved wants the change and controls the process. Change is resisted to the degree that the participant does not want the change and feels that they had no control over the process. Figure 15.6 shows a continuum of ease of change.

The closer we can get the expectations for change to the left of the continuum, the easier the change management process will be. If the change leader crosses the midpoint to the right, resistance and failure are the likely outcomes. Additional factors that affect the probability of a successful change management process are summarized in Figure 15.7.

Figure 15.6   The Continum of Ease of Change

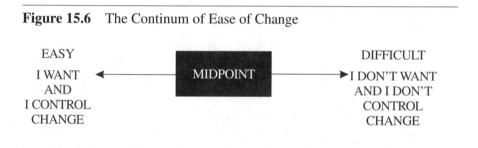

Figure 15.7   Factors that Affect the Possibility that Change Will Be Successful and Prescriptions for Success

DOMAIN	DIAGNOSIS	INTERVENTION
Knowledge	Academic credentials/tests	Education
Skill	Competencies	Training
Attitude	Climate/opinion survey	Recognition practices
Motivation	Culture Assessment	Organizational development
Values	Culture assessment	Organizational development
Capacity	Interview/work performance	Selection
Personality	Personality tests/Myer–Briggs	Therapy/drugs

Many times, the decision to employ and promote is determined by the first two or three domains shown in Figure 15.7. However, the ability to align with vision, strategies, and tactics is much more a function of levels three through seven. A healthcare executive recently said that she believes that all employment decisions are based 90 percent on the tangibles and the firing decisions are based 90 percent on the intangibles. Our focus on the easy-to-measure produces many false hopes and wasted resources.

A great number of change management interventions focus on educational interventions. Such interventions are easy to procure and the amount of time participants are involved with an educational module can be measured easily. The major weakness of this approach as a primary intervention strategy is potent: no relationship exists between knowing something and doing something. Cognitive awareness, or knowledge, is a necessary prerequisite but insufficient condition for behavioral change. A bridge must be built between knowledge and behavior, and the process of building this bridge is called organizational development.

Organizational Development

Organizational development (OD) differs from educational interventions in several fundamental ways. W. Walter Burke (1992, 1) states that, " . . . the practice of OD is more of a process than a step-by-step procedure. That is, OD is a consideration in general of how work is done, what the people who carry out the work believe and feel about their efficiency and effectiveness, rather that a specific, concrete step-by-step procedure for accomplishing something." Peter Senge's breakthrough work *The Fifth Discipline* (1990) supports the use of OD techniques in his powerful concepts about "systematic thinking"and the "learning organization." Unfortunately, some healthcare managers seem to need to oversimplify. When they think of learning in an organization, they think of teaching something in a didactic fashion to a selected group targeted for change. If you ask these managers if they have a learning organization, they will tell you how much they budget for education and training.

Figure 15.7 shows the complexity of change. The most effective change managers have some data and possible interventions for each domain that affects change. However, levels six and seven usually are out of the range of interventions for most leaders of change. The issue of capacity can only be "changed" by placing a person with greater capacity into the role; the issue of personality dysfunction needs to handled with compassion but firmly. Healthcare leaders have a lot of tolerance for low and even dysfunctional behavior. Data-driven change management that uses the appropriate interventions for the desired results always includes approaches to deal with those behaviors that will never respond positively. A wide variety of approaches including changing the individual's job to fit their capacity, employee assistance programs (EAPs), or other therapeutic intervention or separation from the institution can be implemented.

Effective change management incorporates baseline data targeting specific areas for improvement, identifies the most appropriate interventions for the capacity and motivation of the participants, and reassesses the action to determine progress and target the next interventions. Steve Wantz, the OD director for Clarian, is excellent at change management operations. Wantz and a group of high-performing leaders analyzed the Clarian data collected from the initial cultural assessment. Their work resulted in a priority list of 13 behaviors that were deemed to be essential to the evolving culture of the newly merged Clarian Health Partners (see Table 15.2). Wantz created this grid as a blueprint to manage those changes that would have the greatest effect on the development of the new culture, that is, the conversion of values language to behaviors.

Table 15.2 is a good prototype for any change leader. It contains the targeted behaviors, baseline data on each behavior, the desired level to be achieved at the reassessment, and specific interventions that will be used to alter the behaviors. After executive management endorsement, Wantz's group took this "blueprint" to the managers and discussed accountability for action, financial and nonfinancial support systems, and milestones for periodic measurement. This grid served for culturally based change management in the same way that a budget would serve for financial performance. All change processes need a data-based decision tool that drives accountability to action. The other critical element in success is the role Wantz continues to play: the internal champion of the plan.

Kotter (1995) discusses the role of the "guiding coalition." He believes that " . . . in most successful cases (of cultural transformation), the guiding coalition is always pretty powerful—in terms of titles, information and expertise, reputation, and relationships. In both small and large companies, a successful guiding coalition may consist of only three to five people during the first year of a renewal effort. But in big companies, the coalition needs to grow to the 20 to 50 range before much progress can be made" (62). The importance of Kotter's notion of the guiding coalition is unquestionable; however, I believe that the key to the guiding coalition's long-term effectiveness, and to the ultimate success of the change management process, is an internal champion.

In OMHS and Clarian Health Partners and any other healthcare systems with successful change management processes, four immutable components

Table 15.2 Behaviors and Intervention Plan for Culture of Clarian Health Partners (1998–1999)

	Baseline Results (%)	Desired Results (%)	Interventions to Be Used						
			Service Plan	Selection	Diversity	Attitude Survey	Staff and Leadership Development	Communication	Recognition
1. Around here we are encouraged to try new things.	76	94		X	X		X		X
2. Every person at Clarian can invent, create, promote, and solve problems.	48	87		X	X		X		X
3. Employees here receive a lot of attention.	55	83	X			X	X	X	X
4. At Clarian, we hear more about what people do right than the mistakes they make.	28	82	X				X		X
5. Evaluations of my work are tied to how well I do.	49	87	X			X			X
6. I regularly receive information about the quality of my work.	34	66	X					X	X
7. At Clarian, there is respect for each individual worker.	39	85	X		X		X		X
8. Communication at Clarian is very informal and frequent.	43	86						X	
9. People at all levels at Clarian share information about how well we are doing.	40	85					X	X	
10. Clarian cares about me as a person.	31	83	X		X		X		X
11. Everyone at Clarian knows what it stands for.	49	87	X	X			X	X	X
12. Almost everyone has similar values and ideas about what Clarian should be doing.	20	80	X	X					X
13. Everyone at Clarian knows what we value most.	15	79	X	X			X	X	X

Figure 15.8 Essential Components to Manage Change and Strengthen Organizational Culture

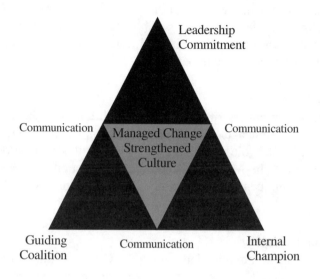

can be observed: (1) CEO leadership; (2) an internal champion; (3) a guiding coalition; and (4) a communication strategy. Figure 15.8 shows the interdependency of these elements.

CEO Leadership

The role of the CEO cannot be overstated. Without continued, visible, genuine, and enthusiastic support, any change process will be weak, fail to work, or in fact create behaviors contraindicative of the professed goals of the change effort. Greg Carlson at OMHS and William Loveday at Clarian are ideal examples for the role of the CEO. Both set the tone for the change process and committed the appropriate personal and institutional resources to its success. Their commitment to the process is impossible to question except by the most cynical observers.

Internal Champion

Carlson and Loveday both identified an internal champion for the process. Sister Jeanette Haas at OMHS is the senior vice president of mission effectiveness and Steve Wantz is the director of organizational development at Clarian Health Partners. Internal champions typically hold positions in mission services, human resources, or organizational development. The CEO cannot be the internal champion. The role of the internal champion is to handle the day-to-day details and work with the guiding coalition to stay on target for periodic measurable achievements. The internal champion needs to be a formal as well as an informal, disciplined leader with a vast array of skills such as facilitation, negotiation, persuasion, and attention to detail.

Guiding Coalition

The role of the members of the guiding coalition is to be the internal consultants for the change process. The selection of these individuals is critical; they must be role models for the behavior that is most desired for the organization. "The Myths of Employee Satisfaction" (Atchison 1999) explains one technique for the selection of the best members for the guiding coalition.

Communication Strategy

The quality of the communication among the CEO, the internal champion, and the guiding coalition holds the change management process together. The three corners of this triangle must design a communication plan that includes performance accountabilities and measurement goals. Too often change management processes break down because of complacency and lack of a disciplined feedback loop characterized by measured achievement and difficulties. The champion manages the frequency and agendas for ongoing, productive communication. Sister Jeanette Haas in OMHS discovered that in the early phases, very frequent—at least weekly—meetings with the guiding coalition and Greg Carlson were needed. In the early phases the CEO must not let the importance of the process be lessened or contaminated. The best way for the CEO to ensure that their leadership in the change process is not weakened is to constantly focus on the organization's vision statement.

Vision Statement

The vision statement answers the question: Where is this organization going and how do we know we have arrived? Visions drive strategy, which leads to tactical (departmental) plans, and, most importantly, tactics define individual performance. Without a clear vision that underpins all decisions, individuals are left with little choice but to repeat previously successful behaviors until someone tells them otherwise. Organizations without visions default to "retrovisioning" and become consumed with what happened yesterday. Because they do not have a picture of where they want to go, they obsess about where they have been and the embedded problems with the way things are done. Their change motif is reaction. CEOs of organizations without a meaningful vision are viewed without trust or respect because unpredictable and many times autocratic impulses are presented as managed change processes. Without a vision to provide the context for change, no progress will be made. In the managed change process the CEO must be the standard bearer for the vision. The criteria and construction of an effective vision is beyond the scope of this article, but I advise readers to ensure that their corporate vision is the most effective one possible to support a managed change process (for assistance on vision statements, see Senge 1990 and Atchison 1990). The internal champion and the guiding coalition communicate with the CEO to ensure that the vision is converted to measurable achievements. This means creating a behavior list or catalog of appropriate behaviors.

The appropriate behavior list is derived from two content areas. An organization's vision advises those behaviors that relate to forward movement. Corporate values advise those behaviors that relate to day-to-day performance. The best, and easiest, way to begin to create a catalog of the behaviors that are the manifestation of the organization's culture is trait analysis combined with gap and force-field analysis.

First, the guiding coalition identifies persons inside or outside of the healthcare system who live the values and seem forward thinking. Once the group of individuals is complete, the internal champion facilitates a discussion of the specific traits each person displayed to be included. The list if traits is analyzed according to two standards: (1) which traits represent which value or vision element; and (2) which of the traits is the most behaviorally specific. The criteria for behavioral specificity is the ability to be measured and observed. Too often words like courtesy, respect, and empathy are used in the belief that they really describe something. Change management programs must have a list of specific, observable, and measurable traits to procede to the next phase of gap analysis.

The technique of gap analysis, used quite frequently in budget variance analysis, works when moving from undesirable behaviors to desirable behaviors. Gap analysis simply says, "Here is where we are, and here is where we want to be—how do we bridge the gap?" The technique of force-field analysis helps manage change by determining the existing drivers (to move forward) and the restrainers (to maintain the status quo). These two techniques can be used in concert or independently. The degree of specificity of the current and desired behaviors determines each technique's success. The final critical success factor to a successful change management process is how the leaders recognize positive change.

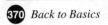

Recognition

The earlier discussion of recognition was in the context of how much internal or external recognition is needed for an individual or a group. Recognition of positive change needs to incorporate personal needs but also must consider the other benefits of recognition. New behaviors require very frequent feedback to replace older behaviors that happen automatically. A simple exercise will demonstrate the fragile nature of new or different behaviors. Pick up a pen/pencil with your nondominant hand and write your name. Now place the writing utensil in your dominant hand and close your eyes and write your name. It is easier to write with your eyes closed with the hand you use all the time. To change this very simple behavior (writing your name) takes a great deal of concentration. You must cognitively override what is easy—subcortical—in your dominant hand. This exercise shows the need for practice and feedback/recognition when attempting something new. In fact, the next time you want someone to change quickly, pick up your pen with your nondominant hand and write the ten reasons why they should change quickly. The guiding principle for the use of feedback and recognition during a change process is that it is very hard to over-recognize but very easy to under-recognize more desirable behaviors.

SUMMARY

The complexity of change management involves the entire sphere of human frailties and potential. More rigor and discipline in data collection and analysis of the many intangibles that affect success are necessary. The role of the CEO cannot be understated. Compelling evidence exists that internal champions and guiding coalitions are necessary to sustain the change process over time. The quality of any of change management process is a function of the degree of specificity and the number of behaviors that define the organization's vision and values.

Change management, when done correctly, results in a committed, proud, and joyful workforce. Anyone can obsess over yesterday's problems and spend time on the easy-to-measure, tangible (financial) elements of the organization. However, it takes courage and discipline to challenge the future and create a work environment that unleashes staff motivation and maximizes the potential of each employee for the benefit of the patients and other customer groups.

REFERENCES

Atchison Consulting Group. 1986. *Healthcare Organizational Assessment.* Champaign, IL: Ameritech.

Atchison, T. A. 1996. "What is Corporate Culture." *Trustee* 49 (Jan): 28.

Atchison, T. A. 1990. *Turning Healthcare Leadership Around: Cultivating Inspired, Empowered, and Loyal Followers.* San Francisco: Jossey-Bass.

Atchison, T. A. 1999. "The Myths of Employee Satisfaction." *Healthcare Executive* 14 (2): 20–21.

Braskamp, L. A., and Maehr, M. M. 1982. *The Motivation Factor: A Theory of Personal Investment.* Lexington, MA: Heath.

Burke, W. W. 1992. *Organization Development: A Process of Learning and Changing,* 2nd ed. Reading, MA: Addison-Wesley.

Clarian Health Partners. 1999. Board Policy Statement.

Deal, T. and Kennedy, A. 1982. *Corporate Cultures.* Reading, MA: Addison-Wesley.

"Ford Rolls Out New Model of Corporate Culture." 1999. *Wall Street Journal* 13 January.

Fromm, E. 1964. *The Heart of Man: Its Genius for Good and Evil.* New York: Harper & Row.

Kotter, J. P. 1995. "Leading Change: Why Transformation Efforts Fail." Harvard Business Review (Mar/Apr).

Kotter, J. P. and Heskett, J. L. 1992. *Corporate Culture and Performance.* New York: The Free Press.

Maslow, A. 1970. *Motivation and Personality,* 2nd ed. New York: Harper & Row.

"Remaking Microsoft." 1999. *Business Week.* 17 May.

Schein, E. H. 1997. *Organizational Culture and Leadership,* 2nd ed. San Francisco: Jossey-Bass.

Schein, E. H. 1995. *Organizational Culture and Leadership: A Dynamic View.* San Francisco: Jossey-Bass.

Senge, P.M. 1990. *The Fifth Discipline: The Art and Practice of The Learning Organization.* New York: Doubleday/Currency.

Thompson, K. R., and Luthans, F. 1990. "Organizational Culture: A Behavioral Perspective." In *Organizational Climate and Culture,* edited by Benjamin Schneider, 319–344. San Francisco: Jossey-Bass.

Working Together

Carson F. Dye, FACHE

COHESIVENESS AND COLLABORATION

Many leadership teams in healthcare strive to capture the "entrepreneurial spirit" that teams in successful businesses possess. The entrepreneurial spirit—or cohesiveness—is a mindset that congeals teams and cheers them on through conception, development, and marketing of new products and services. Unfortunately, this spirit is impermanent and permeable by old-fashioned jealousy and selfish tendencies. When a business expands its operation, it naturally adds new members to its existing team, which is a logical progression but potentially destructive to the cohesiveness of the team. What subsequently occurs between the original members and the newcomers are quarrels over decisions, dissension over leadership issues, and decreased support for the common goal. In essence, although cohesiveness increases productivity, morale, and camaraderie, it does not prevent schism from occurring. Leadership teams, then, should strive to capture not only this spirit but the intricacies of maintaining it.

Collaboration pulls together divided parties to work toward a mutually accepted goal. It transcends traditional compromise in that no exchange of services is necessary to achieve the preferred outcomes of both parties; it only demands equal input and dedication to the cause. Most importantly, collaboration often results in conflict resolution. Conflicting parties typically react by adopting one of the following approaches:

Editors Note: This chapter combines the chapters "Cohesiveness and Collaboration" and "Conflict Management" from the book *Leadership in Healthcare* by Carson F. Dye, 2000, HAP. Other key team values identified by this author are "cooperation and sharing" and "trust."

- Avoid the conflict altogether
- Give in or accommodate the other party
- Compete—drive toward the classic win/lose scenario
- Compromise or strike a deal that gives something to both parties
- Collaborate—drive toward a win/win scenario

Consider the last three approaches. Competition is never an appropriate response because it amplifies the damage and makes it irreversible. Historically, compromise has been recommended, but it leaves both parties only partially satisfied. In compromise, both parties tend to "save" favors, supposedly owed to them, so that they can "cash in" during future conflicts. Note that if neither party anticipates future dealings with one another, then a compromise is usually a better approach than collaboration. Conversely, if the parties continue their relationship and expect further dispute, then collaboration is the only responsible solution. This is the case with senior leadership teams. Cohesiveness begets collaboration and collaboration begets cohesiveness. Although one can exist without the other, one cannot be as effective without the other.

As illustrated by the entrepreneurial-spirit analogy, team cohesiveness has its downsides, including:

1. *Low performance norms.* Performance norms are expected of each member of the team. These norms dictate the quality and quantity of work—how vigorous, how effective, how productive, what goals were achieved, and what contributions were tendered. Because these norms are usually unwritten and solely enforced by the team members, they tend to get overlooked when the team is highly cohesive and cooperative. As a result, the performance norms lower and productivity decreases. Why the contradiction? The reason is twofold: in cohesive teams, (1) highly competent members pick up the slack for members who have less-than-par abilities; therefore, those who need skill enhancement are pardoned and often disregarded; and (2) competent members have become complacent and too polite to subject poor performers to constructive criticisms.

2. *Proliferation of "groupthink."* Groupthink occurs when team members become so enveloped in unanimous thinking that they lose their individual objectivity. As a result, new and creative thoughts are blocked off, objections are stifled, and concurrence becomes the standard. Instead of pursuing the goals of the organization as a whole, keeping the solidarity of the team becomes the team's main purpose. Figure 16.1 lists symptoms of groupthink.

3. *Low tolerance for new members.* Teams that are peopled by "founding members" who abide by tradition and are comfortable with its identity and its mission do not kindly welcome change—particularly in

membership. New members are often viewed as disruptive outsiders and detrimental to the cohesiveness.

4. *Team goals that take precedence over organizational goals.* A highly cohesive leadership teams is fanatical about the welfare of its members. Some teams have been known to reduce clinical and support staff and still maintain excessive administrative support staff. Some organizations still pay executive bonuses even during difficult financial years.

Operationalize the Concept

As we have established, cohesiveness is an important key to collaboration, but its disadvantages must be seriously considered because they sometimes outweigh the advantages. The following are methods that will help you build a cohesive team without building disadvantages.

Minimize selfish behavior. Selfishness is a contagious disease. To prevent it from spreading, you must disinfect yourself first. Demonstrate that you are working on behalf of others' interests, not just on your own. If your

---

Figure 16.1 Symptoms of Groupthink

Groupthink is:

- *An illusion of invulnerability,* which leads to unwarranted optimism and excessive risk taking by the group.
- *Unquestioned assumption of the group's morality* and, therefore, an absence of reflection on the ethical consequences of group action.
- *Collective rationalization* to discount negative information or warnings.
- *Stereotypes of the opposition* as evil, weak, or stupid.
- *Self-censorship* by group members from expressing ideas that deviate from the group consensus due to doubts about their validity or importance.
- *An illusion of unanimity* such that greater consensus is perceived than really exists.
- *Direct pressure on dissenting members,* which reinforces the norm that disagreement represents disloyalty to the group.
- *Mind guards* who protect the group from adverse information.

Source: Reprinted from *Leadership: Enhancing the Lesson of Experience, Third Edition* by Richard L. Hughes, Robert C. Ginnett, and Gordon J. Curphy. 1999. Originally adapted from *Groupthink* by Irving L. Janis, 1982. New York: Irwin/McGraw-Hill.

team members suspect that you are using them or their people, cohesiveness will decline. CEOs and team leaders are responsible for confronting members who display selfish motives and do not contribute to the well-being of the team. Appropriate team behavior must be verbally addressed, possibly at a retreat, and must be written.

Decrease the size of the team. The acquisitions of new service lines and corporate entities of many healthcare systems have greatly widened the reach of leadership teams and expanded their size. This growth has split the focus of the team—some members attend to external functions, while some concentrate on internal operations. As a result, the commonality that used to be so ubiquitous has been replaced by conflict of interest, as the following sentiments from CEOs attest. "We have had more turf battles and less cooperation since our executive council has grown in size and we have picked up additional business lines," admits one CEO. Another stated, "As I saw our senior team grow from 11 members to 18, I saw us lose our camaraderie and team spirit."

Although decreasing team size is difficult because it affects the status—and egos—of existing members, it must be done to preserve cohesiveness. One approach is to divide operations and strategy executives into two teams. Another approach is to hold the meetings of the larger team less frequently, and convene a smaller team more frequently. Some teams seize the opportunity to rebuild or resize when executive turnover occurs; this way, no egos will be harmed and no status is affected.

Dedicate time to get to know one another. Spending time does not imply holding longer meetings to "share" because that can be very counterproductive. What I do suggest is much more fun: socialize with your members! Seize every opportunity presented to you including work parties, lunch periods, before or after meetings, or celebratory gatherings. These interactions not only create a personal bond between you and them, it also communicates a much powerful message: you are interested in them not only as a co-worker but as a person. Consider the following examples practiced by some successful CEOs. One CEO takes her senior team off-location every fourth Friday for a morning "retreat." They cover business during the morning meeting, adjourn for lunch at 11:30, then spend the afternoon just talking about nonwork-related matters. Another CEO takes her team to a local country club the day after their monthly board meetings to enjoy each other's company and catch up. Yet another CEO holds a weekly lunch session that includes no formal agenda but allows informal and often nonwork interactions among the group.

Minimize the influence of cliques. Unfortunately, cliques are not confined to junior high school and they are prevalent in all organizations. The larger the organization, the larger the teams, and the larger the problem of cliques. Cliques are detrimental to any team because they represent dissent and selfishness. Because being in a clique can signal disagreement with the team as a whole, clique members may tend to be less cooperative, more ambitious, and more manipulative. Clique members can influence the team's decisions—whether negatively or positively—because they have solidarity, which is thatched together by each member's personal designs.

The impact of cliques can be minimized several ways:

1. Occasionally recognize the cliques' existence during team meetings, as one CEO does each time: "Well, I know that the operations people (or other identified subteam) have already come to a conclusion on this matter," he begins, "so can we hear from you a synopsis of the discussions that took place before our meeting today?" By making them publicly known, the cliques realize that the team is aware and will not cower to their caprice.

2. Directly confront them privately. The CEO, the team leader, or even peers can address the difficulty that cliques can create, the negativity that they can engender, and the anonymity that they can spread. This confrontational method clearly communicates to cliques that their intentions will not be tolerated.

3. Assign conflicting members to the same task forces wherein they can work toward the same goal. The purpose here is to improve relations and spread out the expertise and knowledge that members withhold only for her/his own clique.

4. Discuss the existence of cliques with the whole team and how this can harm team performance. This is often best done under the expert guidance of a facilitator.

Ensure that the team understands why they exist. All team members must be on the same vehicle that will take them forward. Frequently clarify your goals, your purpose, and expectations. Discuss them with the team and make changes, if necessary. Strive for 100 percent commitment and support by making everyone on the team part of the development of the goals. Nothing inspires cohesiveness more than personal involvement.

Ensure that all team members are equal. Imbalance of power produces divisiveness, which is the mother of cliques. This phenomenon is often caused by the actions of the CEO or team leader. The CEO or team leader must treat all members equally before, during, and after team meetings, inside or outside the meeting room. Personal relationships must be managed to avoid creating the perception—real or imagined—that different levels of influence exist.

Discuss and assign roles to each team member. A specific role in a leadership team heightens the sense of belonging and importance of any member. Roles include being a team spirit leader, devil's advocate, team conscience, team historian, "mom," "dad," or meeting room organizer. Although seemingly simplistic, these roles give the assigned member a reason for attending and actively participating. Some teams use team-building sessions to discuss roles that can be assigned.

Consider a heavier emphasis on team compensation. If the compensation structure of an organization is designed to recognize and reward individual performance, then team behavior will receive less attention. As a result, team members will think and act more selfishly because they are only compensated for their individual merits. While the purview of this chapter is not compensation, attention must be given to the fact that it affects team cohesiveness, hence its effectiveness.

Manage team meetings to ensure equality of interaction. The golden rules of meetings are (1) dedicate ample time for discussion of key issues and (2) dedicate ample time for every team member to provide input. Many examples of these principles exist, including the following. To prevent turf battles, one CEO required his team to wear a generalist operations hat during debate on organizational issues. To get members involved, one CEO calls on team members who have not spoken or taken an active role in discussions, while another assigns members a specific point of view—either devil's advocate or proponent—to take during a debate. To elicit a wider response, some CEOs use Nominal Group Technique (NGT) or other team discussion tools.

Rally the team against an outside threat. Competition, acquisition, and downsizing are only three of the real-world pressures that organizations today face. Many CEOs have used these as outside threats to unite senior and middle management teams and medical staffs, to gain support, and to stretch and strengthen the muscles of cohesiveness and collaboration. A note of caution is appropriate here: too much attention spent watching the activities of a competitor can cause an organization to lose focus on its own core competencies.

Without cohesiveness and collaboration, the greatest victories in sports, the classic symphonies, the most successful peace pacts would never have existed. A healthcare leadership team that lacks these values cannot fulfill its many potentials nor be beneficial to itself, its organization, and its community.

CONFLICT MANAGEMENT

Conflict is the natural byproduct of human complexity and interaction. It is present everywhere, even in seemingly uncomplicated tasks such as deciding what to order at a restaurant. The magnitude and acceleration of a conflict are always dependent on the number of people involved, which is why teams are a breeding ground for volatile disagreements. Complex systems beget complex hierarchical structures beget complex conflicts. As we have discussed, the days of autocratic leadership are dwindling and are being succeeded by team-driven governance. Leaders progress in today's environment by becoming engineers of consent—opening up to others' suggestions and steering them to concur on a common goal—and managing the discord that may potentially arise.

Unfortunately, however, many CEOs continue to stifle conflict, fail to discuss and confront its genesis, and have not established a conflict-management guideline for the entire team. The reasons—or excuses—are varied: some CEOs see conflict as a disease that can destroy the cohesiveness of the team and impede its growth; some are too busy to engage in confrontation and resolution; some simply are afraid to grapple with a subject so menacing; and others are so confident in their abilities to handle a conflict that they handle it only on an as-it-happens basis, rather than establish a preventive plan of action.

The biggest irony is that team conflict is good because it:

- *Ends complacency.* Conflict turns members from being too satisfied with everything to being concerned about everything. Members start to question ingrained, inefficient processes, traditions, and decisions.
- *Initiates discussion.* Although discussion is scarce at the beginning of a conflict as parties strategize, it soon ignites as conflict deepens.
- *Steers action.* Whether or not the subsequent action is beneficial or feasible, conflict inspires action.
- *Demands participation.* Members who are otherwise inactive and silent become involved when conflicts exist because they tend to choose sides that best represent their views.

Although conflicts are inevitable, they are manageable. Teams who do not manage their conflicts are doomed to quick disintegration.

Operationalize the Concept

Assume that you, as a leader or team member, are already convinced that conflict is a necessary evil, the next step you must learn is how to acknowledge and manage it if you cannot completely avoid it.

Discuss and adopt conflict-management guidelines. The first step toward conflict management is acknowledging that conflict inevitably occurs when intelligent, opinionated people converge. The second step is developing

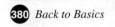

rules so if a conflict does occur, all members can debate, deliberate, and compromise accordingly. These guides should be reviewed regularly by all members of the team and new members must be informed of its existence. Figure 16.2 is an example of a conflict-management guideline.

Develop a common approach. Minimize conflict by discussing, and possibly adopting, a working style that can benefit all. For example, if the

---

Figure 16.2   Conflict Management Guideline

1. *Declare the conflict*. Not all discussions during group interaction are conflict-oriented. When a struggle ensues, however, someone must inform everyone that a conflict has arisen so that proper procedures can be followed. Although this may sound trite, it can become a powerful tool for managing conflict appropriately.

2. *Give reason for the conflict*. Although disagreements and arguments are normal and necessary, they cannot be initiated out of caprice or malice. Strife, hostility, and animosity must still be avoided at all cost, but if they do surface the reason(s) must be stated.

3. *Clarify the issues of conflict*. A neutral group member or one who is not directly embroiled in the conflict must be elected to clarify contentions and interpret ambiguities. All members must actively participate in the dispute and specify in detail their issues. Although members are entitled to express their concerns based on their emotional ties, facts must govern the debate, not opinions.

4. *Address one conflict at a time*. To ensure appropriate and thoughtful consideration of all issues, only one issue at a time will be considered. Although many people tend to save their issues and raise them all during debates, it will not be allowed or tolerated. All members should address their concerns as they occur.

5. *All members must participate*. No party in the dispute will be allowed to "pull in their heads" during the conflict. All must give their opinion and not cower behind their given parties.

6. *Be fair*. Members must keep their weapons appropriate to the level of the fight. In other words, a member cannot keep attacking without giving the other a chance to retort and defend.

7. *Declare that the conflict is over*. All members must know that the debate has ended and an outcome has been reached. The outcome agreement should be specifically defined so that no confusion, which could escalate into another conflict, arise later.

team's size makes quick, thoughtful decision making impossible, divide the team into several subteams or have every member volunteer for them. The subteams can be assigned a specific agenda for which its members are accountable.

Be careful with *directspeak* technique. *Directspeak* is the straightforward manner of communication without being insensitive. *Directspeak* does not work everywhere, but it thrives in team settings in which trust prevails because every member of these teams knows that confrontations are never meant to be personal attacks. CEOs or team leaders must be aware that some team members are uncomfortable with this technique, toe the line to avoid offending others, and are not active participants in debates. Conversely, some members are strong-willed and more verbal, which may intimidate the mild-spoken members. What results is another conflict: a personality conflict. One way to minimize personality conflict is to emphasize the greater good of the team or to focus on the goals during debate. When certain debates among his senior team become too fierce, one CEO jots down the goals of the debate on a flip chart to help the team focus on the issue and not on attacks.

Strengthen the team dynamic. One of the fundamental ways to build a stronger team is to revamp the compensation system. Team-based compensation maximizes the willingness of members to serve and stay because if team members were paid according to what they accomplish for the team, then they are more likely to believe in and work harder toward the goal. Another way to reinforce teams is by creating a culture in which members are accountable for the results of each decision and responsible for reaching the team's objective. Often the only way that this team culture or attitude can be created is when the CEO or team leader, who has the most power within the team, enforces it.

Teach and reiterate conflict-management approaches. The five approaches to conflict are avoidance, collaboration, compromise, accommodation, and competition. These approaches are typical in that they illustrate the sink-or-swim mindset of many teams.

Unfortunately, avoidance is always one of the first approaches, but it is valid only when the conflict is too minor to merit full-time consideration. When major conflicts are sidestepped, they will absolutely escalate in intensity and meaning. Although collaboration lasts longer and builds strong relationships among parties involved, it is seldom a practical response. The reason for this is that trust cannot be earned quickly so breaking down barriers and ambiguities is time consuming and does not fit the quick-solution pattern. Compromise is the most democratic and most satisfying approach because it works for both parties, but it is also the most overused. It also stalls decision making because too much consideration and not enough action are taken to satisfy everyone's demands. Accommodation is the most temporary and dangerous approach because it is based on giving and receiving favors. When members start "accommodating" or giving in to the demands of others, they do it not because of some heartfelt belief in the other member's causes but because they expect the favor back. This trading perpetuates distrust, bureaucracies, and fear. Competition, which is sometimes called "forcing," is the classic win/lose approach. The win column refers to some arguments won and the lose column refers to everything else. Competition serves only to create an environment in which members posture for authority and influence and misuse team meetings as personal battlefields. Perhaps the only time this approach is appropriate is when tough decisions have to be made and competing against each other will yield a faster, possibly more efficient result.

Identify and eliminate the antecedents of conflict. As does everything in the universe, conflict has a beginning and an end. And as with many things in the universe, the beginning and the end are controllable. The ideal end of conflict is a solution that not only suits everyone but is lasting. The ideal beginning is insight to know what will work and what will not. In the book, *Organizational Behavior,* authors Robert Kreitner and Angelo Kinicki (1998) list the following warning signs:

- Incompatible personalities or values systems
- Overlapping or unclear job boundaries
- Competition for limited resources
- Inadequate communication
- Interdependent tasks (e.g., one person cannot complete his or her assignment until others have competed their work)
- Organizational complexity (i.e., conflict tends to increase as the number of hierarchical layers and specialized tasks increase)
- Unreasonable or unclear policies, standards, or rules
- Unreasonable deadlines or extreme time pressure
- Collective decision making (i.e., the greater the number of people participating in a decision, the greater the potential for conflict)
- Decision making by consensus
- Unmet expectations (i.e., employees who have unrealistic expectations about job assignments, pay, or promotions are more prone to conflict)
- Unresolved or suppressed conflicts

As healthcare systems continue to become more intricate and as quick decision making becomes the norm, conflict can only keep pace and become as complex, or even more so. Although conflict can exist alone, it thrives within teams. To a strong team, it is a temporary foe but a permanent ally. To a weak team, it is a predator. What role does conflict play on your team?

17

Managing Your Career in the Era of Uncertainty

J. Larry Tyler, FACHE

O ne of the best attributes of the healthcare field for the past 30 years was that it was predictable, and because of this, one was able to make long-term plans—especially career plans. Career planning was helped by an abundance of mentors and an ever-expanding set of opportunities for hospital administrators. Even the marginally competent could find work. Career planning was enhanced even more because the government, through the Medicare program's cost-based reimbursement, paid us even when we made a mistake. You had to foul up pretty badly under these circumstances to be fired.

The role of a hospital administrator was a pretty comfortable one: the field was literally and figuratively a gentleman's profession. You came into the field as an assistant administrator with a few departments, and after a few years you would be promoted to Vice President of Support Services, then Vice President of Professional Services, then Senior Vice President, then COO, and finally CEO. From there, one could move into a larger facility or perhaps to a multihospital system in either a corporate or a regional setting. Wednesday afternoon was spent playing golf with doctors or board members, and there was plenty of time to be involved in association work or to travel to educational conferences. When retirement finally came, there would be a big to-do, a gold watch, a testimonial dinner, and perhaps some compensated consulting to help fill the time. It was a nice life and held wonderful satisfaction for anyone entering the field.

Editor's Note: This chapter is from Chapter 18 of *Tyler's Guide* by J. Larry Tyler, 1998, HAP

Then, in the 1980s, all of this began to change. Society became disenchanted with the continual increases in the cost of healthcare. Expenditures were far outpacing the rate of inflation and consuming an ever-increasing portion of the gross national product. As Americans matured and retired, Medicare expenditures started to consume so much of the nation's budget that deficits ballooned and other programs vital to our nation had to be cut back. General Motors complained that healthcare costs were more than the cost of steel in the automobiles sold to the American public. Clearly, something had to change. Society no longer would tolerate the most expensive healthcare money could buy.

HELLO, MANAGED CARE!

By the mid-1980s, managed care began to expand from its traditional roots as business tried to control its healthcare costs. The government accommodated the shift to managed care by changing the reimbursement system to one based on paying a set amount for an illness, regardless of the cost. Hospitals reacted first by shifting the costs to the other payors. The natural result was for the affected corporations to adopt managed care programs that shifted healthcare to the least costly providers, which caused providers to organize themselves into larger entities to have clout in the marketplace and in the delivery of services. A second strategy was to downsize the organization, flattening layers of management and outsourcing major departments. All of this meant accelerated change in the healthcare field. Hospitals no longer can execute five- and ten-year plans; the best they can hope for is that assumptions are still valid after three years. Healthcare organizations can now neither rely on their traditional allies nor shy away from doing business with their traditional competitors. Hospital administrators can no longer view themselves as "brick and mortar" people. They must now concern themselves with contractual arrangements, joint ventures, networks, and a host of systems such as PHOs, MSOs, PSOs, HMOs, and whatever the latest system may be.

All of this has had a tremendous effect on the ability of a healthcare executive to plan a career. Career planning is something that we can't do anymore because all of our assumptions have been rendered meaningless. The only assumption we *can* make is that change will be with us for the duration of our careers; we are therefore going to have to make constant changes in the direction our careers take, the way we look at our careers, and the way that we look at our lives. This chapter is devoted to helping you understand how change is going to affect you and what you can do about it.

THE OLD SKILL SET

Back when we could help people predict careers and career paths, there was a common set of skills that we looked for in healthcare executives, because these skills were necessary to succeed in the job and reach the position of CEO in a hospital.

Social Skills

We required healthcare executives to be able to get along. This included courting the board members and community leaders, as well as having the ability to deal with employees. Healthcare is not noted for producing the no-nonsense hard-driving leaders that we often find in general industry. Usually, when one of these does get through, he or she can only go so far before being dismissed. Healthcare has long rewarded the "kinder, gentler" leader and the one who is mission driven. Even for-profit healthcare companies can only tolerate so much drive and ambition.

Management

We used to look for good managers. Many aspects of day-to-day administration needed to be coordinated and overseen. We needed people who could "manage" government programs, "manage" the medical staff, and "manage" the board. We rewarded good management and hired executives who understood control. We had lots of managers for lots of departments and lots of people standing in line for their turn to manage. We managed to manage ourselves into managed care.

Operations

The people that really succeeded in the old days were those who had an operations background and really knew how to get things done. These were people who could organize large groups of employees or systems to deliver a service or a product. Those who planned or developed strategy were relegated to staff jobs and not necessarily given any glory by the operating folks. You were judged by how many people were in the departments reporting to you, and because operations had the most, operations people were at the top of the pyramid.

Physician Relations

This was often a skill associated with giving the physicians anything they requested, whether it fit within the strategic plan or was even necessary.

Physician recruiting was a necessary part of a hospital administrator's job and was expected by the board. Revenues increased each time a physician decided to practice at your hospital instead of your competitor's, and physicians became experienced in playing one administrator against the other. While there is an art in telling a physician "no" when it comes to an unreasonable request, in some organizations you were criticized and ostracized for not giving physicians exactly what they desired. Administrators socialized with doctors and entertained them as much as possible to add admissions to their facility. Being a successful physician recruiter and having strong physician relations was a prime asset. But the healthcare world as we knew it changed. Out of this change and restructure there developed a group of winners and losers, a list that may surprise you.

LOSERS IN HEALTHCARE RESTRUCTURING

Hospital CEOs

It may be hard to believe that a hospital CEO could be a loser in healthcare restructuring. After all, this is the position to which most aspired when entering the healthcare profession. The CEO—with the most prestige and highest compensation of all of the healthcare executives—was at the top of the healthcare career ladder. Although hospital CEOs are still at the top in prestige and compensation, there are unfortunately not many places for them to go in the new healthcare environment. If they are forced out of a job or leave for any reason, they find a terrible job market and have a hard time landing a similar opportunity, regardless of their competence.

What caused all of this? Healthcare restructuring, of course. Mergers of hospital organizations has caused the number of CEO positions to decline. Few new hospitals are being built, thus no new CEO slots are opening up. In the 1970s and 1980s as healthcare expanded, other organizations helped to soak up the surplus of CEOs. For example, American Medical International (AMI) by the early 1980s had 13 regional offices across the United States. In each regional office a number of the executives were former hospital CEOs who had been promoted. By the early 1990s, however, AMI had eliminated all of its regional offices and the corresponding executive positions associated with these offices. Nonprofit systems and associations such as the VHA also had numerous positions that were filled by former hospital CEOs. All of these organizations have reduced the number of posts that former CEOs can fill. In addition, many multihospital organizations, especially those that have multiple facilities in the same city or region, have elected to eliminate the CEO position at the hospital. Product-line management has been one of the instigators of this trend, but the desire to run a tighter and leaner organization has also contributed. Boards of directors have also been eliminated at these facilities, resulting in less need for a CEO. There has also been a trend to "shoot the messenger." With all of the change that is taking place, the CEO sometimes becomes the lightning rod for discontent among the medical staff and the board. Hospital CEOs who are out of work often cannot find a comparable job and end up taking a cut in pay and a step backwards to remain in the field.

Operations Personnel

Remember the old skill set? Operations personnel, who managed others, were once highly prized. Unfortunately, the new healthcare environment doesn't value these people the same way. Downsizing and restructing has caused hospitals to operate with fewer people, and department heads are now responsible for numerous departments—so not as many heads are required. Vice Presidents of This and That are no longer needed. Management layers have been eliminated, and streamlining has resulted in fewer jobs for those who are primarily in operations. The watershed year for the lack of opportunities in hospital operations was 1994, when not a single graduate of the University of Minnesota's hospital administration program took a job in a hospital.

Physician Specialists

The elite of medicine in recent history has been the physician specialist, whose extra training guaranteed additional income and prestige. Primary care physicians were not especially valued by either the hospitals or the specialists. Hospitals made lots of money from specialty care, and specialists were powerful physicians on the medical staff. Healthcare restructuring and the rise of managed care caused a tremendous upheaval in the specialist category. In most specialties, compensation is being scaled back and surpluses of physician specialists have begun to occur.

WINNERS IN HEALTHCARE RESTRUCTURING

While the losers in healthcare restructuring have been licking their wounds, some winners have emerged that are changing the face of healthcare and causing excitement in the careers of people who are lucky enough to be among them.

Managed Care Executives

Almost everyone having *any* managed care experience has seen their incomes rise significantly in the last few years. The managed care arena has been extremely dynamic and fast paced. Evolution from discounted fee-for-service to "capitated" plans has been accomplished in record time—and managed care is still evolving. Whether an executive is developing provider networks, point-of-service plans, or fully capitated health plans or is merely processing claims, managed care is an exciting place to be.

Physician Executives

Perhaps one of the fastest-growing positions is that of the physicians executive. As hospitals have tried to deal with the changes in healthcare, they have often employed physicians in advisory and staff roles either on a permanent or part-time basis. Most often this employment took the form of medical director for some program or for the entire hospital. This has been the traditional role for the physician executive and many positions have been created that allow physicians at least some role in management and leadership. In many ways supply has also created demand. Many physicians are now disenchanted with the practice of medicine and want to have more say in the system and how it works. They wish to exit clinical medicine and enter the executive ranks. The leadership for training in this area has been assumed by the American College of Physician Executives, which functions as a professional organization for those already practicing administrative medicine and as a training ground for those interested in redirecting their careers. It has a little over 12,000 members and is growing at about 10–15 percent per year. Physician executives have now begun to move beyond the medical director position and into operating jobs. They are becoming an alternative to the lay administrator in some hospitals.

Financial Executives

"Bean counter" is a pejorative term often associated with financial executives. I am not talking about "bean counters" when I mention financial executives. I am talking about executives from the financial ranks who have transcended the tendency of accountants to be more interested in dealing with numbers than with people. Financial executives have learned how to be both accountants and communicators at the same time. Healthcare is now placing such an emphasis on finance that financial executives have seen their careers move into almost every aspect of the healthcare field. This trend started in the hospitals with the advent of the prospective payment system: To deal with diagnosis-related groups and ICD-9-CM coding, we made the financial executives in charge of medical records and admitting, which were not their traditional departments. Those who succeeded were then given other departments to operate. After a while it was hard to tell whether the financial executive was the accountant or the operating person. Now that hospitals have begun to operate MSOs and manage physician practices, financial executives are being called on to involve themselves in these endeavors because of the large sums being lost by the physician practices. Financial considerations are driving the healthcare system, and financial executives often find themselves in the driver's seat.

Practice Managers

Perhaps no group has done so well as the practice managers. Physicians have begun to organize themselves better and to consolidate their practices into larger groups. Thus, they need executive talent to deal with the headaches and challenges of running a modern physician practice. Multipractice organizations such as MedPartners and PhyCor also have caused a tremendous growth in this area. Hospitals have bought physician practices by the scores and have created a demand for practice administrators. With all of this activity, salaries have soared—and so have career opportunities. As an example, membership in the Medical Group Management Association grew from 11,030 in 1990 to 19,600 in 1997—a growth rate of 78 percent.

Primary Care Physicians

The Health Care Financing Administration started the revolution by implementing the Relative Value Scale, which changed the way that primary care physicians were compensatd vis-à-vis specialists. HMOs and managed care plans added their ideas regarding gatekeepes. When all was said and done, the balance of power shifted to the primary care doctors, and life has never been the same. Primary care physicians have seen their incomes, prestige, and power increase. They are now always in demand, and therefore their careers are on the move.

PARADIGM CHANGE

For most of the 1990s we talked about "paradigm change" in general business. Well, the paradigm changed in healthcare, as well. Here is a list of some of the paradigm changes that affect the careers of healthcare executives.

Old Paradigm vs. New Paradigm
- From manager to leader
- From barriers to opportunities
- From control of staff to processes that yield results
- From competition to collaboration

- From compliance to commitment
- From controlling to coaching
- From directing to participating
- From either/or linear to generative, inclusive thinking
- From exclusionary to inclusionary
- From extrinsic rewards to intrinsic motivations
- From premature problem solving to consultation
- From holding information and power to sharing knowledge and power
- From internal standards to customer specifications
- From managing behavior to generating results
- From motivation to self-responsibility
- From perfection to customer expectations
- From power plays to persuasion
- From projects, tasks, and responsibilities to meeting customer needs
- From quality control to continuous improvement
- From clear roles and rules to whatever it takes to serve customers
- From spending or downsizing to investigating
- From structure to facilitation (Bearley and Jones 1996)

Because of the structural changes in healthcare and the general changes in how business is run, the new skill set came into being, along with a new set of requirements for anyone willing to succeed in healthcare. Here are some skills that will be needed beyond the year 2000.

THE NEW SKILL SET FOR THE YEAR 2000

Be Flexible and Adaptable!

The new age requires executives to be able to accept new ideas and ways of accomplishing objectives. As healthcare executives we have new, emerging business partners, new types of employees, and new challenges. We can no longer be held to a rigid set of thoughts; we now have to think the unthinkable. We can no longer have control, we have to collaborate. *Those who resist change will be left by the wayside of healthcare.*

Communicate

With change, comes the need to communicate what is happening to boards, medical staff, employees, and customers. We have always valued good communication in executives but its priority was usually toward the bottom of the list. When we talked of communication skills, we usually spoke of written and verbal communications. These two are still held in high regard, but to this list I add the following: listening and visually communicating. The ability to listen to what is being said before responding is especially important with all of the tension surrounding change in healthcare. Some people still follow the axiom "ready, fire . . . aim" and thus speak before comment is necessary or appropriate. People under stress need more time to vent and talk out the issues. A good communicator will give them the opportunity to release tension before proceeding into the hard issues. Visual communications has been added to my list because our generation has been brought up with the idea that a presentation must have visual effects if it is to be believed. It is no longer appropriate to get up and give a speech. One must also have charts, graphs, color, cartoons, and animation. People bore easily and now we must use all of our resources to communicate the message; what used to be impressive "high-tech" presentations have now become the norm.

Provide Visionary Leadership!

Remember that under the old skill set I put management. Well, the new skill set relegates management to the second tier. We no longer manage as tightly as we once did. In fact, executives are rarely able to control what is happening. We have to set parameters and expectations, then get out of the way. About five years ago, I started seeing the term *visionary leader* come up every time I interviewed boards regarding what they wanted in their next CEO. Leaders who feel they must command and control are having a hard time in the new healthcare environment. Organizations are seeking individuals who:

- have a vision;
- can articulate that vision;
- can achieve "buy-in"; and
- can then implement change through leadership.

Be Financially Astute!

One of the essential skill sets for the new era is the ability to be able to understand financial statements. Healthcare has become more focused on the bottom line, even in the nonprofit sector. Budget preparation and information is now freely disseminated into the organization and is no longer held under lock and key in a closet by the accounting staff. Each healthcare executive must now possess a working knowledge of the accounting and budgetary process and make decisions based on financial data—reasons why the MBA has become such a popular degree. It is no longer acceptable for candidates to rely heavily on the chief financial officer for financial decisions. All executives *must* have a functional knowledge of financial statements.

Be Physician Friendly!

Although it is hard to believe, in the past there were successful hospital administrators who didn't like dealing with physicians. Fortunately, they are migrating out of the field. Once you could operate a hospital or other healthcare organization and still be at war with the medical staff. This is no longer the case. Successful institutions have integrated physicians into the decision-making process, and physicians are assuming ever-higher leadership positions in healthcare organizations. In this new environment the successful healthcare executive is the one who enjoys working with physicians to improve the system.

Assume Risk Wisely!

For the most part, healthcare is a field adverse to risk, especially for nonprofit organizations. Some boards will push the CEO to assume risk on a project, but if it loses money, they will turn on and then fire the CEO. Unfortunately, almost everything that a healthcare organization undertakes nowadays involves risk, and healthcare executives are being required to assume more risk than ever before. Because of the downside of risk assumption and failure, some healthcare executives have become virtually paralyzed in their decision making, which will eventually jeopardize their jobs. Others, who have no clue about how much risk they are assuming, may rashly plunge their organizations into contracts and new ways of doing business with a "bet the firm" attitude. The new healthcare environment will reward those who take risks prudently and knowledgeably and who are comfortable making the decision to assume risk.

Build Teams!

The paradigm shift from control to collaboration and the commensurate growth in the number of direct reports has caused the concept of team building to be extremely important. It is nearly impossible for the healthcare executive to make all of the decisions in the organization. Decisions, responsibility, authority, and accountability all have to be delegated. Correspondingly, glory, reward, and respect have to be shared. A healthcare executive who is good at team building will enjoy a successful career.

Resolve Conflicts!

In the old healthcare environment it was much easier to please everyone. There were enough resources available to buy most of the equipment requested by the medical staff. Healthcare organizations would go along to get along, and most interests could be aligned easily. Nowadays, it is a different story. Conflicts arise constantly as the healthcare environment changes, and almost any decision made by a healthcare organization has the opportunity of making one or more constituents really angry. Saying "No!" is something that healthcare executives must learn how to do continually and diplomatically as resources become scarce and competition heats up. Those who are able to resolve the inevitable conflicts without making everyone angry and irrational have a rare talent that is necessary for survival in the new environment.

Learn Negotiation Skills!

Managed care has caused negotiation skills to be more important than ever. Most progressive organizations will have many opportunities for healthcare executives to exercise their negotiating skills. Negotiations with other organizations, with doctors, with unions, with managed care plans, with joint venture partners, with acquisition targets, and with the government have been added to the traditional negotiations with vendors. Every strategic initiative requires negotiating, and courses teaching negotiating skills have been popular with healthcare executives. Negotiate your way into taking one of these courses now!

Gain Computer Skills!

Healthcare executives can no longer function without the ability to use the computer. Computers are showing up in the CEO's office, and the PC has made its way onto almost every desk. Communication by e-mail allows information to flow not only throughout the organization but throughout the world via the Internet. Beyond e-mail skills, management information systems that provide up-to-the-hour data allow the healthcare executive to make timely decisions and to understand trends. When communicating to constituencies, executives are replacing the overhead projector and its black and white transparencies with the computer data projector and its "whiz-bang" animation and color. PowerPoint has taken the place of the chalkboard. Having computer skills puts a healthcare executive one step ahead of other competitors in this ever-changing field.

SO WHAT ARE YOU PLANNING TO DO?

I wrote this chapter to give you my ideas about what is happening in careers and to stimulate you to take action. *The healthcare field has changed and you are going to have to change with it.* The following are my suggestions on dealing with these changes and their effects on your career.

Redefine Your Definition of Success

We now have less control over our careers. As I stated in the beginning of this chapter, I no longer believe in career planning in the traditional sense. In addition, modern life is taking its toll on our private lives at home. It is becoming very common for executives to make career decisions that are motivated by family considerations. We are moving away from a definition of our success as one characterized by career achivement and money to one characterized by life achievement and happiness. Family life is becoming more important than corporate life. Balance is more important than maximization. My favorite publication, the *Wall Street Journal*, will often run a front-page story of an executive who stepped down, stepped away, or changed careers because of family considerations. If all you are needing is some encouragement or someone saying to you that it is okay to change your direction, I just did it. I hope you have the courage to do what is best for both you and your family.

Acquire New Skills

This entire chapter has been devoted to discussing the skills you need in the new healthcare environment, and now is the time to acquire them. Continuing education courses are available in many different venues to allow you to do so. If you need to go back to college full- or part-time, then do it! If you need different experiences to acquire the skills, go see your boss now to set up a development plan with other work assignments. If you can't get new skills at your place of employment, change jobs. Don't sit back and be overwhelmed by the changes in healthcare. Do something about it. Prepare yourself.

Be Prepared to Take a Lateral Career Move or to Take a Step Backward

The convention was that if you made a job change that it would always be for a higher position, which is no longer the case. Many healthcare executives are having to take a lateral position or a step backwards to remain in the field. This lack of advancement may be hard on the psyche but it is realistic given the times and the situations. Unfortunately, some executives begin their job searches thinking that they are going to move up and come to the reality of the situation only in the later stages of the job search. At that point, they may have turned down perfectly good opportunities that would have made them happy but their expectations were too high. At this point in healthcare "a bird in the hand is worth fifteen in the bush." As you begin your job search, do lots of homework and talk to lots of people about your job prospects. If you are on my list of winners in healthcare restructuring, your prospects should be good. If you are on the list of losers, your prospects are dimmer.

Consider a Healthcare-Related Job

Executives are looking closer these days at opportunities outside of healthcare provision. Managed care has generated lots of opportunities for many people. Consulting has been seen tremendous growth, allowing executives to remain in the field and continue to advance. Suppliers are also hiring executives for various positions because of their contacts, and numerous joint ventures have given displaced executives the opportunity to do something related to healthcare. Most of these jobs are good positions that you might leverage into more security or income than you currently have while allowing you to remain connected to healthcare.

Leave the Field

This may be the hardest move to make, but it is worth considering. The thought of leaving healthcare was once never considered by healthcare executives. They thought leaving the field was admitting that they could no longer "cut it" in the executive ranks, and the loss of income was inevitable when changing fields. Unfortunately, job opportunities may no longer be available even for the competent executive. With diminished opportunities, getting into a field that is growing dramatically may revive your career or contribute to your overall happiness. Furthermore, who says that staying in the same field for an entire career is the right thing to do? What did buggy-whip makers do when the automobile came along? They changed fields. The new healthcare environment is not for everyone. If it is not for you, then get into something that you can be good at and enjoy. In my other life—before working in executive searches—I was an accountant. But I was not made to be an accountant. I enjoyed being around people and having conversations. My bosses at Price Waterhouse told me that they enjoyed reviewing my work papers. They loved the way I wrote, but they always worried whether I had done the work correctly. I was lucky. I changed fields before I had committed a lifetime to something that I didn't like and at which I would never have been more than average. A number of my friends have left healthcare, and I talk to them occasionally. They are all enjoying what they are doing. There are other worlds out there that need exploring.

PREPARING YOURSELF FOR UNCERTAINTY

Put Your Financial House in Order

Too many people are living beyond their means and are not prepared for the financial disruptions that occur when one is without work. If you live below your means, then you have a head start on some of the decisions and circumstances you may face in a job change. You will be able to consider jobs that you might like but that may not initially compensate you at your current level. Desperation is not a good feeling for enhanced career decision making. Get the bills paid off and have six months' worth of cash available to cover expenses. You will sleep better at night, and your job search will be less frantic.

Try Your Hand at Creating New Business Opportunities

If you can create a new business either at work or during your spare time, you will always have something to fall back on. You can then use those skills to do the same for another employer or do it for yourself. Having created a new business gives you an immense degree of self confidence that will come across during an interview. Healthcare organizations are creating new businesses every day. Be the one in your institution who is known as the new-business developer. One day, you may do so well that you'll have a free-standing business with you as the CEO. The new healthcare environment encourages and rewards entrepreneurship and risk taking.

Prepare Yourself to Find a New Job

The chances for being displaced as healthcare restructures are enormous. Unfortunately, some people sit back and do nothing until they actually have to find a new job. The best time to prepare for finding a new job is when you really don't have to find one. Accept first of all the reality that you might be displaced and that displacement might come tomorrow. Accepting reality and dealing with it now can remove the dread of impending doom. Second, update your resume so that when an unsought opportunity comes along you are prepared to move head without having to update your resume. Third, have candid dicussions with your family. They need to understand the volatility of the healthcare field and your job prospects within it. Sometimes executives don't want to worry the children or spouse, preferring to keep them secure by keeping them in the dark. Unfortunately, when the reality of a job change comes about they are unprepared to deal with it and the reality can then be doubly traumatic. Fourth, make sure you are maintaining your network and compiling the names and addresses of potential contacts to help you when the need arises.

Find a Job that Makes You Happy

Happiness is one of the real keys to success. People who enjoy their jobs enjoy going to work. There is a lot of unhappiness in healthcare as we move to a new environment. As you change jobs you should be careful to look first for something that you think you will enjoy as opposed to something that would pay you your current compensation. What good is money if you hate going to work? Remember: *Find a job you like, and you'll never have to work the rest of your life.*

REFERENCE

Bearley, W. L., and J. E. Jones. 1996. *360 Degree Feedback: Strategies, Tactics, and Techniques for Developing Leaders.* Amherst, MA, and Minneapolis, MN: HRD Press & Lakewood Publications.

Index

About the Authors

Thomas A. Atchison, Ed.D., is president of the Atchison Consulting Group based in Oak Park, Illinois.

Charles J. Austin, Ph.D., is professor in the Department of Health Administration and Policy in the College of Health Professions at the Medical University of South Carolina.

Eric N. Berkowitz, Ph.D., is professor of marketing at the Isenberg School of Management, The University of Massachusetts at Amherst.

Errol Biggs, Ph.D., FACHE, is director, Programs in Health Administration, University of Colorado at Denver.

Stuart B. Boxerman, D.Sc., is associate professor and deputy director of the Health Administration Program at Washington University School of Medicine.

Carson F. Dye, FACHE, is a management and search consultant for Witt/ Kieffer Ford Hadelman and Lloyd, a healthcare and education executive search organization. He also teaches at Ohio State University.

Steven T. Fleming, Ph.D., is an associate professor of health services management at the University of Kentucky. He also teaches in the Martin School of Public Policy and Administration and the Kentucky School of Public Health.

Louis C. Gapenski, Ph.D., is a professor in health services administration and finance at the University of Florida.

John R. Griffith, FACHE, is the Andrew Pattullo Collegiate Professor in the Department of Health Management and Policy, School of Public Health at the University of Michigan.

Craig E. Holm, CHE, is a director of Health Strategies & Solutions, Inc., a healthcare management consulting firm.

Arnold D. Kaluzny, Ph.D., is a professor of health policy and administration at the School of Public Health at the University of North Carolina at Chapel Hill.

Joel M. Lee, Dr.P.H., is a professor and director of undergraduate studies in the Division of Health Services Management with the University of Kentucky College of Allied Health Professions. He is also the director of the Doctor of Public Health program in the Kentucky School of Public Health and a faculty associate with the Center for Health Services Management and Research.

Beaufort B. Longest, Jr., Ph.D., FACHE, is professor of health services administration in the Graduate School of Public Health, a professor of business administration in Katz Graduate School of Business, and the founding director of the Health Policy Institute at the University of Pittsburgh.

Thomas C. Ricketts III, Ph.D., is the deputy director for Health Policy Analysis at the Cecil G. Sheps Center for Health Services Research and an assistant professor, Department of Health Policy and Administration, School of Public Health at the University of North Carolina at Chapel Hill

F. Douglas Scutchfield, M.D., is the Peter P. Bosomworth Professor of health services research and policy, and professor of preventive medicine and environmental health at the University of Kentucky. He is director of the Division of Health Services Management and director of the Kentucky School of Public Health.

J. Stuart Showalter, J.D., is director of compliance at the Orlando Regional Health System. He taught health law and public policy in the health administration program at Washington University School of Medicine, St. Louis.

J. Larry Tyler, FACHE, is president and CEO of Tyler & Company, executive search consultants.

James E. Veney, Ph.D., is a professor of health policy and administration at the School of Public Health at the University of North Carolina, Chapel Hill. He is the director of the doctoral program in the Department of Health Policy and Administration.

Alan M. Zuckerman, FACHE, is a founding partner and director of Health Strategies & Solutions, Inc., a healthcare management consulting firm.

Howard S. Zuckerman, Ph.D., is professor, Department of Health Services, School of Public Health and Community Medicine, University of Washington, Seattle.